Breast Pathology

Editor

LAURA C. COLLINS

SURGICAL PATHOLOGY CLINICS

www.surgpath.theclinics.com

Consulting Editor
JASON L. HORNICK

March 2018 • Volume 11 • Number 1

ELSEVIER

1600 John F. Kennedy Boulevard • Suite 1800 • Philadelphia, Pennsylvania, 19103-2899

http://www.theclinics.com

SURGICAL PATHOLOGY CLINICS Volume 11, Number 1
March 2018 ISSN 1875-9181, ISBN-13: 978-0-323-58176-9

Editor: Stacy Eastman
Developmental Editor: Donald Mumford

Surgical Pathology Clinics (ISSN 1875-9181) is published quarterly by Elsevier Inc., 360 Park Avenue South, New York, NY 10010. Months of issue are March, June, September, and December. Business and Editorial Office: Elsevier Inc., 1600 John F. Kennedy Blvd., Ste. 1800, Philadelphia, PA 19103-2899. Accounting and Circulation Offices: Elsevier Inc., 3251 Riverport Lane, Maryland Heights, MO 63043. Periodicals postage paid at New York, NY and at additional mailing offices. Subscription prices are $206.00 per year (US individuals), $279.00 per year (US institutions), $100.00 per year (US students/residents), $258.00 per year (Canadian individuals), $318.00 per year (Canadian Institutions), $258.00 per year (foreign individuals), $318.00 per year (foreign institutions), and $120.00 per year (international & Canadian students/residents). Foreign air speed delivery is included in all *Clinics'* subscription prices. All prices are subject to change without notice. **POSTMASTER:** Send address changes to *Surgical Pathology Clinics*, Elsevier, 3251 Riverport Lane, Maryland Heights, MO 63043. **Customer Service: 1-800-654-2452 (US). From outside the United States, call 1-314-447-8871. Fax: 1-314-447-8029. E-mail: JournalsCustomerServiceusa@elsevier.com (for print support)** and **JournalsOnlineSupport-usa@elsevier.com (for online support)**.

Reprints. For copies of 100 or more, of articles in this publication, please contact the Commercial Reprints Department, Elsevier Inc., 360 Park Avenue South, New York, NY 10010-1710. Tel. 212-633-3874; Fax: 212-633-3820; E-mail: reprints@elsevier.com.

Surgical Pathology Clinics of North America is covered in *MEDLINE/PubMed (Index Medicus)*.

Contributors

CONSULTING EDITOR

JASON L. HORNICK, MD, PhD
Director of Surgical Pathology and
Immunohistochemistry, Brigham and
Women's Hospital, Professor of Pathology,
Harvard Medical School, Boston,
Massachusetts, USA

EDITOR

LAURA C. COLLINS, MD
Vice Chair of Anatomic Pathology, Director of
Breast Pathology, Beth Israel Deaconess
Medical Center, Professor of Pathology,
Harvard Medical School, Boston,
Massachusetts, USA

AUTHORS

KIMBERLY H. ALLISON, MD
Director of Breast Pathology and
Breast Pathology Fellowship Program,
Director of Pathology Residency Training
Program, Professor of Pathology, Stanford
University School of Medicine, Stanford,
California, USA

VEERLE BOSSUYT, MD
Department of Pathology, Yale University, New
Haven, Connecticut, USA

EDI BROGI, MD, PhD
Department of Pathology, Memorial Sloan
Kettering Cancer Center, New York, New York,
USA

BENJAMIN C. CALHOUN, MD, PhD
Director of Breast Pathology, Associate
Professor, Department of Pathology
and Laboratory Medicine, Women's and
Children's Hospital, The University of North
Carolina at Chapel Hill, Chapel Hill, North
Carolina, USA

ASHLEY CIMINO-MATHEWS, MD
Associate Professor of Pathology and
Oncology, The Johns Hopkins Hospital,
Baltimore, Maryland, USA

LAURA C. COLLINS, MD
Vice Chair of Anatomic Pathology, Director of
Breast Pathology, Beth Israel Deaconess
Medical Center, Professor of Pathology,
Harvard Medical School, Boston,
Massachusetts, USA

DEBORAH A. DILLON, MD
Assistant Professor of Pathology, Department
of Pathology, Brigham and Women's Hospital,
Boston, Massachusetts, USA

BETH T. HARRISON, MD
Instructor, Department of Pathology, Brigham
and Women's Hospital, Boston,
Massachusetts, USA

GAETANO MAGRO, MD, PhD
Professor, Department of Medical and Surgical
Sciences and Advanced Technologies, G.F.
Ingrassia, Anatomic Pathology, University of
Catania, Catania, Italy

JONATHAN D. MAROTTI, MD
Assistant Professor of Pathology,
Department of Pathology and Laboratory
Medicine, Dartmouth-Hitchcock Medical
Center, Lebanon, New Hampshire, USA; Geisel
School of Medicine at Dartmouth, Hanover,
New Hampshire, USA

STUART J. SCHNITT, MD
Chief of Breast Oncologic Pathology,
Dana-Farber/Brigham and Women's Cancer
Center, Professor, Department of Pathology,
Harvard Medical School, Boston,
Massachusetts, USA

**BENJAMIN YONGCHENG TAN, MBBS,
FRCPath**
Consultant, Department of Anatomical
Pathology, Singapore General Hospital,
Singapore

PUAY HOON TAN, MBBS, FRCPA, FRCPath
Senior Consultant and Chairman, Division of
Pathology, Singapore General Hospital,
Singapore

HANNAH Y. WEN, MD, PhD
Department of Pathology, Memorial Sloan
Kettering Cancer Center, New York, New York,
USA

Contents

Benign and atypical lesions associated with breast cancer risk are often encountered in core needle biopsies (CNBs) of the breast. For these lesions, the rate of upgrade to carcinoma in excision specimens varies widely in the literature. Many CNB studies are limited by a lack of radiologic-pathologic correlation, consistent criteria for excision, and clinical follow-up for patients who forego excision. This article highlights contemporary diagnostic criteria and outcome data that would support an evidence-based approach to the management of these nonmalignant lesions of the breast diagnosed on CNB.

Fibroepithelial breast lesions encompass a heterogeneous group of neoplasms that range from benign to malignant, each exhibiting differing degrees of stromal proliferation in relation to the epithelial compartment. Fibroadenomas are common benign neoplasms that may be treated conservatively. Phyllodes tumors are relatively rare lesions and classified as benign, borderline, or malignant based on histologic evaluation of various parameters. The diagnostic interpretation of "gray-zone" fibroepithelial lesions often imposes formidable demands on a pathologist's skills. This article offers practical recommendations for the diagnostic workup of these lesions, including the appropriate utilization of ancillary investigations and the approach to core needle biopsies.

Lymph node inclusions can occur in axillary lymph nodes, where they can mimic metastatic breast carcinoma. This article provides an overview of epithelial and non-epithelial lymph node inclusions, including mammary-type glandular inclusions, Mullerian-type glandular inclusions, squamous inclusions, mixed glandular-squamous inclusions, and nodal nevi. The discussion emphasizes the histologic and immunophenotypic features and differential diagnoses of each entity.

Mucinous lesions of the breast include a variety of benign and malignant epithelial processes that display intracytoplasmic or extracellular mucin, including mucocele-like lesions, mucinous carcinoma, solid papillary carcinoma, and other rare subtypes of mucin-producing carcinoma. The most important diagnostic challenge is the finding of free-floating or stromal mucin accumulations for which the significance depends on the clinical, radiologic, and pathologic context. This article emphasizes the differential diagnosis between mucocelelike lesions and mucinous carcinoma, with a brief consideration of potential mimics, such as biphasic and mesenchymal lesions with myxoid stroma ("stromal mucin") and foreign material.

Gaetano Magro

Spindle cell lesions of the breast cover a wide spectrum of diseases ranging from reactive tumorlike lesions to high-grade malignant tumors. The recognition of the benign spindle cell tumorlike lesions (nodular fasciitis; reactive spindle cell nodule after biopsy, inflammatory pseudotumor/inflammatory myofibroblastic tumor; fascicular variant of pseudoangiomatous stromal hyperplasia) and tumors (myofibroblastoma, benign fibroblastic spindle cell tumor, leiomyoma, schwannoma, spindle cell lipoma, solitary fibrous tumor, myxoma) is crucial to avoid confusion with morphologically similar but more aggressive bland-appearing spindle cell tumors, such as desmoid-type fibromatosis, low-grade (fibromatosis-like) spindle cell carcinoma, low-grade fibrosarcoma/myofibroblastic sarcoma, and dermatofibrosarcoma protuberans.

Hannah Y. Wen and Edi Brogi

Lobular carcinoma in situ (LCIS) is a risk factor and a nonobligate precursor of breast carcinoma. The relative risk of invasive carcinoma after classic LCIS diagnosis is approximately 9 to 10 times that of the general population. Classic LCIS diagnosed on core biopsy with concordant imaging and pathologic findings does not mandate surgical excision, and margin status is not reported. The identification of variant LCIS in a needle core biopsy specimen mandates surgical excision, regardless of radiologic-pathologic concordance. The presence of variant LCIS close to the surgical margin of a resection specimen is reported, and reexcision should be considered.

Kimberly H. Allison

Ancillary testing in breast cancer has become standard of care to determine what therapies may be most effective for individual patients with breast cancer. Single-marker tests are required on all newly diagnosed and newly metastatic breast cancers. Markers of proliferation are also used and include both single-marker tests like Ki67 as well as panel-based gene expression tests, which have made more recent contributions to prognostic and predictive testing in breast cancers. This article focuses on pathologist interpretation of these ancillary test results, with a focus on expected versus unexpected results and troubleshooting borderline, unusual, or discordant results.

Laura C. Collins

The nonobligate precursor lesions columnar cell change/hyperplasia and flat epithelial atypia, atypical ductal hyperplasia and atypical lobular hyperplasia, lobular carcinoma in situ, and low-grade ductal carcinoma in situ share morphologic, immunophenotypic, and molecular features supporting the existence of a low-grade breast neoplasia pathway. The practical implication for pathologists is that the identification of one of these lesions should prompt careful search for others. From a clinical management perspective, however, their designation as "precursor lesions" should not be overemphasized, as the risk of progression among the earliest lesions is exceedingly low. Factors determining which lesions will progress remain unknown.

Jonathan D. Marotti and Stuart J. Schnitt

Only a few breast cancer histologic subtypes harbor distinct genetic alterations that are associated with a specific morphology (genotype-phenotype correlation). Secretory carcinomas and adenoid cystic carcinomas are each characterized by recurrent translocations, and invasive lobular carcinomas frequently have *CDH1* mutations. Solid papillary carcinoma with reverse polarity is a rare breast cancer subtype with a distinctive morphology and recently identified *IDH2* mutations. The authors review the clinical and pathologic features and underlying genetic alterations of those breast cancer subtypes with established genotype-phenotype correlations and discuss the phenotypes associated with germline mutations in genes associated with hereditary breast cancer.

Veerle Bossuyt

Standardization of quantification of residual disease in the breast and lymph nodes with routine pathologic macroscopic and microscopic evaluation leads to accurate and reproducible measures of response to neoadjuvant treatment. Multidisciplinary collaboration and correlation of clinical, imaging, gross, and microscopic findings is essential. The processing approach to post-neoadjuvant breast cancer surgical specimens and the elements needed in the pathology report are the same regardless of breast cancer subtype or type of neoadjuvant treatment. The residual cancer burden incorporates response in the breast and in the lymph nodes into a score that can be combined with other emerging prognostic factors.

SURGICAL PATHOLOGY CLINICS

RELATED INTEREST

Clinics in Laboratory Medicine, September 2016 (Vol. 36, No. 3)
Pharmacogenomics and Precision Medicine
Kristen K. Reynolds and Roland Valdes Jr, *Editors*

THE CLINICS ARE AVAILABLE ONLINE!
Access your subscription at:
www.theclinics.com

Preface
Contemporary Topics in Breast Pathology

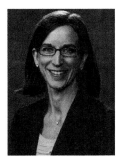

Laura C. Collins, MD
Editor

Breast pathology can be one of the more challenging areas for all involved in diagnostic surgical pathology, and there are several areas of breast pathology that are particularly difficult or problematic. In this Breast Pathology issue of *Surgical Pathology Clinics*, experts in the field have provided comprehensive reviews of commonly encountered problematic lesions in breast pathology, including fibroepithelial lesions, spindle cell lesions, mucinous lesions, and lobular carcinoma in situ, as well as the less frequently encountered, but nonetheless problematic, phenomenon of lymph node inclusions. In addition, there are state-of-the-art reviews on the processing and reporting of breast specimens in the setting of neoadjuvant systemic therapy and ancillary prognostic and predictive testing in breast cancer. Articles discussing the low-grade breast neoplasia pathway and recent discoveries in special-type breast cancers with specific genotypic-phenotypic features present new ways to think about molecular mechanisms and breast tumor progression. Finally, a contemporary review of the data on upgrade rates associated with nonmalignant breast lesions sampled by core needle biopsy aims to move us in the direction of fewer excisions of benign breast lesions.

In each article, high-quality photomicrographs or diagrams complement the text where appropriate to further illustrate the points being discussed.

It is hoped that the reviews presented in this issue of *Surgical Pathology Clinics* will be a useful resource to all pathologists involved in diagnostic breast pathology.

Laura C. Collins, MD
Vice Chair of Anatomic Pathology
Director of Breast Pathology
Beth Israel Deaconess Medical Center
Harvard Medical School
330 Brookline Avenue
Boston, MA 02215, USA

E-mail address:
lcollins@bidmc.harvard.edu

Surgical Pathology 11 (2018) ix
https://doi.org/10.1016/j.path.2017.12.001
1875-9181/18/© 2017 Published by Elsevier Inc.

Core Needle Biopsy of the Breast
An Evaluation of Contemporary Data

Benjamin C. Calhoun, MD, PhD

KEYWORDS

- Atypical ductal hyperplasia • Atypical lobular hyperplasia • Lobular carcinoma in situ
- Lobular neoplasia • Flat epithelial atypia • Radial scar • Papilloma

---

Key points

- Most patients with atypical breast lesions diagnosed on core biopsy are referred for immediate surgical excision.

- Recent studies indicate that, for many of these lesions, the rate of upgrade to carcinoma may be lower than initially reported in studies that lacked radiologic-pathologic correlation.

- Careful clinical-pathologic and radiological–pathologic correlation may identify subsets for whom excision is not required.

ABSTRACT

Benign and atypical lesions associated with breast cancer risk are often encountered in core needle biopsies (CNBs) of the breast. For these lesions, the rate of "upgrade" to carcinoma in excision specimens varies widely in the literature. Many CNB studies are limited by a lack of radiological–pathological correlation, consistent criteria for excision, and clinical follow-up for patients who forego excision. This article highlights contemporary diagnostic criteria and outcome data that would support an evidence-based approach to the management of these nonmalignant lesions of the breast diagnosed on CNB.

OVERVIEW: SCREENING AND DETECTION

Changes in imaging techniques for breast cancer screening and diagnosis have had an impact on the types of specimens in which pathologists encounter risk-associated lesions. In the past 2 decades, it has become much more common for atypical ductal hyperplasia (ADH) and atypical lobular hyperplasia (ALH) to be diagnosed on core needle biopsy (CNB) versus an excisional biopsy.[1] The widespread adoption of digital mammography has resulted in more CNBs for microcalcifications with more diagnoses of columnar cell lesions and ADH.[2] Digital breast tomosynthesis appears to identify more atypical lesions and radial scars, including some that are occult on conventional digital mammography.[3,4]

In the largest case-control studies of open biopsies, atypical hyperplasia (ADH and ALH), flat epithelial atypia (FEA), papillomas, and radial scars were identified in approximately 4%, 2%, 5% to 6%, and 5% to 9%, respectively[5–12] The frequency of atypical hyperplasia in CNBs also appears to be approximately 4%.[13,14] In vacuum-assisted stereotactic CNBs specifically, the frequency of ADH, and ALH and lobular carcinoma in situ (LCIS) may be as high as 10% to 15%.[15–17] FEA and benign papillomas

---

Disclosure Statement: B.C. Calhoun does not have any relationships with a commercial company with a direct financial interest in subject matter or materials discussed in this article.

Department of Pathology and Laboratory Medicine, University of North Carolina, Women's and Children's Hospitals, 3rd Floor, Room 30212, 101 Manning Drive, Chapel Hill, NC 27514, USA

E-mail address: ben.calhoun@unc.edu

appear to account for 1% and 2% to 3% of CNBs, respectively.[14,18,19] The frequency of radial scars in recent studies of CNBs is approximately 1% to 2%.[14,20,21] If an estimated 1.5 million image-guided CNBs are performed annually in the United States[22] and 8% contain ADH, ALH, LCIS, FEA, or a radial scar,[14] approximately 120,000 women could be referred for surgical excision for these diagnoses each year.

In the vast majority of cases, risk-associated lesions cannot be recognized grossly. The discussion in this article focuses on the assessment of microscopic features, the selected application of immunohistochemistry, and the risk of carcinoma associated with these lesions when diagnosed on CNB.

ATYPICAL DUCTAL HYPERPLASIA

The definition of ADH is essentially based on a histologic comparison to ductal carcinoma in situ (DCIS) and is discussed in full in the article on the low-grade breast neoplasia pathway by Laura C. Collins's article, "Precursor Lesions of the Low Grade Breast Neoplasia Pathway," elsewhere in this issue. ADH fulfills some, but not all, of the criteria for a diagnosis of low-grade DCIS (Fig. 1).[5] A combination of cytologic and architectural features are required for the diagnosis of ADH,[23] whereas cytologic (nuclear) atypia alone may satisfy criteria for a diagnosis of FEA (discussed later in this article).[24]

In CNBs with borderline features of ADH versus low-grade DCIS, many experts recommend reporting the CNB as ADH or "atypical intraductal proliferative lesion" and referral for an excisional biopsy for further evaluation, rather than diagnosing low-grade DCIS before more thorough examination of the area with the imaging abnormality.[25,26] A conservative approach to the diagnosis of low-grade DCIS on CNB may mitigate overtreatment (eg, mastectomy or even bilateral mastectomy) in cases with atypia of limited extent on the CNB and no carcinoma in the excision specimen.

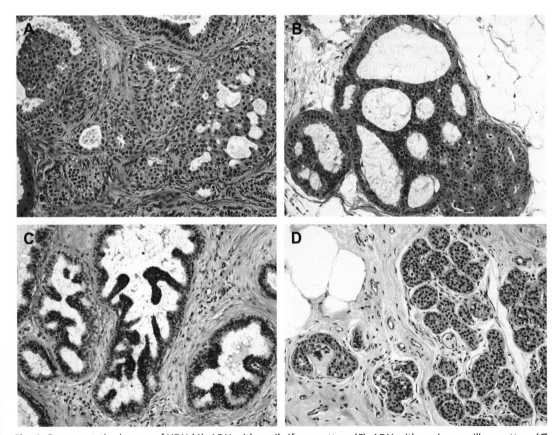

Fig. 1. Representative images of UDH (*A*), ADH with a cribriform pattern (*B*), ADH with a micropapillary pattern (*C*), and ALH with microcalcifications (*D*). H&E, original magnification ×200 (*A–D*).

Key Features
ATYPICAL DUCTAL HYPERPLASIA

- Monomorphic epithelial cell population with distinct cell borders and low-grade nuclear atypia

- Architectural atypia includes cribriform patterns with well-developed secondary spaces bounded by rigid arcades or bridges as well as micropapillary and solid patterns

- Involvement of at least 2 duct spaces or an area ≥2 mm usually required for a diagnosis of low-grade DCIS versus ADH, but a more conservative approach is recommended for lesions encountered in CNB specimens

- ADH (and low-grade DCIS) is typically uniformly negative for high-molecular-weight cytokeratins whereas USH shows a heterogeneous "mosaic" staining pattern

---

IMMUNOPHENOTYPE

The diagnosis of ADH is primarily based on evaluation of the hematoxylin-eosin (H&E) histologic features mentioned previously. However, in selected cases, the absence of immunoreactivity for high-molecular-weight cytokeratins may be helpful in distinguishing ADH from usual ductal hyperplasia (UDH) (**Fig. 1**A),[27–29] or in evaluating limited or fragmented core biopsy specimens with detached atypical epithelial cell groups. It is important to remember that immunohistochemistry studies cannot be used to distinguish ADH from DCIS, both of which are negative for high-molecular-weight cytokeratins.

OUTCOME FOLLOWING CORE NEEDLE BIOPSY

For ADH diagnosed on CNB, the rate of upgrade to DCIS or invasive carcinoma has been reported to be as high as 33% to 56%.[30–33] Two recent large series of CNB reported upgrade rates of 18%[14] and 39.8%[34] for ADH. In studies that explicitly include radiological–pathologic correlation, the average rate of upgrade to carcinoma is approximately 20%.[13,35–38] CNBs obtained under ultrasound guidance with a 14-gauge device are more likely to be upgraded.[31,39] This may be related to the smaller volume of tissue obtained with a 14-gauge device versus a 12-gauge vacuum-assisted CNB. Another factor is the likelihood that most 14-gauge ultrasound-guided CNBs are performed to evaluate a mass or mass with calcifications rather than suspicious calcifications alone. The upgrade rate for ADH does not appear to be significantly lower with larger 9-gauge versus 11-gauge vacuum-assisted stereotactic core biopsy devices.[33,40]

Some studies suggest that the pattern of atypia (eg, micropapillary pattern) and the number of foci of ADH on CNB influence the likelihood of upgrade at excision.[15,35,36,38,41,42] It may be possible to identify subsets of patients with ADH (eg, those with only focal ADH and no residual calcifications after CNB) who could safely forego immediate excision,[37] but this is not a standard practice. Most upgrades after a CNB diagnosis of ADH are DCIS,[43] but upgrades to invasive carcinoma do occur, and most experts recommend excision for all diagnoses of ADH on CNB.[44]

In addition to the risk of upgrade on excision in the immediate setting, ADH is associated with an increased risk for the subsequent development of carcinoma.[5,6,45] In large case-control studies of open biopsies, the cumulative breast cancer incidence after a diagnosis of atypical hyperplasia (ADH and ALH), is approximately 25% to 30% at 25 years (ie, approximately 1% per year).[46–48] In a recent large series of patients in the Breast Cancer Surveillance Consortium, those diagnosed with ADH on CNB had a 5% risk of developing an invasive carcinoma in the first 10 years of follow-up.[1]

ATYPICAL LOBULAR HYPERPLASIA AND LOBULAR CARCINOMA IN SITU

Lobular breast lesions were originally described as "lobular" based on their location in breast terminal ducts and lobules.[49] It has been well established for some time that intraductal proliferations in the breast arise in the terminal duct-lobular unit (TDLU) and the descriptors "ductal" and "lobular" do not indicate different sites (or cells) of origin.[50] However, these terms remain in use because ductal and lobular lesions are morphologically, clinically, and biologically distinct in many ways.[51]

ALH and LCIS are usually incidental findings in CNBs, accounting for fewer than 1% of cases in some studies.[13,14] However, ALH and LCIS occasionally may be associated with microcalcifications detected by screening mammography.[52–55]

Some investigators use the term lobular neoplasia to collectively refer to ALH and classic LCIS.[47,56,57]

LCIS is the subject of Hannah Y Wen and Edi Brogi's article, "Lobular Carcinoma in Situ," elsewhere in this issue.[57,58] In brief, ALH and LCIS are characterized by a monomorphic epithelial cell population with minimal nuclear atypia that lacks cellular cohesion and contains frequent intracytoplasmic vacuoles (**Fig. 1**D).[57,58]

Key Features
ATYPICAL LOBULAR HYPERPLASIA AND CLASSIC LOBULAR CARCINOMA IN SITU

- Monomorphic epithelial cell population with minimal nuclear atypia that lacks cellular cohesion and contains frequent intracytoplasmic vacuoles

- The cytologic features of ALH and classic LCIS are similar with cases with minimal expansion (<50%) of the TDLU diagnosed as ALH

- E-cadherin is usually (but not always!) negative in ALH and classic LCIS

- Cytoplasmic staining for p120 catenin and loss of beta catenin expression may be helpful in cases with aberrant E-cadherin staining patterns

---

IMMUNOPHENOTYPE

ALH and LCIS are usually negative for E-cadherin due to somatic alterations of the CDH1 gene on the long arm of chromosome 16.[59,60] Use of E-cadherin as well as p120 catenin and beta catenin can be helpful in classifying low-grade solid intraductal proliferations on CNB with a differential diagnosis of ADH (or low-grade DCIS) versus ALH (or LCIS)[61–65]. ALH and LCIS are also negative for high-molecular-weight cytokeratins, similar to ADH and DCIS.[65]

OUTCOME FOLLOWING CORE NEEDLE BIOPSY

The upgrade rate for ALH and LCIS was reported to be as high as 15% to 33% in earlier studies.[66–70] In 2 recently published studies, the upgrade rates for ALH, LCIS, and the combined category of ALH/LCIS were 9%,[14] 28%,[14] and 23.6%,[34] respectively. However, with radiological–pathologic correlation, the upgrade rate for incidental ALH and classic LCIS appears to be 3%.[14,69,71–74] The variability in

upgrade rates has led some investigators to recommend caution in the interpretation of the data for (classic) LCIS.[75] Buckley and colleagues[75] pointed out that many studies are retrospective from single institutions that suffer from small sample size and a lack follow-up for patients who do not undergo excision (ie, selection bias). These potential limitations also may apply to the CNB literature in general as pathologists, radiologists, and surgeons seek to determine which patients may safely forego excision.[76] However, a recent study of a series of CNB with LCIS in a prospective multi-institutional registry indicated an upgrade rate of only 3% with local pathology review and 1% with central pathology review.[77] Thus, observation may be appropriate for incidental classic LCIS on CNB in cases that lack other indications for excision[44,54,55,72,73,78]

The data on the upgrade rate for malignancy associated with the less common (nonclassic) variants of LCIS, including pleomorphic LCIS and florid LCIS with comedo necrosis are limited. Pleomorphic and florid LCIS are more likely to be associated with suspicious microcalcifications and therefore less likely to be incidental findings.[79–83] In current practice, patients with these nonclassic forms of LCIS should be referred for surgical excision because of the greater reported association with invasive carcinoma[79,81–84] and the uncertainty about clinical management.[85] Pleomorphic and florid LCIS should not be diagnosed as lobular neoplasia, not otherwise specified, on CNB.

Although the risk of upgrade on excision drives short-term clinical management of screen-detected lesions, ALH and LCIS also confer an increased risk for the subsequent development of breast cancer. In the Nashville Cohort, the cumulative incidence of invasive breast cancer after a diagnosis of LCIS was 17% at 15 years.[47] In a more recent study, the cumulative breast cancer incidence for patients diagnosed with LCIS was 26% at 15 years.[86] In studies of ALH and LCIS diagnosed on core biopsy with clinical–radiological follow-up only (ie, not immediately excised), approximately 2% (or fewer) of patients developed carcinoma near the core biopsy site within 3 to 5 years; although this number should be interpreted with caution, as some cases may represent undersampling rather than short-term progression.[71,74,87]

FLAT EPITHELIAL ATYPIA

Columnar cell lesions (CCL) of the breast are frequently encountered in CNB performed to evaluate mammographically indeterminate calcifications. The current World Health Organization (WHO) classification provides 3 diagnostic categories: columnar cell change, columnar cell hyperplasia, and FEA.[24] FEA is frequently associated with ADH, low-grade DCIS, tubular carcinomas, and lobular neoplasia (see discussion of the low-grade neoplasia pathway)[88,89] Many patients with FEA on CNB are offered local excision to exclude coexisting carcinoma, but management recommendations vary (see Laura C Collins's article, "Precursor Lesions of the Low Grade Breast Neoplasia Pathway", in this issue for further details).[90]

Columnar cell change and columnar cell hyperplasia are typically recognized as dilated acinar spaces of the TDLU that may have irregular contours and are lined by columnar epithelial cells with oval nuclei (Fig. 2A, B).[91] In columnar cell hyperplasia there may be multilayering of the epithelium with the formation of mounds or tufts suggestive of a micropapillary pattern.[92]

FEA differs in that the dilated acini of the TDLU are lined by 3 to 5 layers of epithelial cells with low-grade monomorphic cytology, increased nuclear/cytoplasmic ratios, and loss of polarity (Fig. 2C, D).[24]

Key Features
FLAT EPITHELIAL ATYPIA

- TDLUs are enlarged with dilated acini that may have smooth contours

- One or more layers of epithelial cells with low-grade monomorphic cytology, increased nuclear/cytoplasmic ratios, and loss of polarity

- Apical snouts and blebs as well as flocculent eosinophilic luminal secretions with concentric lamellar calcifications

- Complex architectural patterns are absent

- FEA is frequently associated with ADH, low-grade DCIS, tubular carcinoma, and lobular neoplasia

- CCL and FEA are positive for estrogen receptor (ER) and negative for high-molecular-weight cytokeratins

IMMUNOPHENOTYPE

There is little role for immunohistochemistry in CNB specimens of CCLs. All CCLs are positive for ER and bcl-2 and negative for high-molecular-weight cytokeratins.[93] In cases for which the differential diagnosis is FEA versus apocrine change, immunoreactivity for ER would favor FEA.[93]

OUTCOME FOLLOWING CORE NEEDLE BIOPSY

In a meta-analysis that included studies without radiological–pathologic correlation, 13% to 67% of cases of FEA diagnosed on CNB were upgraded to carcinoma on excision.[94] Some studies of pure FEA diagnosed on CNB with radiological–pathologic correlation have reported upgrade rates of up to 13%.[95–102] However, other studies have shown much lower upgrade rates, ranging from 0% to 7%, especially when all microcalcifications were removed[18,101,103,104]; and, 2 more recent studies that included radiological–pathologic correlation and assessment of residual microcalcifications reported upgrade rates for FEA of 2% to 3%.[103,105] In a study of 50 cases of pure FEA managed with observation only, no patients developed carcinoma after a median follow-up of 5 years.[98] The WHO Working Group recommends radiological–pathologic correlation for patients with pure FEA diagnosed on core biopsy, and, in the absence of any other indications for excision, observation may be appropriate.[24,44]

PAPILLOMAS

The spectrum of morphology in the broadly defined category of papillary lesions includes intraductal papilloma, papillomas involved by ADH or DCIS, encapsulated (intracystic) papillary carcinomas, and solid papillary carcinomas.[106] The CNB diagnosis of an atypical papillary lesion or papillary carcinoma should lead to referral for surgical excision. The more common and problematic issue is the management of histologically benign papillomas diagnosed on CNB.

Intraductal papillomas[107] grow out the duct wall with arborizing fibrovascular cores that protrude into the lumen (Fig. 3A). The fibrovascular cores are lined by a layer of epithelial cells and a myoepithelial cell layer (Fig. 3B). In other cases, usual-type hyperplasia may fill and expand the spaces between the fibrovascular cores in benign papillomas.[108] Apocrine change is also frequently seen in benign papillomas. Sclerosed papillomas are relatively common and may be associated with calcifications. The pattern of entrapped epithelium in sclerosed papillomas may mimic the appearance of (nodular) sclerosing adenosis or invasive carcinoma.

Key Features
INTRADUCTAL PAPILLOMAS

- Arborizing fibrovascular cores that may be lined by one or more layers of epithelial cells and a myoepithelial cell layer
- Apocrine change and UDH are frequently seen
- Stromal sclerosis calcifications are relatively common
- The epithelial component of atypical papillary lesions will be positive for ER and negative for high-molecular-weight cytokeratins

IMMUNOPHENOTYPE

Immunohistochemistry may aid in distinguishing benign intraductal papillomas (with or without sclerosis and florid UDH) from papillomas with ADH or DCIS, papillary DCIS, and encapsulated (intracystic) papillary carcinomas.[109–112]

A combination of high-molecular-weight cytokeratin and ER studies may be particularly helpful in CNB of papillary lesions with a cellular epithelial component that raises the possibility of ADH or DCIS.[110,113] In a papilloma with florid UDH, immunohistochemistry for high-molecular-weight cytokeratins should show a heterogeneous ("mosaic") staining pattern and immunoreactivity for ER should be variable (as opposed to strong and diffuse). High-molecular-weight cytokeratin stains also may highlight an intact myoepithelial cell layer.

In atypical papillary lesions, the epithelial component is at least focally monomorphic and shows low-grade cytologic atypia. A myoepithelial cell layer may or may not be demonstrable on the fibrovascular cores or lining the duct wall at the periphery of the lesion. The atypical epithelial component will be negative for high-molecular-weight cytokeratins. As was discussed for ADH (previously in this article), immunohistochemistry for high-molecular-weight cytokeratins aids in the distinction between (florid) UDH and ADH/DCIS. A negative high-molecular-weight cytokeratin stain does

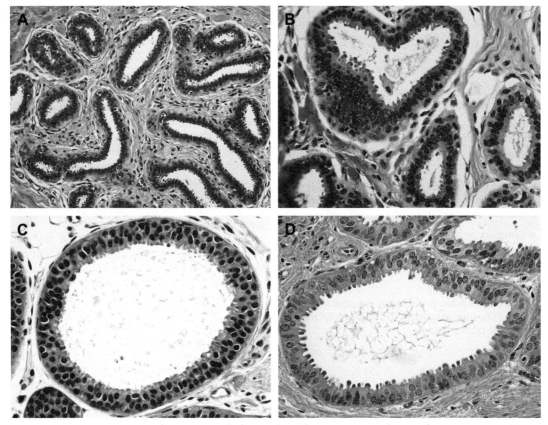

Fig. 2. Representative images of columnar cell change (*A* and *B*, H&E, original magnification ×100 and ×200, respectively) and FEA (*C* and *D*, H&E, original magnification ×400).

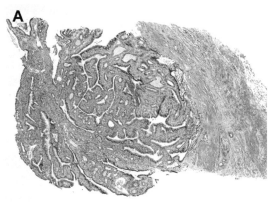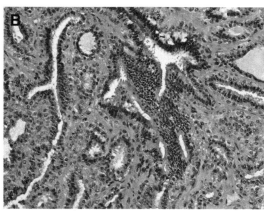

Fig. 3. Representative images of a benign intraductal papilloma (*A* and *B*, H&E, original magnification ×40 and ×200, respectively).

not distinguish ADH from DCIS or an encapsulated papillary carcinoma. For a subset of CNBs, it may be best to report them as "atypical papillary lesions" or "atypical papillary neoplasms." Classification as a papilloma with ADH or DCIS versus papillary DCIS versus an encapsulated papillary carcinoma may be deferred to the excision specimen.

Differential Diagnosis
INTRADUCTAL PAPILLOMAS

- Papilloma with ADH or DCIS
- Papillary DCIS
- Encapsulated (or intracystic) papillary carcinoma
- H&E features
  - Florid UDH contains a mixed epithelial cell population with streaming and overlapping of nuclei
  - ADH/DCIS contains a monomorphic population with low-grade cytologic atypia and distinct cell-cell borders
  - ADH and DCIS in a papilloma may show complex architecture (eg, cribriform pattern)
- Immunohistochemistry
  - Florid UDH shows a mixed staining pattern for high-molecular-weight cytokeratins
  - ADH and DCIS are negative for high-molecular-weight cytokeratins
  - UDH shows variable immunoreactivity for ER with weak to moderate intensity

  - ADH, low-grade DCIS, and encapsulated papillary carcinoma usually strongly, diffusely positive for ER
  - Benign papillomas and papillomas with ADH or DCIS should show immunoreactivity for myoepithelial cell markers
  - Encapsulated papillary carcinomas may be negative for myoepithelial cell markers

OUTCOME FOLLOWING CORE NEEDLE BIOPSY

A meta-analysis of 34 CNB studies reported an overall upgrade rate of 15.7% for nonmalignant papillary lesions with an upgrade rate for benign papillomas of 7.0% versus 36.9% for atypical papillary lesions.[114] A review of 15 studies published in 2009 or later of benign papillomas diagnosed on CNB with excision follow-up showed an overall upgrade rate of approximately 6% with DCIS accounting for most upgrades.[43] More recently, in a series of 224 solitary, benign, radiologically concordant intraductal papillomas diagnosed on CNB, Swapp and colleagues[115] reported no upgrades in the 77 patients who underwent immediate excision. Jaffer and colleagues[116] reported no upgrades in a series of 46 CNBs with incidental benign papillomas measuring smaller than 2 mm ("micropapillomas") and recommended radiological follow-up for these patients rather than excision. Conversely, a study that included 146 benign papillomas measuring ≤15 mm did not find a size threshold below which there were no upgrades to carcinoma.[117] One limitation of that study was that the data for benign papillomas and papillary lesions with atypia and carcinoma on CNB were combined, making it difficult to assess the outcome for benign papillomas alone.[117]

In studies reporting the clinical and radiological follow-up of benign papillomas that were observed rather than excised, the rate of developing carcinoma within 3 to 5 years of the core biopsy ranged from 0% to 4%.[115,118–124] Based on the short time interval (eg, 4 months) to the development of DCIS and invasive carcinoma in some cases, the possibility that some of these carcinomas represent tumors missed at the time of the original CNB (ie, false-negative CNB) cannot be excluded.[118]

The subsequent breast carcinoma risk associated with a diagnosis of papilloma was evaluated in 2 large case-control studies of open biopsies.[8,9] Benign (solitary) papillomas were associated with an relative risk (RR) of approximately 2, similar to proliferative breast disease without atypia.[8,9] The presence of atypical hyperplasia increased the risk for the subsequent development of breast cancer in both studies.[8,9] Multiple papillomas,[9,125] especially those associated with atypical hyperplasia,[9] appear to confer increased risk for the subsequent development of breast cancer.

RADIAL SCAR

Radial scars are an important subset of sclerosing lesions of the breast. They are relatively uncommon and the frequency with which they are diagnosed in CNBs specifically is not well established. Radial scars accounted for approximately 5% to 9% of cases in the largest case-control studies of open biopsies.[10–12] In 2 recent CNB studies, radial scars accounted for approximately 1% to 2% of cases over a 16-year to 17-year period.[20,21] Early studies suggested that radial scars were more common in women with breast cancer,[126] but those findings were not confirmed in subsequent studies.[127,128]

The observation that radial scars are colocalized with carcinoma in some cases also suggested a potential relationship between radial scars and breast cancer.[129–132] The term complex sclerosing lesion was originally proposed for radial scars measuring more than 10 mm.[133] In current practice, the terms radial scar and complex sclerosing lesion are often used interchangeably. Some pathologists use a diagnosis of complex sclerosing lesion to convey suspicion of a radial scar in CNBs that show features suggestive but not definitely diagnostic for a radial scar.

Radial scars of the breast typically have a central focus of fibroelastotic stroma with epithelial elements entrapped in the stroma (Fig. 4A, B).[134] The stellate appearance and the distortion or compression of entrapped glands may mimic carcinoma radiologically and histologically.[135,136] A variety of proliferative fibrocystic changes may extend from the central sclerotic focus in a radial pattern.[136] UDH, sclerosing adenosis, columnar cell change and papillomas may be seen in association with radial scars and are often associated with mammographically detected calcifications.

Key Features
RADIAL SCARS

- Central focus of fibroelastotic stroma with epithelial elements entrapped in the stroma

- Proliferative fibrocystic changes extend from the center in a radial pattern

- UDH, sclerosing adenosis, columnar cell change and papillomas may be present and associated with calcifications

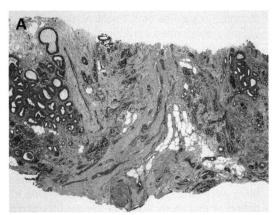
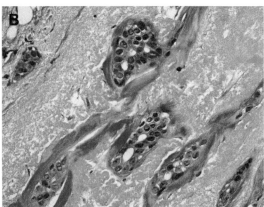

Fig. 4. Representative images of a radial scar (*A* and *B*, H&E, original magnification ×40 and ×400, respectively).

IMMUNOPHENOTYPE

There is no established role for immunohisto-chemistry in the identification of radial scars. If myoepithelial cells are not easily identified on H&E slides, immunohistochemical studies for myoepithelial cell markers (eg, a combination of p63 and smooth muscle myosin heavy chain) can be helpful in differentiating radial scars from low-grade, tubular-type invasive carcinomas,[137,138] especially in limited or fragmented CNBs. Discontinuity of the myoepithelial cell layer on immunohistochemistry studies must be interpreted with caution, particularly in the context of a lesion that otherwise has benign histologic features, as the staining pattern for myoepithelial cells may be disrupted by attenuation of the myoepithelial cell layer and/or alterations in the phenotype of the myoepithelial cells in benign sclerosing lesions.[136,137] If atypical hyperplasia is suspected, the immunohistochemical evaluation could include E-cadherin and high-molecular-weight cytokeratins as discussed for ALH and ADH previously.

Differential Diagnosis
RADIAL SCARS

- Sclerosing adenosis
- Low-grade ductal or tubular-type invasive carcinoma
- H&E features
  - Radial scars lack the lobulocentric pattern and distribution of sclerosing adenosis
  - Sclerosing adenosis lacks the elastotic change typical of radial scars
  - Myoepithelial cells are often visible on H&E slides in the entrapped glands of radial scars
  - The distorted or compressed glands in radial scars do not infiltrate the fat in the irregular pattern characteristic of infiltrative carcinoma
- Immunohistochemistry
  - The glands in radial scars usually show immunoreactivity for myoepithelial cell markers
  - Invasive carcinoma will be negative for myoepithelial cell markers
  - Caveat: the myoepithelial cell layer may be attenuated in radial scars and the myoepithelial cell in radial scars may show loss of expression of some myoepithelial cell markers

OUTCOME FOLLOWING CORE NEEDLE BIOPSY

The reported upgrade rates for radial scars diagnosed on CNB have ranged from 0% to 40%.[130,139–147] Studies with radiological–pathologic correlation indicate that the upgrade rate for radial scars without atypia is ≤2%.[20,21,148] In a recent series of 77 small (ie, ≤5 mm), incidental radial scars diagnosed on CNB, there were no upgrades to carcinoma.[148] In another series of 48 CNBs, only 1 case (2%) was upgraded based on a 2-mm focus of low-grade DCIS in a background of ADH in the excision specimen.[21] In a meta-analysis including 21 published studies of radial scars diagnosed on CNB, the overall upgrade rate for radial scars without atypia was 7.5%,[21] with most of the upgrades being DCIS. The upgrades to invasive carcinoma were of tumors with low-grade ductal or tubular histology.

The published data on the follow-up for patients with radial scars diagnosed on CNB that were not excised is limited. In a series of 25 patients with radial scars that were not immediately excised with a median follow-up of 79 months, Miller and colleagues[20] reported that 1 patient (4%) was found to have a 3-mm low-grade DCIS on a later excision, but that patient had atypia associated with the radial scar at the time of CNB. Other studies with short-term follow-up for radial scars that were not excised have shown no subsequent upgrades.[143]

Some experts recommend a size threshold of greater than 10 mm for requiring excision of radial scars.[149,150] However, the correlation between the size of the radial scar and the likelihood of upgrade on excision is not always observed.[143] In current practice, there is no clear consensus on which patients with radial scars may be observed and most patients are still referred for surgical consultation. Excision for incidental radial scars and radial scars without atypia that measure ≤5 mm may not be necessary. Excision is recommended for larger radial scars and those associated with ADH, ALH, or LCIS.[20]

There are conflicting data on the subsequent breast cancer risk associated with radial scars diagnosed on excisional biopsies. In the Nurses' Health Study, radial scars appear to be an independent risk factor for the subsequent development of carcinoma.[12,151] However, the data from the Mayo Clinic Benign Breast Disease Cohort and the Nashville Cohort indicate that the proliferative disease (benign or atypical) frequently associated with radial scars appears to account for any breast cancer risk that could attributed to radial scars.[10,11]

> **Key Points**
> MANAGEMENT OF SELECTED
> BENIGN AND ATYPICAL LESIONS
> DIAGNOSED ON CNB
>
> - ADH: All patients referred for surgical consultation and excision
> - ALH: Surveillance may be appropriate for incidental ALH
> - LCIS: Surveillance may be appropriate for incidental classic LCIS
> - FEA: Surveillance may be appropriate for FEA if all calcifications removed
> - Papilloma: Surveillance may be appropriate for benign solitary and incidental papillomas
> - Radial scar: Surveillance may be appropriate for incidental radial scars without atypia

SUMMARY

Approximately 5% of patients with screen-detected breast abnormalities and nonmalignant CNB lesions undergo immediate excision and the ratio of benign-to-malignant diagnoses in the excision specimens may be as high as 3:1.[34] Patients with a diagnosis of DCIS are known to be likely to undergo multiple additional imaging studies and biopsies in the 10 years following diagnosis.[152] Comparable data are not available for patients diagnosed with atypical hyperplasia and the other lesions discussed herein, but based on current practice patterns, it seems likely that many of these patients will undergo additional imaging studies and biopsies.

The data from contemporary CNB studies, especially those that document radiological–pathologic correlation and concordance, suggest that not all patients with FEA, ALH, LCIS, benign papilloma, or radial scars require surgery. The National Comprehensive Cancer Network (NCCN) Breast Cancer Screening and Diagnosis Guidelines (Version 2.2016) include a provision that selected patients with these CNB diagnoses may be offered surveillance as an alternative to immediate excision.[153] Future studies of larger, single-institution cohorts with prospective multidisciplinary evaluation should continue to provide more guidance on which patients may safely forego immediate excision.[87,154] Given the relatively low frequency of some of these risk-associated lesions in CNBs, multi-institutional registries may be required to provide adequate data for guiding future management.[77,155]

REFERENCES

1. Menes TS, Kerlikowske K, Lange J, et al. Subsequent breast cancer risk following diagnosis of atypical ductal hyperplasia on needle biopsy. JAMA Oncol 2017;3(1):36–41.
2. Verschuur-Maes AH, van Gils CH, van den Bosch MA, et al. Digital mammography: more microcalcifications, more columnar cell lesions without atypia. Mod Pathol 2011;24(9):1191–7.
3. Partyka L, Lourenco AP, Mainiero MB. Detection of mammographically occult architectural distortion on digital breast tomosynthesis screening: initial clinical experience. AJR Am J Roentgenol 2014;203(1):216–22.
4. Ray KM, Turner E, Sickles EA, et al. Suspicious findings at digital breast tomosynthesis occult to conventional digital mammography: imaging features and pathology findings. Breast J 2015;21(5):538–42.
5. Dupont WD, Page DL. Risk factors for breast cancer in women with proliferative breast disease. N Engl J Med 1985;312(3):146–51.
6. Hartmann LC, Sellers TA, Frost MH, et al. Benign breast disease and the risk of breast cancer. N Engl J Med 2005;353(3):229–37.
7. Said SM, Visscher DW, Nassar A, et al. Flat epithelial atypia and risk of breast cancer: a Mayo cohort study. Cancer 2015;121(10):1548–55.
8. Page DL, Salhany KE, Jensen RA, et al. Subsequent breast carcinoma risk after biopsy with atypia in a breast papilloma. Cancer 1996;78(2):258–66.
9. Lewis JT, Hartmann LC, Vierkant RA, et al. An analysis of breast cancer risk in women with single, multiple, and atypical papilloma. Am J Surg Pathol 2006;30(6):665–72.
10. Sanders ME, Page DL, Simpson JF, et al. Interdependence of radial scar and proliferative disease with respect to invasive breast carcinoma risk in patients with benign breast biopsies. Cancer 2006;106(7):1453–61.
11. Berg JC, Visscher DW, Vierkant RA, et al. Breast cancer risk in women with radial scars in benign breast biopsies. Breast Cancer Res Treat 2008;108(2):167–74.
12. Aroner SA, Collins LC, Connolly JL, et al. Radial scars and subsequent breast cancer risk: results from the Nurses' Health Studies. Breast Cancer Res Treat 2013;139(1):277–85.
13. Menes TS, Rosenberg R, Balch S, et al. Upgrade of high-risk breast lesions detected on mammography in the Breast Cancer Surveillance Consortium. Am J Surg 2014;207(1):24–31.

14. Mooney KL, Bassett LW, Apple SK. Upgrade rates of high-risk breast lesions diagnosed on core needle biopsy: a single-institution experience and literature review. Mod Pathol 2016;29(12):1471–84.

15. Sneige N, Lim SC, Whitman GJ, et al. Atypical ductal hyperplasia diagnosis by directional vacuum-assisted stereotactic biopsy of breast microcalcifications: considerations for surgical excision. Am J Clin Pathol 2003;119(2):248–53.

16. Houssami N, Ciatto S, Bilous M, et al. Borderline breast core needle histology: predictive values for malignancy in lesions of uncertain malignant potential (B3). Br J Cancer 2007;96(8):1253–7.

17. Eby PR, Ochsner JE, DeMartini WB, et al. Is surgical excision necessary for focal atypical ductal hyperplasia found at stereotactic vacuum-assisted breast biopsy? Ann Surg Oncol 2008;15(11): 3232–8.

18. Calhoun BC, Sobel A, White RL, et al. Management of flat epithelial atypia on breast core biopsy may be individualized based on correlation with imaging studies. Mod Pathol 2015;28(5):670–6.

19. Rosen EL, Bentley RC, Baker JA, et al. Imaging-guided core needle biopsy of papillary lesions of the breast. AJR Am J Roentgenol 2002;179(5): 1185–92.

20. Miller CL, West JA, Bettini AC, et al. Surgical excision of radial scars diagnosed by core biopsy may help predict future risk of breast cancer. Breast Cancer Res Treat 2014;145(2):331–8.

21. Conlon N, D'Arcy C, Kaplan JB, et al. Radial scar at image-guided needle biopsy: is excision necessary? Am J Surg Pathol 2015;39(6):779–85.

22. Liberman L. Clinical management issues in percutaneous core breast biopsy. Radiol Clin North Am 2000;38(4):791–807.

23. Page DL, Rogers LW. Combined histologic and cytologic criteria for the diagnosis of mammary atypical ductal hyperplasia. Hum Pathol 1992; 23(10):1095–7.

24. Schnitt SJ, Collins L, Lakhani SR, et al. Flat epithelial atypia. In: Lakhani SR, Ellis IO, Schnitt SJ, et al, editors. World Health Organization classification of tumours of the breast. 4th edition. Lyon (France): International Agency for Research on Cancer (IARC); 2012. p. 87.

25. Vandenbussche CJ, Khouri N, Sbaity E, et al. Borderline atypical ductal hyperplasia/low-grade ductal carcinoma in situ on breast needle core biopsy should be managed conservatively. Am J Surg Pathol 2013;37(6):913–23.

26. Simpson JF, Schnitt SJ, Visscher D, et al. Atypical ductal hyperplasia. In: Lakhani SR, Ellis IO, Schnitt SJ, et al, editors. World Health Organization Classificaiton of tumours of the breast. 4th edition. Lyon (France): International Agency for Research on Cancer; 2012. p. 88–9.

27. Moinfar F, Man YG, Lininger RA, et al. Use of keratin 35betaE12 as an adjunct in the diagnosis of mammary intraepithelial neoplasia-ductal type–benign and malignant intraductal proliferations. Am J Surg Pathol 1999;23(9):1048–58.

28. Otterbach F, Bankfalvi A, Bergner S, et al. Cytokeratin 5/6 immunohistochemistry assists the differential diagnosis of atypical proliferations of the breast. Histopathology 2000;37(3):232–40.

29. Schnitt SJ, Collins LC. Intraductal proliferative lesions. In: Biopsy interpretation of the breast. 2nd edition. Philadelphia: Lippincott Williams & Wilkins; 2013. p. 58–79.

30. Youn I, Kim MJ, Moon HJ, et al. Absence of residual microcalcifications in atypical ductal hyperplasia diagnosed via stereotactic vacuum-assisted breast biopsy: is surgical excision obviated? J Breast Cancer 2014;17(3):265–9.

31. Mesurolle B, Perez JC, Azzumea F, et al. Atypical ductal hyperplasia diagnosed at sonographically guided core needle biopsy: frequency, final surgical outcome, and factors associated with underestimation. AJR Am J Roentgenol 2014;202(6):1389–94.

32. Caplain A, Drouet Y, Peyron M, et al. Management of patients diagnosed with atypical ductal hyperplasia by vacuum-assisted core biopsy: a prospective assessment of the guidelines used at our institution. Am J Surg 2014;208(2):260–7.

33. Eby PR, Ochsner JE, DeMartini WB, et al. Frequency and upgrade rates of atypical ductal hyperplasia diagnosed at stereotactic vacuum-assisted breast biopsy: 9-versus 11-gauge. AJR Am J Roentgenol 2009;192(1):229–34.

34. Farshid G, Gill PG. Contemporary indications for diagnostic open biopsy in women assessed for screen-detected breast lesions: a ten-year, single institution series of 814 consecutive cases. Breast Cancer Res Treat 2017;162(1):49–58.

35. Wagoner MJ, Laronga C, Acs G. Extent and histologic pattern of atypical ductal hyperplasia present on core needle biopsy specimens of the breast can predict ductal carcinoma in situ in subsequent excision. Am J Clin Pathol 2009;131(1):112–21.

36. Kohr JR, Eby PR, Allison KH, et al. Risk of upgrade of atypical ductal hyperplasia after stereotactic breast biopsy: effects of number of foci and complete removal of calcifications. Radiology 2010; 255(3):723–30.

37. McGhan LJ, Pockaj BA, Wasif N, et al. Atypical ductal hyperplasia on core biopsy: an automatic trigger for excisional biopsy? Ann Surg Oncol 2012;19(10):3264–9.

38. Khoury T, Chen X, Wang D, et al. Nomogram to predict the likelihood of upgrade of atypical ductal hyperplasia diagnosed on a core needle biopsy in mammographically detected lesions. Histopathology 2015;67(1):106–20.

39. Lacambra MD, Lam CC, Mendoza P, et al. Biopsy sampling of breast lesions: comparison of core needle- and vacuum-assisted breast biopsies. Breast Cancer Res Treat 2012;132(3):917–23.

40. Lourenco AP, Mainiero MB, Lazarus E, et al. Stereotactic breast biopsy: comparison of histologic underestimation rates with 11- and 9-gauge vacuum-assisted breast biopsy. AJR Am J Roentgenol 2007;189(5):W275–9.

41. Ely KA, Carter BA, Jensen RA, et al. Core biopsy of the breast with atypical ductal hyperplasia: a probabilistic approach to reporting. Am J Surg Pathol 2001;25(8):1017–21.

42. Nguyen CV, Albarracin CT, Whitman GJ, et al. Atypical ductal hyperplasia in directional vacuum-assisted biopsy of breast microcalcifications: considerations for surgical excision. Ann Surg Oncol 2011;18(3):752–61.

43. Calhoun BC, Collins LC. Recommendations for excision following core needle biopsy of the breast: a contemporary evaluation of the literature. Histopathology 2016;68(1):138–51.

44. Morrow M, Schnitt SJ, Norton L. Current management of lesions associated with an increased risk of breast cancer. Nat Rev Clin Oncol 2015;12(4):227–38.

45. London SJ, Connolly JL, Schnitt SJ, et al. A prospective study of benign breast disease and the risk of breast cancer. JAMA 1992;267(7):941–4.

46. Hartmann LC, Radisky DC, Frost MH, et al. Understanding the premalignant potential of atypical hyperplasia through its natural history: a longitudinal cohort study. Cancer Prev Res (Phila) 2014;7(2):211–7.

47. Page DL, Kidd TE Jr, Dupont WD, et al. Lobular neoplasia of the breast: higher risk for subsequent invasive cancer predicted by more extensive disease. Hum Pathol 1991;22(12):1232–9.

48. Page DL, Schuyler PA, Dupont WD, et al. Atypical lobular hyperplasia as a unilateral predictor of breast cancer risk: a retrospective cohort study. Lancet 2003;361(9352):125–9.

49. Foote FW, Stewart FW. Lobular carcinoma in situ: a rare form of mammary cancer. Am J Pathol 1941;17(4):491–6, 3.

50. Wellings SR, Jensen HM, Marcum RG. An atlas of subgross pathology of the human breast with special reference to possible precancerous lesions. J Natl Cancer Inst 1975;55(2):231–73.

51. Dabbs DJ, Schnitt SJ, Geyer FC, et al. Lobular neoplasia of the breast revisited with emphasis on the role of E-cadherin immunohistochemistry. Am J Surg Pathol 2013;37(7):e1–11.

52. Simpson PT, Gale T, Fulford LG, et al. The diagnosis and management of pre-invasive breast disease: pathology of atypical lobular hyperplasia and lobular carcinoma in situ. Breast Cancer Res 2003;5(5):258–62.

53. Esserman LE, Lamea L, Tanev S, et al. Should the extent of lobular neoplasia on core biopsy influence the decision for excision? Breast J 2007;13(1):55–61.

54. Middleton LP, Grant S, Stephens T, et al. Lobular carcinoma in situ diagnosed by core needle biopsy: when should it be excised? Mod Pathol 2003;16(2):120–9.

55. D'Alfonso TM, Wang K, Chiu YL, et al. Pathologic upgrade rates on subsequent excision when lobular carcinoma in situ is the primary diagnosis in the needle core biopsy with special attention to the radiographic target. Arch Pathol Lab Med 2013;137(7):927–35.

56. Haagensen CD, Lane N, Lattes R, et al. Lobular neoplasia (so-called lobular carcinoma in situ) of the breast. Cancer 1978;42(2):737–69.

57. Lakhani SR, Schnitt SJ, O'Malley F, et al. Lobular neoplasia. In: Lakhani SR, Ellis IO, Schnitt SJ, et al, editors. World Health Organization classification of tumours of the breast. Lyon (France): International Agency for Resarch on Cancer; 2012. p. 78–80.

58. Page DL, Dupont WD, Rogers LW, et al. Atypical hyperplastic lesions of the female breast. A long-term follow-up study. Cancer 1985;55(11):2698–708.

59. Vos CB, Cleton-Jansen AM, Berx G, et al. E-cadherin inactivation in lobular carcinoma in situ of the breast: an early event in tumorigenesis. Br J Cancer 1997;76(9):1131–3.

60. Mastracci TL, Tjan S, Bane AL, et al. E-cadherin alterations in atypical lobular hyperplasia and lobular carcinoma in situ of the breast. Mod Pathol 2005;18(6):741–51.

61. Sarrio D, Perez-Mies B, Hardisson D, et al. Cytoplasmic localization of p120ctn and E-cadherin loss characterize lobular breast carcinoma from preinvasive to metastatic lesions. Oncogene 2004;23(19):3272–83.

62. Dabbs DJ, Bhargava R, Chivukula M. Lobular versus ductal breast neoplasms: the diagnostic utility of p120 catenin. Am J Surg Pathol 2007;31(3):427–37.

63. Geyer FC, Lacroix-Triki M, Savage K, et al. beta-Catenin pathway activation in breast cancer is associated with triple-negative phenotype but not with CTNNB1 mutation. Mod Pathol 2011;24(2):209–31.

64. Dabbs DJ, Kaplai M, Chivukula M, et al. The spectrum of morphomolecular abnormalities of the E-cadherin/catenin complex in pleomorphic lobular carcinoma of the breast. Appl Immunohistochem Mol Morphol 2007;15(3):260–6.

65. Bratthauer GL, Moinfar F, Stamatakos MD, et al. Combined E-cadherin and high molecular weight cytokeratin immunoprofile differentiates lobular,

ductal, and hybrid mammary intraepithelial neoplasias. Hum Pathol 2002;33(6):620–7.

66. Brem RF, Lechner MC, Jackman RJ, et al. Lobular neoplasia at percutaneous breast biopsy: variables associated with carcinoma at surgical excision. AJR Am J Roentgenol 2008;190(3):637–41.

67. Cangiarella J, Guth A, Axelrod D, et al. Is surgical excision necessary for the management of atypical lobular hyperplasia and lobular carcinoma in situ diagnosed on core needle biopsy? A report of 38 cases and review of the literature. Arch Pathol Lab Med 2008;132(6):979–83.

68. Bianchi S, Bendinelli B, Castellano I, et al. Morphological parameters of lobular in situ neoplasia in stereotactic 11-gauge vacuum-assisted needle core biopsy do not predict the presence of malignancy on subsequent surgical excision. Histopathology 2013;63(1):83–95.

69. Subhawong AP, Subhawong TK, Khouri N, et al. Incidental minimal atypical lobular hyperplasia on core needle biopsy: correlation with findings on follow-up excision. Am J Surg Pathol 2010;34(6): 822–8.

70. Hussain M, Cunnick GH. Management of lobular carcinoma in-situ and atypical lobular hyperplasia of the breast–a review. Eur J Surg Oncol 2011; 37(4):279–89.

71. Nagi CS, O'Donnell JE, Tismenetsky M, et al. Lobular neoplasia on core needle biopsy does not require excision. Cancer 2008;112(10):2152–8.

72. Rendi MH, Dintzis SM, Lehman CD, et al. Lobular in-situ neoplasia on breast core needle biopsy: imaging indication and pathologic extent can identify which patients require excisional biopsy. Ann Surg Oncol 2012;19(3):914–21.

73. Murray MP, Luedtke C, Liberman L, et al. Classic lobular carcinoma in situ and atypical lobular hyperplasia at percutaneous breast core biopsy: outcomes of prospective excision. Cancer 2013; 119(5):1073–9.

74. Shah-Khan MG, Geiger XJ, Reynolds C, et al. Long-term follow-up of lobular neoplasia (atypical lobular hyperplasia/lobular carcinoma in situ) diagnosed on core needle biopsy. Ann Surg Oncol 2012;19(10):3131–8.

75. Buckley ES, Webster F, Hiller JE, et al. A systematic review of surgical biopsy for LCIS found at core needle biopsy—do we have the answer yet? Eur J Surg Oncol 2014;40(2):168–75.

76. Georgian-Smith D, Lawton TJ. Controversies on the management of high-risk lesions at core biopsy from a radiology/pathology perspective. Radiol Clin North Am 2010;48(5):999–1012.

77. Nakhlis F, Gilmore L, Gelman R, et al. Incidence of adjacent synchronous invasive carcinoma and/or ductal carcinoma in-situ in patients with lobular neoplasia on core biopsy: results from a prospective multi-institutional registry (TBCRC 020). Ann Surg Oncol 2016;23(3):722–8.

78. Renshaw AA, Derhagopian RP, Martinez P, et al. Lobular neoplasia in breast core needle biopsy specimens is associated with a low risk of ductal carcinoma in situ or invasive carcinoma on subsequent excision. Am J Clin Pathol 2006;126(2): 310–3.

79. Flanagan MR, Rendi MH, Calhoun KE, et al. Pleomorphic lobular carcinoma in situ: radiologic-pathologic features and clinical management. Ann Surg Oncol 2015;22(13):4263–9.

80. Georgian-Smith D, Lawton TJ. Calcifications of lobular carcinoma in situ of the breast: radiologic-pathologic correlation. AJR Am J Roentgenol 2001;176(5):1255–9.

81. Carder PJ, Shaaban A, Alizadeh Y, et al. Screen-detected pleomorphic lobular carcinoma in situ (PLCIS): risk of concurrent invasive malignancy following a core biopsy diagnosis. Histopathology 2010;57(3):472–8.

82. Bagaria SP, Shamonki J, Kinnaird M, et al. The florid subtype of lobular carcinoma in situ: marker or precursor for invasive lobular carcinoma? Ann Surg Oncol 2011;18(7):1845–51.

83. Alvarado-Cabrero I, Picon Coronel G, Valencia Cedillo R, et al. Florid lobular intraepithelial neoplasia with signet ring cells, central necrosis and calcifications: a clinicopathological and immunohistochemical analysis of ten cases associated with invasive lobular carcinoma. Arch Med Res 2010;41(6):436–41.

84. Chivukula M, Haynik DM, Brufsky A, et al. Pleomorphic lobular carcinoma in situ (PLCIS) on breast core needle biopsies: clinical significance and immunoprofile. Am J Surg Pathol 2008;32(11): 1721–6.

85. Masannat YA, Bains SK, Pinder SE, et al. Challenges in the management of pleomorphic lobular carcinoma in situ of the breast. Breast 2013;22(2): 194–6.

86. King TA, Pilewskie M, Muhsen S, et al. Lobular carcinoma in situ: a 29-year longitudinal experience evaluating clinicopathologic features and breast cancer risk. J Clin Oncol 2015;33(33):3945–52.

87. Middleton LP, Sneige N, Coyne R, et al. Most lobular carcinoma in situ and atypical lobular hyperplasia diagnosed on core needle biopsy can be managed clinically with radiologic follow-up in a multidisciplinary setting. Cancer Med 2014;3(3): 492–9.

88. Abdel-Fatah TM, Powe DG, Hodi Z, et al. High frequency of coexistence of columnar cell lesions, lobular neoplasia, and low grade ductal carcinoma in situ with invasive tubular carcinoma and invasive lobular carcinoma. Am J Surg Pathol 2007;31(3): 417–26.

89. Collins LC, Achacoso NA, Nekhlyudov L, et al. Clinical and pathologic features of ductal carcinoma in situ associated with the presence of flat epithelial atypia: an analysis of 543 patients. Mod Pathol 2007;20(11):1149–55.

90. Georgian-Smith D, Lawton TJ. Variations in physician recommendations for surgery after diagnosis of a high-risk lesion on breast core needle biopsy. AJR Am J Roentgenol 2012;198(2):256–63.

91. Schnitt SJ, Vincent-Salomon A. Columnar cell lesions of the breast. Adv Anat Pathol 2003;10(3):113–24.

92. Schnitt SJ, Collins LC. Columnar cell lesions and flat epithelial atypia of the breast. Semin Breast Dis 2005;8(2):100–11.

93. Schnitt SJ, Collins LC. Columnar cell lesions and flat epithelial atypia. In: Biopsy interpretaiton of the breast. Philadelphia: Lippincott Williams & Wilkins; 2013. p. 107–35.

94. Verschuur-Maes AH, van Deurzen CH, Monninkhof EM, et al. Columnar cell lesions on breast needle biopsies: is surgical excision necessary? A systematic review. Ann Surg 2012;255(2):259–65.

95. Lavoue V, Roger CM, Poilblanc M, et al. Pure flat epithelial atypia (DIN 1a) on core needle biopsy: study of 60 biopsies with follow-up surgical excision. Breast Cancer Res Treat 2011;125(1):121–6.

96. Bianchi S, Bendinelli B, Castellano I, et al. Morphological parameters of flat epithelial atypia (FEA) in stereotactic vacuum-assisted needle core biopsies do not predict the presence of malignancy on subsequent surgical excision. Virchows Arch 2012;461(4):405–17.

97. Peres A, Barranger E, Becette V, et al. Rates of upgrade to malignancy for 271 cases of flat epithelial atypia (FEA) diagnosed by breast core biopsy. Breast Cancer Res Treat 2012;133(2):659–66.

98. Uzoaru I, Morgan BR, Liu ZG, et al. Flat epithelial atypia with and without atypical ductal hyperplasia: to re-excise or not. Results of a 5-year prospective study. Virchows Arch 2012;461(4):419–23.

99. Ceugnart L, Doualliez V, Chauvet MP, et al. Pure flat epithelial atypia: is there a place for routine surgery? Diagn Interv Imaging 2013;94(9):861–9.

100. Villa A, Chiesa F, Massa T, et al. Flat epithelial atypia: comparison between 9-gauge and 11-gauge devices. Clin Breast Cancer 2013;13(6):450–4.

101. Dialani V, Venkataraman S, Frieling G, et al. Does isolated flat epithelial atypia on vacuum-assisted breast core biopsy require surgical excision? Breast J 2014;20(6):606–14.

102. Prowler VL, Joh JE, Acs G, et al. Surgical excision of pure flat epithelial atypia identified on core needle breast biopsy. Breast 2014;23(4):352–6.

103. Yu CC, Ueng SH, Cheung YC, et al. Predictors of underestimation of malignancy after image-guided core needle biopsy diagnosis of flat epithelial atypia or atypical ductal hyperplasia. Breast J 2015;21(3):224–32.

104. Becker AK, Gordon PB, Harrison DA, et al. Flat ductal intraepithelial neoplasia 1A diagnosed at stereotactic core needle biopsy: is excisional biopsy indicated? AJR Am J Roentgenol 2013;200(3):682–8.

105. Acott AA, Mancino AT. Flat epithelial atypia on core needle biopsy, must we surgically excise? Am J Surg 2016;212(6):1211–3.

106. Collins LC, Schnitt SJ. Papillary lesions of the breast: selected diagnostic and management issues. Histopathology 2008;52(1):20–9.

107. Mulligan AM, O'Malley FP. Papillary lesions of the breast: a review. Adv Anat Pathol 2007;14(2):108–19.

108. Wei S. Papillary lesions of the breast: an update. Arch Pathol Lab Med 2016;140(7):628–43.

109. Tse GM, Ni YB, Tsang JY, et al. Immunohistochemistry in the diagnosis of papillary lesions of the breast. Histopathology 2014;65(6):839–53.

110. Grin A, O'Malley FP, Mulligan AM. Cytokeratin 5 and estrogen receptor immunohistochemistry as a useful adjunct in identifying atypical papillary lesions on breast needle core biopsy. Am J Surg Pathol 2009;33(11):1615–23.

111. Collins LC, Carlo VP, Hwang H, et al. Intracystic papillary carcinomas of the breast: a reevaluation using a panel of myoepithelial cell markers. Am J Surg Pathol 2006;30(8):1002–7.

112. Hill CB, Yeh IT. Myoepithelial cell staining patterns of papillary breast lesions: from intraductal papillomas to invasive papillary carcinomas. Am J Clin Pathol 2005;123(1):36–44.

113. Tse GM, Tan PH, Lui PC, et al. The role of immunohistochemistry for smooth-muscle actin, p63, CD10 and cytokeratin 14 in the differential diagnosis of papillary lesions of the breast. J Clin Pathol 2007;60(3):315–20.

114. Wen X, Cheng W. Nonmalignant breast papillary lesions at core-needle biopsy: a meta-analysis of underestimation and influencing factors. Ann Surg Oncol 2013;20(1):94–101.

115. Swapp RE, Glazebrook KN, Jones KN, et al. Management of benign intraductal solitary papilloma diagnosed on core needle biopsy. Ann Surg Oncol 2013;20(6):1900–5.

116. Jaffer S, Bleiweiss IJ, Nagi C. Incidental intraductal papillomas (<2 mm) of the breast diagnosed on needle core biopsy do not need to be excised. Breast J 2013;19(2):130–3.

117. Glenn ME, Throckmorton AD, Thomison JB 3rd, et al. Papillomas of the breast 15 mm or smaller: 4-year experience in a community-based dedicated breast imaging clinic. Ann Surg Oncol 2015;22(4):1133–9.

118. Yamaguchi R, Tanaka M, Tse GM, et al. Management of breast papillary lesions diagnosed in ultrasound-guided vacuum-assisted and core needle biopsies. Histopathology 2015;66(4):565–76.

119. Wyss P, Varga Z, Rossle M, et al. Papillary lesions of the breast: outcomes of 156 patients managed without excisional biopsy. Breast J 2014;20(4):394–401.

120. Cyr AE, Novack D, Trinkaus K, et al. Are we over-treating papillomas diagnosed on core needle biopsy? Ann Surg Oncol 2011;18(4):946–51.

121. Nayak A, Carkaci S, Gilcrease MZ, et al. Benign papillomas without atypia diagnosed on core needle biopsy: experience from a single institution and proposed criteria for excision. Clin Breast Cancer 2013;13(6):439–49.

122. Bennett LE, Ghate SV, Bentley R, et al. Is surgical excision of core biopsy proven benign papillomas of the breast necessary? Acad Radiol 2010;17(5):553–7.

123. Holley SO, Appleton CM, Farria DM, et al. Pathologic outcomes of nonmalignant papillary breast lesions diagnosed at imaging-guided core needle biopsy. Radiology 2012;265(2):379–84.

124. Sohn V, Keylock J, Arthurs Z, et al. Breast papillomas in the era of percutaneous needle biopsy. Ann Surg Oncol 2007;14(10):2979–84.

125. Haagensen CD. Intraductal papilloma. In: Haagensen CD, editor. Diseases of the breast. 2nd edition. Philedelphia: W. B. Saunders Company; 1971. p. 276–90.

126. Wellings SR, Alpers CE. Subgross pathologic features and incidence of radial scars in the breast. Hum Pathol 1984;15(5):475–9.

127. Nielsen M, Jensen J, Andersen JA. An autopsy study of radial scar in the female breast. Histopathology 1985;9(3):287–95.

128. Anderson TJ, Battersby S. Radial scars of benign and malignant breasts: comparative features and significance. J Pathol 1985;147(1):23–32.

129. Frouge C, Tristant H, Guinebretiere JM, et al. Mammographic lesions suggestive of radial scars: microscopic findings in 40 cases. Radiology 1995;195(3):623–5.

130. Douglas-Jones AG, Denson JL, Cox AC, et al. Radial scar lesions of the breast diagnosed by needle core biopsy: analysis of cases containing occult malignancy. J Clin Pathol 2007;60(3):295–8.

131. Sloane JP, Mayers MM. Carcinoma and atypical hyperplasia in radial scars and complex sclerosing lesions: importance of lesion size and patient age. Histopathology 1993;23(3):225–31.

132. Doyle EM, Banville N, Quinn CM, et al. Radial scars/complex sclerosing lesions and malignancy in a screening programme: incidence and histological features revisited. Histopathology 2007;50(5):607–14.

133. Page DL, Anderson TJ. Radial scars and complex sclerosing lesions. In: Page DL, Anderson TJ, editors. Diagnostic histopathology of the breast. Edinburgh (United Kingdom): Churchill Livingstone; 1987. p. 89–103.

134. Linell F, Ljungberg O, Andersson I. Breast carcinoma. Aspects of early stages, progression and related problems. Acta Pathol Microbiol Scand Suppl 1980;(272):1–233.

135. Troupin RH, Orel SG. New insights into mammographic correlations in breast pathology. Curr Opin Radiol 1991;3(4):593–601.

136. Rabban JT, Sgroi DC. Sclerosing lesions of the breast. Semin Diagn Pathol 2004;21(1):42–7.

137. Hilson JB, Schnitt SJ, Collins LC. Phenotypic alterations in myoepithelial cells associated with benign sclerosing lesions of the breast. Am J Surg Pathol 2010;34(6):896–900.

138. de Moraes Schenka NG, Schenka AA, de Souza Queiroz L, et al. p63 and CD10: reliable markers in discriminating benign sclerosing lesions from tubular carcinoma of the breast? Appl Immunohistochem Mol Morphol 2006;14(1):71–7.

139. Brenner RJ, Jackman RJ, Parker SH, et al. Percutaneous core needle biopsy of radial scars of the breast: when is excision necessary? AJR Am J Roentgenol 2002;179(5):1179–84.

140. Becker L, Trop I, David J, et al. Management of radial scars found at percutaneous breast biopsy. Can Assoc Radiol J 2006;57(2):72–8.

141. Cawson JN, Malara F, Kavanagh A, et al. Fourteen-gauge needle core biopsy of mammographically evident radial scars: is excision necessary? Cancer 2003;97(2):345–51.

142. Lopez-Medina A, Cintora E, Mugica B, et al. Radial scars diagnosed at stereotactic core-needle biopsy: surgical biopsy findings. Eur Radiol 2006;16(8):1803–10.

143. Resetkova E, Edelweiss M, Albarracin CT, et al. Management of radial sclerosing lesions of the breast diagnosed using percutaneous vacuum-assisted core needle biopsy: recommendations for excision based on seven years' of experience at a single institution. Breast Cancer Res Treat 2011;127(2):335–43.

144. Linda A, Zuiani C, Furlan A, et al. Radial scars without atypia diagnosed at imaging-guided needle biopsy: how often is associated malignancy found at subsequent surgical excision, and do mammography and sonography predict which lesions are malignant? AJR Am J Roentgenol 2010;194(4):1146–51.

145. Andacoglu O, Kanbour-Shakir A, Teh YC, et al. Rationale of excisional biopsy after the diagnosis of benign radial scar on core biopsy: a single institutional outcome analysis. Am J Clin Oncol 2013;36(1):7–11.

146. Bianchi S, Giannotti E, Vanzi E, et al. Radial scar without associated atypical epithelial proliferation on image-guided 14-gauge needle core biopsy: analysis of 49 cases from a single-centre and review of the literature. Breast 2012;21(2):159–64.

147. Osborn G, Wilton F, Stevens G, et al. A review of needle core biopsy diagnosed radial scars in the Welsh Breast Screening Programme. Ann R Coll Surg Engl 2011;93(2):123–6.

148. Matrai C, D'Alfonso TM, Pharmer L, et al. Advocating nonsurgical management of patients with small, incidental radial scars at the time of needle core biopsy: a study of 77 cases. Arch Pathol Lab Med 2015;139(9):1137–42.

149. Neal L, Sandhu NP, Hieken TJ, et al. Diagnosis and management of benign, atypical, and indeterminate breast lesions detected on core needle biopsy. Mayo Clin Proc 2014;89(4):536–47.

150. Nassar A, Conners AL, Celik B, et al. Radial scar/complex sclerosing lesions: a clinicopathologic correlation study from a single institution. Ann Diagn Pathol 2015;19(1):24–8.

151. Jacobs TW, Byrne C, Colditz G, et al. Radial scars in benign breast-biopsy specimens and the risk of breast cancer. N Engl J Med 1999;340(6):430–6.

152. Nekhlyudov L, Habel LA, Achacoso N, et al. Ten-year risk of diagnostic mammograms and invasive breast procedures after breast-conserving surgery for DCIS. J Natl Cancer Inst 2012;104(8):614–21.

153. NCCN Clinical Practice Guidelines in Oncology (NCCN Guidelines). Breast cancer screening and diagnosis. Version 2.2016 2017. Available at: https://www.nccn.org/professionals/physician_gls/pdf/breast-screening.pdf. Accessed May 22, 2017.

154. Krishnamurthy S, Bevers T, Kuerer H, et al. Multidisciplinary considerations in the management of high-risk breast lesions. AJR Am J Roentgenol 2012;198(2):W132–40.

155. Esserman LJ, Thompson IM Jr, Reid B. Overdiagnosis and overtreatment in cancer: an opportunity for improvement. JAMA 2013;310(8):797–8.

A Diagnostic Approach to Fibroepithelial Breast Lesions

Benjamin Yongcheng Tan, MBBS, FRCPath[a],
Puay Hoon Tan, MBBS, FRCPA, FRCPath[b],*

KEYWORDS

- Breast • Fibroepithelial lesion • Fibroadenoma • Phyllodes tumor • Periductal stromal tumor

---

Key points

- Fibroadenomas are common benign neoplasms of the breast. In comparison, phyllodes tumors are relatively rare and possess potential for recurrence.

- Phyllodes tumors are graded as benign, borderline, or malignant based on histologic evaluation of various parameters. A nomogram based on stromal atypia, mitotic activity, stromal overgrowth, and surgical margin status (AMOS criteria) can individualize recurrence risk.

- Distinction of cellular fibroadenoma from phyllodes tumor can be challenging, especially on limited samples such as core needle biopsies.

- The major differential diagnoses of a malignant spindle cell breast tumor are metaplastic spindle cell carcinoma, malignant phyllodes tumor, and (rarely) sarcoma.

- Recent work has generated new insights into the genetic underpinning of this group of neoplasms, including the prevalence of somatic *MED12* exon2 mutations in fibroadenomas and phyllodes tumors, with additional genomic aberrations observed in borderline and malignant phyllodes tumors.

ABSTRACT

Fibroepithelial breast lesions encompass a heterogeneous group of neoplasms that range from benign to malignant, each exhibiting differing degrees of stromal proliferation in relation to the epithelial compartment. Fibroadenomas are common benign neoplasms that may be treated conservatively. Phyllodes tumors are relatively rare lesions, and classified as benign, borderline, or malignant based on histologic evaluation of various parameters. The diagnostic interpretation of "gray-zone" fibroepithelial lesions often imposes formidable demands on a pathologist's skills. This article offers practical recommendations for the diagnostic workup of these lesions, including the appropriate utilization of ancillary investigations and the approach to core needle biopsies.

Fibroepithelial breast lesions encompass a heterogeneous group of biphasic neoplasms that range from benign to malignant, each of which exhibits differing degrees of epithelial and stromal proliferation.

FIBROADENOMA

CLINICAL FEATURES

A fibroadenoma usually presents as a painless, firm, mobile breast lump, often in younger women aged 20 to 35 years. Multiple and bilateral fibroadenomas occur less commonly. Increasingly, nonpalpable fibroadenomas of smaller size are detected by screening mammography. In adolescents, fibroadenomas may attain significant

---

Disclosure Statement: The authors have no financial conflicts of interest to disclose.
[a] Department of Anatomical Pathology, Singapore General Hospital, Level 10, Diagnostics Tower, Academia, 20 College Road, Singapore 169856, Singapore; [b] Division of Pathology, Singapore General Hospital, Level 7, Diagnostics Tower, Academia, 20 College Road, Singapore 169856, Singapore
* Corresponding author.
E-mail address: tan.puay.hoon@singhealth.com.sg

Surgical Pathology 11 (2018) 17–42
https://doi.org/10.1016/j.path.2017.09.003

dimensions. Patients treated with cyclosporin A immunosuppressive therapy have a propensity for development of fibroadenomas, which may be multiple, bilateral, and of larger size than usual.[1,2] In this patient population, lesional regression and/or stability were observed on substitution of tacrolimus for cyclosporin as an alternative immunosuppressive agent.[3]

GROSS FEATURES

Fibroadenomas are ovoid, circumscribed, white, firm-to-rubbery masses. Although generally 3 cm or smaller, larger fibroadenomas (>4 cm) may occur, especially in younger women. The cut surface, which is typically whitish in color, shows a solid, lobulated appearance that can reveal slender slitlike spaces. Areas of calcification may be present.

MICROSCOPIC FEATURES

A balanced, biphasic proliferation of glandular and stromal elements characterizes fibroadenomas. Although the relative amount of each element may vary, an evenly distributed gland-stroma ratio is usually seen throughout a given lesion. Lesional borders are circumscribed and pushing, without infiltration into surrounding tissue. Of note, fibroadenomas may rarely infarct, especially in gravid patients; the remnant "ghost" architecture of a characteristically balanced biphasic proliferation will suggest the diagnosis.

The stroma of fibroadenomas is typically low in cellularity, shows no significant nuclear atypia, lacks appreciable mitotic activity (except in young or pregnant women), and does not exhibit overgrowth. It frequently has a loose, myxoid quality, especially in younger patients. Myxoid stromal foci may wreathe epithelial elements as prominent cuffs. In older women, the stroma tends to be hypocellular and densely hyalinized. Not infrequently, multinucleated stromal giant cells with nuclear atypia may be found[4–6]; the presence of these cells has not been shown to carry prognostic significance, and should not detract from the correct classification of an otherwise typical lesion. Stromal dystrophic calcifications, often coarse, may be identified. Rarely, ossification may occur, especially in a postmenopausal setting. Pseudoangiomatous stromal hyperplasia (PASH), a benign myofibroblastic proliferation, can on occasion be identified[7] (Fig. 1).

The epithelial component of fibroadenomas comprises ductal epithelial cells supported on an intact myoepithelial layer. An intracanalicular pattern of stromal growth compresses associated epithelium into curvilinear, slitlike spaces, whereas a pericanalicular stromal growth pattern circumferentially surrounds epithelial-lined spaces without luminal distortion.[8] Tangential sectioning may impart an appearance of festooning epithelial "beads" describing the underlying glandular arc. Many fibroadenomas demonstrate both intracanalicular and pericanalicular patterns.

A full spectrum of benign and malignant epithelial changes may be seen in fibroadenomas. Benign processes include lactational change, simple cysts, usual ductal hyperplasia, apocrine metaplasia, and sclerosing adenosis. Atypical ductal hyperplasia (ADH) and atypical lobular hyperplasia may be present within fibroadenomas; furthermore, ductal carcinoma-in-situ (DCIS), lobular carcinoma-in-situ, and invasive carcinomas may arise in or secondarily involve fibroadenomas from adjacent breast tissue.

CYTOLOGIC FINDINGS IN FIBROADENOMA

Cytologic preparations of needle-aspirated fibroadenomas typically yield cellular sheets and "staghorn" clusters of epithelial cells, admixed with numerous bare myoepithelial nuclei.[9,10] Background stromal material, including myxoid stroma, also can be seen (Fig. 2). Rarely, multinucleated giant cells may be discerned.[11,12] The presence of significant epithelial atypia may suggest the concomitant presence of in situ or invasive epithelial malignancy. It is important to note that aspirates of fibroadenoma represent one of the major pitfalls in overdiagnosis of malignancy on breast cytology due to the accompaniment by occasional nuclear atypia and intact cells.

FIBROADENOMA VARIANTS

Cellular Fibroadenoma

The stroma of a cellular fibroadenoma displays conspicuous cellularity (Fig. 3), which may raise the diagnostic possibility of a phyllodes tumor (PT). The distinction of a cellular fibroadenoma from a PT is discussed in detail in a separate section ("Core biopsy of fibroepithelial lesions: challenges and practical recommendations") later in this article.

Complex Fibroadenoma

Defined as a fibroadenoma with at least 1 of the following features: sclerosing adenosis, cysts ≥3 mm in size, papillary apocrine metaplasia, and epithelial calcifications, these tumors tend to present at an older age and are of smaller size than conventional fibroadenomas.[13,14] Florid changes may obscure the underlying fibroadenomatous nature of the lesion, especially on limited core biopsy material.

Fig. 1. (A) Fibroadenoma with a characteristic low-magnification appearance of epithelial and stromal proliferation arranged in a predominantly intracanalicular growth pattern whereby the stroma stretches the epithelium. (B) Pseudoangiomatous stromal hyperplasia with slitlike spaces lined by myofibroblasts is present within the fibroadenoma.

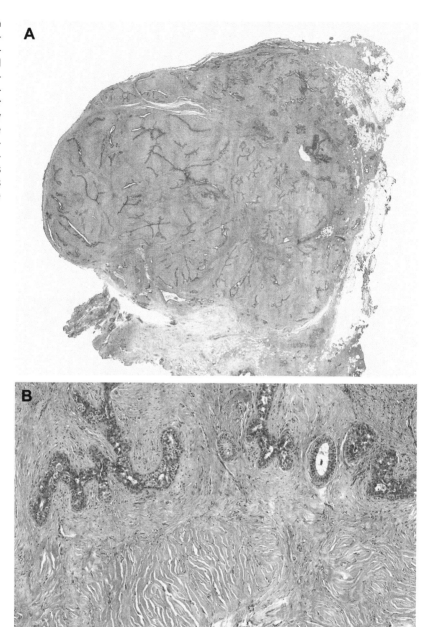

Juvenile Fibroadenoma

Juvenile fibroadenomas, which can exhibit relatively rapid growth in young women, display increased stromal cellularity and epithelial hyperplasia. The stroma, which tends to grow in a pericanalicular fashion, may assume fascicular arrays. Florid epithelial proliferation, often in the form of delicate micropapillary projections reminiscent of gynecomastoid change, can mimic epithelial atypia (ADH or DCIS). The ability of juvenile fibroadenoma to attain a significant size, with resultant breast distortion, has attracted the appellation "giant fibroadenoma,"

although some investigators reserve the application of this term to lesions >5 cm in dimension.[15,16]

Despite the presence of mild intratumoral heterogeneity in some juvenile fibroadenomas, a uniform distribution of stromal cellularity, well-defined lesional borders, and lack of significant stromal atypia should point away from a PT diagnosis.[17]

Myxoid Fibroadenoma

Marked and widespread stromal myxoid change is the hallmark of this lesion (Fig. 4). Extensive

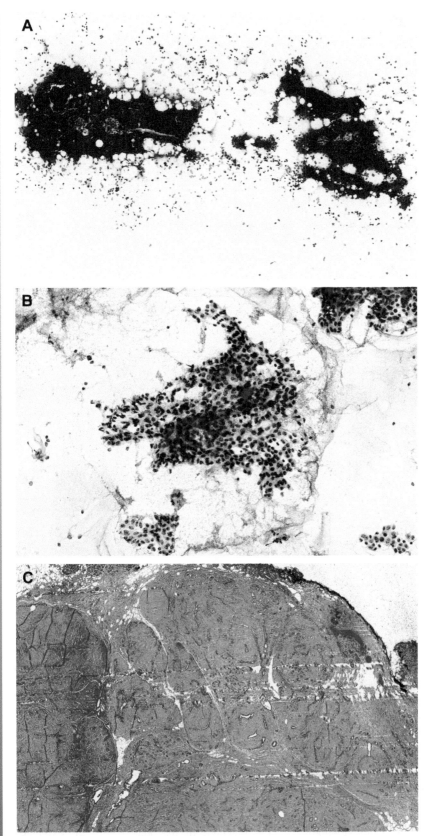

Fig. 2. Fine needle aspiration cytology of a fibroadenoma. (*A*) Diff-Quik smear shows cohesive branched epithelial aggregates punctuated by secondary luminal spaces, with scattered naked ovoid nuclei in the background. (*B*) Papanicolaou stain shows a bimodal population of epithelial cells with interspersed ovoid myoepithelial nuclei. Nuclear atypia may be seen, which can lead to a false-positive diagnosis. (*C*) Excision shows a fibroadenoma.

Fig. 3. Cellular fibroadenoma. (*A*) At low magnification, there is increased stromal cellularity that is variably distributed. (*B*) At higher magnification, stromal cells appear to be more densely aggregated.

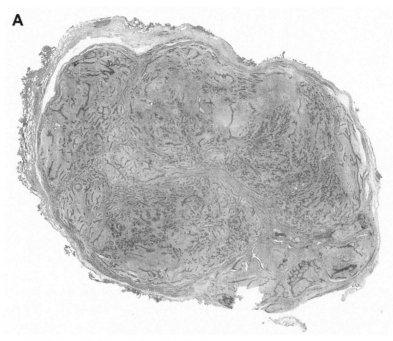

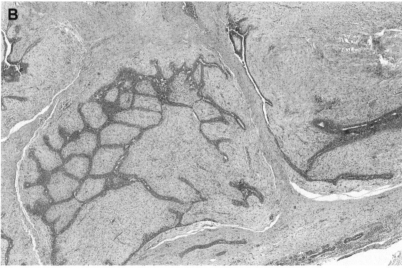

myxoid change contributes to an overall impression of stromal hypocellularity, and may in limited samples convey an erroneous impression of a mucin-predominant process, such as myxoma or mucinous carcinoma. Myxoid fibroadenoma is associated with Carney syndrome, an autosomal dominant condition characterized by a complex of myxomas, spotty skin pigmentation, endocrine overactivity, and psammomatous melanotic schwannomas; in the breasts of these patients, multiple and bilateral myxoid fibroadenomas may be found.[18] However, most cases of myxoid fibroadenomas are seen in patients without known systemic genetic aberrations.

ANCILLARY INVESTIGATIONS

Ancillary testing is not generally required for the diagnosis of fibroadenoma. Immunohistochemical interrogation with CD34 highlights the stromal cells of fibroadenomas,[19,20] which have also been shown to exhibit weak-to-strong nuclear beta-catenin staining.[21] Ki67 typically shows low (<5%) proliferation; however, considerable overlap with PTs, which may also exhibit low proliferative activity, limits the diagnostic utility of this marker.[22–24] Variable estrogen receptor (ER)-beta expression has been reported within the stroma of fibroepithelial lesions, with ER-alpha restricted

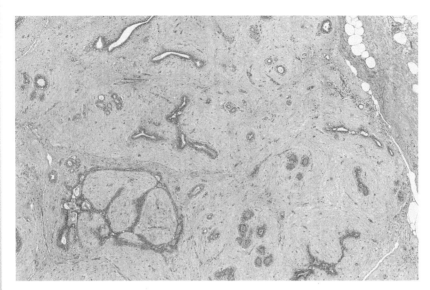

Fig. 4. Myxoid fibroadenoma shows a paucicellular myxoid stroma.

to epithelial cells[25–32]; determination of hormone receptor status is not routine practice in the diagnostic evaluation of these lesions.

DIFFERENTIAL DIAGNOSIS

The major differential diagnosis of a cellular fibroadenoma is with PT. Points of distinction, including the challenges of core needle biopsy diagnosis, are discussed in a separate section ("Core biopsy of fibroepithelial lesions: challenges and practical recommendations") later in this article.

Fibroadenomatoid Change

This descriptor is used when there are appearances that are histologically similar to a fibroadenoma, without formation of a discrete nodule. The stroma, which lacks hypercellularity, overgrowth, and atypia, may be hyalinized.

Tubular Adenoma

A tubular adenoma may be considered to represent the utmost manifestation of adenotic pericanalicular growth, with numerous round-to-oval glandular profiles evenly dispersed within relatively scant stroma (Fig. 5). On occasion, a lesion may demonstrate features of both tubular adenoma and conventional fibroadenoma.

Nodular Pseudoangiomatous Stromal Hyperplasia

The myofibroblastic proliferation associated with stromal clefting that characterizes PASH surrounds rather than distorts epithelium. Spindled cells lining the clefted spaces in PASH are highlighted by CD34 immunohistochemical staining, but are negative for CD31 and Factor VIII. Of note, PASH may be found within the stroma of fibroadenomas and PTs.

Mammary Hamartoma

As compared with a fibroadenoma, the epithelial elements in a mammary hamartoma are more haphazardly distributed. Adipose tissue, a frequent finding within a hamartoma, is rarely seen in a fibroadenoma.[33]

PROGNOSIS

Fibroadenomas are benign tumors, although recent work indicates that similar mutagenic events may underlie development of both fibroadenomas and PTs. In general, fibroadenomas do not recur after complete surgical removal; however, some adolescent patients may experience the growth of new lesions postexcision.[34] Complex fibroadenomas appear to confer an increased relative risk (3.1x) of subsequent breast cancer development,[14] with the risk amplified by a family history of breast carcinoma. No definite increased cancer risk has been found for patients with juvenile fibroadenomas.

Key Features
FIBROADENOMA

- Circumscribed, biphasic proliferation of epithelial and stromal elements
- Mixed intracanalicular and pericanalicular growth patterns
- Stroma shows low cellularity, no significant nuclear atypia, no overgrowth, and absent to rare mitoses

ΔΔ

Differential Diagnosis
FIBROADENOMA

PT	• Exaggerated intracanalicular growth with leaflike fronds
	• Permeative stromal borders, stromal hypercellularity, stromal nuclear atypia, increased stromal mitoses, stromal overgrowth, and malignant heterologous elements may be present
Fibroadenomatoid change	• Does not form a discrete nodule
Tubular adenoma	• Numerous rounded glandular profiles densely disposed within relatively sparse stroma
Nodular PASH	• Myofibroblastic proliferation surrounds rather than distorts epithelial elements
	• Spindled cells positive for CD34, and negative for CD31 and Factor VIII
Mammary hamartoma	• Constituent elements are haphazardly distributed
	• Adipose tissue often present, which is rare in fibroadenomas
	• Typified by "breast within a breast" appearance

PHYLLODES TUMORS

CLINICAL FEATURES

PTs account for 0.3% to 1.0% of all breast tumors in Western countries, constituting 2.5% of breast fibroepithelial tumors, occurring predominantly in middle-aged women. These tumors are reported at a higher frequency and younger age in Asian women.[35,36] Malignant PTs, which usually occur 2 to 5 years later than benign PTs, have been reported more frequently in Hispanic women, especially those from Central and South America.[37,38]

Usually presenting as a firm-to-hard breast mass, large PTs may dramatically stretch the overlying skin, which in exceptional cases can ulcerate. Multifocal or bilateral PTs have been rarely described.[39–42] Paraneoplastic syndromes, including hypoglycemia secondary to insulinlike growth factor II secretion, have been reported in association with large PTs.[43–47]

No clinical features reliably distinguish between PTs and fibroadenomas, or among the different categories of PT.

GROSS FEATURES

PTs generally form circumscribed, solid masses. Characteristically, PTs show tan, gray, or pink cut surfaces with discernible fleshy, leaflike buds bulging into clefts, although this classic gross appearance may not be obvious in smaller lesions. Large tumors can show foci of necrosis and/or hemorrhage (**Fig. 6**).

MICROSCOPIC FEATURES

PTs display an exaggerated pattern of intracanalicular stromal growth, with leaflike stromal fronds protruding into elongated, variably distended clefts lined by a double layer of myoepithelial and epithelial cells.[8] Based on combinatorial analysis of various histologic parameters, PTs are categorized as benign, borderline, or malignant.

The epithelial component of PTs may, as in fibroadenomas, exhibit a full spectrum of benign and malignant changes. PASH has been found to be more common in PTs compared with fibroadenomas.[23]

Benign Phyllodes Tumor

Benign PTs show well-defined tumor borders (**Fig. 7**). Small tumor "nubbins" may bulge into adjacent breast parenchyma; these protuberant buds have delimited, "pushing" contours, without finger- or lacelike permeation of surrounding tissue. The stroma, which is usually more cellular than that of fibroadenomas, contains relatively monomorphic nuclei with few mitoses (<5 per 10 high-power fields [HPFs]). Cellularity is often accentuated just adjacent to the epithelial component, apparent on low-power examination as zones of stromal condensation around epithelial lumina. The stromal cells exhibit at most mild nuclear atypia, although scattered giant cells, akin to those occasionally detected in fibroadenomas, may be found. Stromal myxoid change and hyalinization are a manifestation of tumoral heterogeneity.

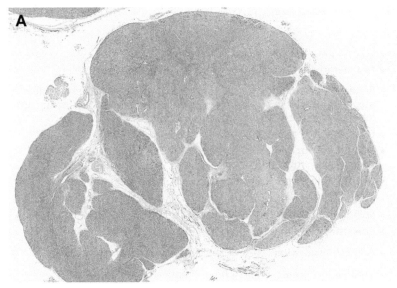

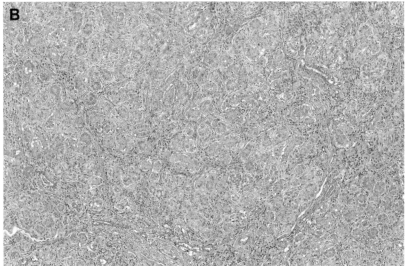

Fig. 5. Tubular adenoma at low (*A*) and higher magnification (*B*) shows a lobulated circumscribed lesion composed of closely placed bilayered tubules.

Malignant Phyllodes Tumor

Malignant PTs, which account for 10% to 20% of all PTs,[36,42] are diagnosed in the presence of permeative stromal extension into surrounding breast tissue, pronounced stromal cellularity, marked stromal nuclear atypia, brisk stromal mitotic activity (≥10 per 10 HPFs), and stromal overgrowth (defined as the absence of epithelial elements in 1 low-power field). Identification of malignant heterologous element(s), such as liposarcoma, chondrosarcoma, osteosarcoma, or rhabdomyosarcoma, relegates a tumor into the malignant category outright, without the requirement for other criteria (Fig. 8).

Borderline Phyllodes Tumor

A borderline PT, as implied by the designation, exhibits histologic features insufficient for an outright diagnosis of malignancy. It may show focally infiltrative borders, moderately increased stromal cellularity (which may be diffusely or patchily distributed), mild-to-moderate stromal nuclear atypia, frequent mitoses (5–9 per 10 HPFs), and at most focal stromal overgrowth

Fig. 6. Macroscopic appearance of a large phyllodes tumor shows a brownish gray mass with whitish and yellowish areas of necrosis. Histologic assessment revealed a malignant phyllodes tumor.

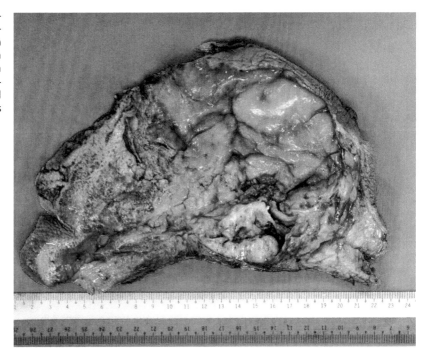

(**Fig. 9**). No malignant heterologous elements should be present.

CYTOLOGIC FINDINGS IN PHYLLODES TUMOR

PT may yield cytologic findings indistinguishable from that of fibroadenoma, comprising an admixture of variably cellular stromal fragments and benign epithelial cells.[48,49] A relative abundance of spindled cells, which may be individually scattered over the aspirate background, nestled in fibromyxoid material, and/or aggregated as hypercellular sheets, is a clue to the correct diagnosis[50–54] (**Fig. 10**). Significant stromal nuclear atypia (including nuclear pleomorphism,

Fig. 7. Benign phyllodes tumor shows a pushing circumscribed border, with leafy fronds composed of hypercellular stroma bounded by benign epithelium.

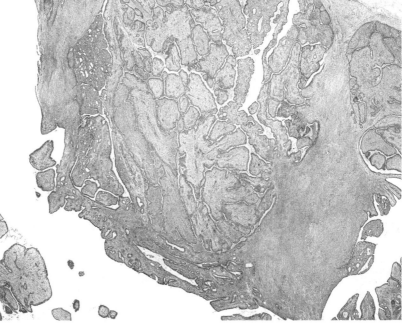

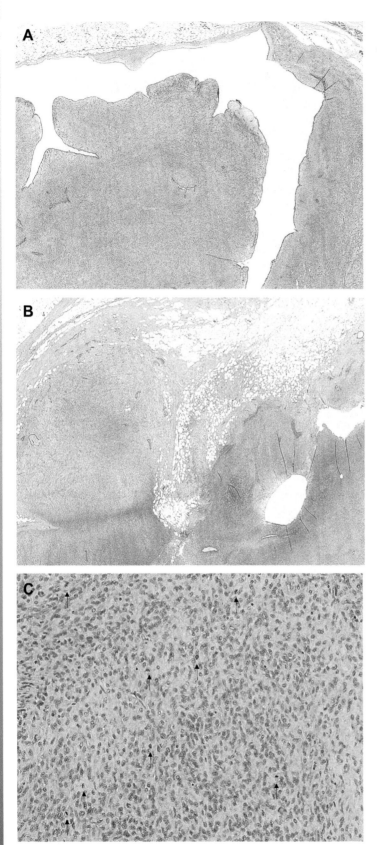

Fig. 8. Malignant phyllodes tumor. (*A*) Low magnification shows a typical fronded appearance of a phyllodes tumor. (*B*) Areas with stromal overgrowth and widely permeative borders are present. (*C*) Brisk mitotic activity is observed (*arrows*).

Fig. 9. Borderline phyllodes tumor. (*A*) Macroscopic specimen shows a lobulated mass with whitish firm and yellowish myxoid areas with a semblance of a cauliflower appearance. (*B*) Low magnification shows patulous fronds of stroma capped by benign epithelium, separated by elongated clefted spaces. (*C*) At higher magnification, a permeative margin is seen, where the stromal component extends into the surrounding adipose tissue.

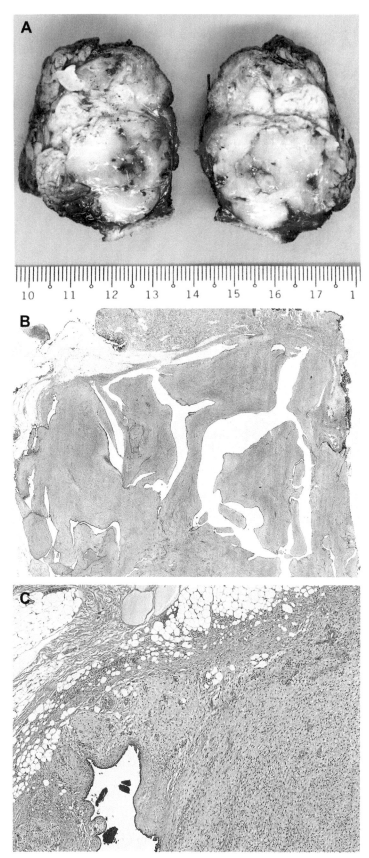

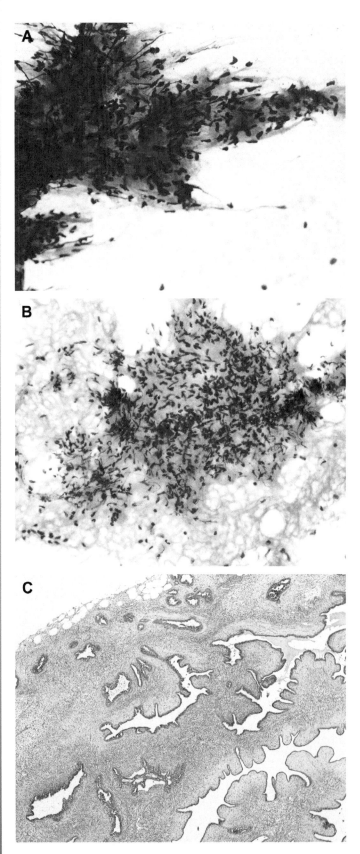

Fig. 10. Fine needle aspiration cytology of a phyllodes tumor. (A) Diff-Quik smear shows a cellular stromal clump with spindled cells displaying narrow elongated nuclei. (B) Papanicolaou smear shows a similar appearance of overlapping spindled stromal cells in a cellular aggregate. (C) Excision specimen confirming a phyllodes tumor.

hyperchromasia, coarse nuclear chromatin, and irregular nuclear contours), prominent spindle cell mitotic activity, and sarcomatous elements are features of malignant PT in the appropriate context[51,55]; for example, lipoblasts imply the presence of liposarcomatous differentiation.[56] Due to morphologic heterogeneity in many PTs, sampling adequacy directly influences diagnostic certainty. A paucity of epithelial elements may be an indication of PT stromal overgrowth[57]; however, in such cases, the differential diagnostic list should incorporate other spindle cell proliferations of the breast, including reactive/inflammatory conditions and neoplasms, such as nodular fasciitis, myofibroblastoma, fibromatosis, metaplastic carcinoma, and primary or metastatic sarcoma.[51]

A NOTE ON SAMPLING

Due to the intratumoral heterogeneity inherent in PTs, areas with high-grade histology may exist only as minor foci within an ostensibly lower-grade tumor. On the other hand, marked overgrowth of malignant stroma in a malignant PT may mask the fibroepithelial nature of the lesion; in such cases, extensive sampling is required to evince the typical epithelial structures crucial to the diagnosis. All PTs should therefore be adequately sampled for accurate histologic classification. At least 1 block per centimeter of maximum tumor dimension is recommended, with additional sampling of grossly heterogeneous areas as indicated.[58]

ANCILLARY INVESTIGATIONS

These are not generally required or useful for grade classification. Although some studies have demonstrated grade-correlated increases of Ki67 (MIB1) expression in PTs,[59] the degree of overlap in benign, borderline and malignant PTs, which exist along a biologic continuum, precludes functional use of Ki67 as a discriminatory marker in any given case.[23,60–64]

DIFFERENTIAL DIAGNOSIS

At the benign morphologic extreme, a PT may resemble a cellular fibroadenoma or mammary fibromatosis, whereas a malignant PT can simulate a metaplastic carcinoma, sarcoma, or melanoma. The differentials of a borderline PT include benign and malignant PTs. Distinction of cellular fibroadenoma from benign PT is discussed in a separate section ("Core biopsy of fibroepithelial lesions: challenges and practical recommendations") later in this article.

Fibromatosis

An ill-circumscribed, variably cellular proliferation of long, sweeping spindle cells characterizes fibromatosis. The constituent cells usually reveal bland nuclear features with rare mitoses. Prominent collagen deposition may be seen. Focal lymphocytic aggregates may be discerned at the lesional periphery. Although fibromatosis can show infiltrative growth around duct-lobular units, an epithelial component is not an inherent element of this tumor. Typically negative for ER, PR, CD34, cytokeratins, and p63, most cases of fibromatosis exhibit aberrant nuclear β-catenin staining.

Metaplastic Carcinoma

A spindle cell metaplastic breast carcinoma contains, in addition to a high-grade spindle cell component, variable proportions of a malignant epithelial element, which may be squamous, glandular, or mixed adenosquamous in morphology (Fig. 11). Occasionally, spindle cell metaplastic carcinomas can lack obvious epithelial elements. Keratin and p63 immunohistochemistry will decorate, at least focally, the spindle cells in these tumors. Identification of DCIS in spatial proximity lends weight to the diagnosis of metaplastic carcinoma.

Sarcoma

Sarcomas of the breast, both primary and metastatic, are exceptional occurrences. PT and metaplastic breast carcinoma should be thoroughly excluded. Angiosarcoma may be a consideration in patients with prior history of radiation therapy. Clinical and radiological correlation, alongside appropriate immunohistochemical investigations, will be of aid in securing the diagnosis.

Malignant Melanoma

In the appropriate clinical context, malignant melanoma with spindled morphology may enter the list of differentials, which should prompt appropriate immunohistochemical investigations, such as with S100, HMB45, and Melan-A.

Periductal Stromal Tumor

Previously referred to as periductal stromal "sarcoma," periductal stromal tumor (PST)[34] is histologically similar to PT, except for the absence of leaflike stromal fronds. The tumor, which may show a multinodular growth pattern,[65–67] comprises noncircumscribed, localized cuffs of spindle cells surrounding epithelium-lined spaces (Fig. 12). Focal liposarcomatous differentiation has been documented in a case report.[66] An occurrence of PST in a male patient of pediatric

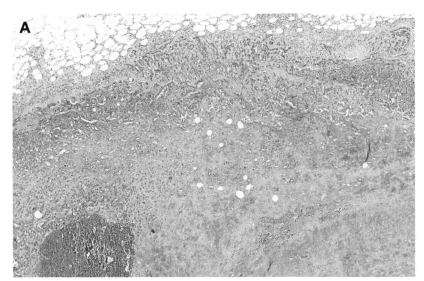

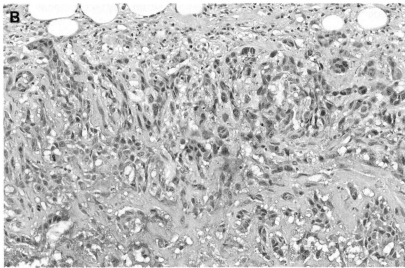

Fig. 11. (*A*) Metaplastic carcinoma shows a chondromyxoid appearance with more cohesive nests of tumor cells at the periphery. (*B*) High magnification reveals pleomorphic tumor cells with mitoses. Immunohistochemistry shows diffuse positive reactivity of tumor cells for p63 (*C*) and the high molecular weight keratin CK5/6 (*D*).

age has been described.[68] The histologic similarity of PST to PT, in addition to observations of its evolution to classic PT,[69] suggest that it may well occupy a position on the spectrum of PT morphology.

PROGNOSIS

Reported recurrence rates for benign, borderline, and malignant PTs are 10% to 17%, 14% to 25%, and 23% to 30%, respectively.[34] A review of the literature yielded summative metastatic rates of 0.13% (2 cases, 0%–3.2%), 1.62% (0%–11.1%), and 16.71% (9.7%–35.3%) for benign, borderline, and malignant PTs, respectively. No

detailed pathologic analysis of the 2 singular cases of apparently metastatic benign PTs was available from the original reports.[70,71] It is not known if exhaustive sampling would have uncovered a higher-grade tumor component in either of these cases. Metastases of PTs almost invariably comprise malignant stromal or heterologous elements without accompanying epithelium.[36,72] Exceptions have been documented in isolated reports[73,74]; in one such case, the epithelial component seen within the metastatic deposit was eventually determined to represent incorporation of pulmonary alveolar tissue, rather than originating from the primary PT. In a study of 952 PTs by Koh and colleagues,[75] large tumor

Fig. 11. (*continued*).

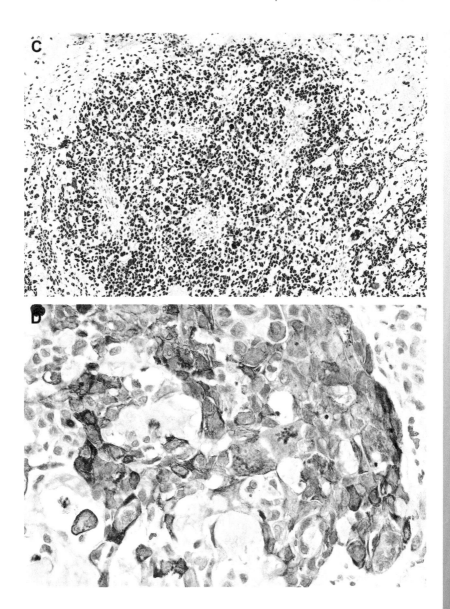

size (≥9 cm) and the presence of malignant heterologous elements predicted for metastasis in malignant PTs.

Although histologic features may, to a certain extent, predict the biologic behavior of PTs, there are limitations to morphologic classification. The problem of interobserver variability is compounded by the fact that each of the 5 histologic parameters key to PT grading exists along a continuum; each parameter contains 2 to 3 categories, giving a total of 108 permutations, from which the pathologist is required to assign 1 of 3 grades. Although diagnostic certainty is achievable at the frankly benign and malignant ends, this is often not the case for the many lesions that fall between the 2 extremes.

In a bid to clarify the impact of each histologic parameter in disease recurrence, Tan and colleagues[42] analyzed 605 PTs in which stromal atypia, mitoses, overgrowth, and surgical margins (the so-called AMOS criteria) were found to significantly predict for recurrence risk, with surgical margin status carrying the most weight. From these results, a nomogram was mathematically derived that could be used to counsel patients with excised PTs on their individual risk of recurrence. The nomogram has been validated in diverse populations.[76–79]

Key Features
PHYLLODES TUMOR

- Biphasic neoplasm with exaggerated intracanalicular growth, resulting in leaflike stromal fronds protruding into epithelium-lined clefts

- Classified as *benign, borderline,* or *malignant* based on a constellation of histologic features:

  1. Stromal borders: circumscribed or permeative

  2. Stromal cellularity: mildly increased, moderately increased, markedly increased

  3. Stromal nuclear atypia: absent/mild, moderate, severe

  4. Stromal mitoses per 10 HPFs: 0 to 4, 5 to 9, $\geq$10

  5. Stromal overgrowth: absent or present

  6. Malignant heterologous element(s): absent or present

- Borderline PT is diagnosed when some, but not all, features favoring malignancy are present

- Presence of a malignant heterologous element classifies a PT as malignant, without the requirement for other parameters

CORE BIOPSY OF FIBROEPITHELIAL LESIONS: CHALLENGES AND PRACTICAL RECOMMENDATIONS

In the context of a core biopsy sample, whereby tissue available for pathologic appraisal embodies only a small proportion of the whole tumor, a histologically equivocal fibroepithelial breast lesion with features of benignity may represent a cellular fibroadenoma or a PT.[80] Precise distinction may be extremely challenging in an individual case. A unanimously accepted criterion drawing the line between degrees of cellularity does not exist.[58] Practically, a pathologist may elect to focus on the most cellular areas of a given tumor. Mild cellularity is characterized by a slight, evenly distributed increase in stromal cell density as compared with perilobular stroma; stromal nuclei are close but do not touch each other. Moderate cellularity may show some overlapping of nuclei. Marked cellularity exhibits pronounced, confluent areas of overlapping nuclear density.[58]

Even among experienced pathologists, it may be no easy task to achieve diagnostic consensus on core biopsy material,[81] although the accurate definition of histologic criteria has been shown to improve interobserver agreement.[82] Histologic attributes found to be predictive of PT on core

Differential Diagnosis
PHYLLODES TUMOR

Cellular fibroadenoma	• Circumscribed borders
	• Mixed intracanalicular and pericanalicular growth patterns
	• Lacks significant stromal hypercellularity, stromal nuclear atypia, increased stromal mitoses, stromal overgrowth, and malignant heterologous elements
PST	• Lacks leaflike fronds
	• Noncircumscribed
	• Multinodular growth may be present
Fibromatosis	• Lacks epithelial component
	• Highlighted by nuclear β-catenin staining
Metaplastic carcinoma	• Lacks leaflike fronds
	• Malignant epithelial component usually present, which may be glandular, squamous, or adenosquamous
	• DCIS may be present adjacent to tumor
	• Spindled cells highlighted by keratin and/or p63 immunohistochemistry
Sarcoma	• Lacks epithelial component
	• May show sarcoma-specific genetic aberrations
	• Important to rule out malignant PT, metaplastic carcinoma, and metastasis before diagnosing a primary breast sarcoma

Fig. 12. Periductal stroma tumor shows a hypercellular wreath of stromal cells around benign bilayered epithelium.

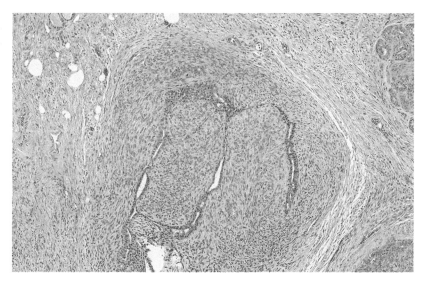

biopsy[22,23,33,83,84] are summarized in the Table "Core Biopsy of Cellular Fibroepithelial Breast Lesions." Among these, increased stromal cellularity and mitotic activity were common key features of PTs, which also exhibited elevated Ki67, topoisomerase IIα (a cell proliferation-related enzyme), and reduced CD34 immunohistochemistry staining.[22,23] Tsang and colleagues,[85] in a study of 118 core needle biopsy specimens of fibroepithelial breast lesions, concluded that PTs demonstrated "more consistent" stromal cellular changes (overall cellularity, variation in cellularity, nuclear pleomorphism, mitotic count) than fibroadenomas. Interestingly, Jara-Lazaro and colleagues[23] found that of 23 core biopsy samples of fibroepithelial breast lesions exhibiting PASH, 19 (83%) were from PTs, a statistically significant association (*P* = .043).

Given the challenge of separating these 2 lesions, it is natural to question if fibroadenomas and benign PTs pose significant differences in risk of recurrence and malignant transformation. Fibroadenomas are benign. Isolated reports document fibroadenoma recurrence risks of 15% to 17%,[86–88] comparable to that for benign PTs, which fall in the range of 10% to 17%.[36,42,89] However, although a recurrence rate of 10.9% was observed in benign PTs in 1 study, with most of the recurrent tumors retaining benign histology, 35% were upgraded to borderline PT and 8% to malignant PT; overall, this amounted to a benign-to-malignant PT upgrade rate of 1%.[42] The critical difference therefore lies in the fact that a benign PT poses a small likelihood of malignant progression. Substantial intratumoral genetic heterogeneity

exists within PTs, with the implication that subclones in benign tumors may acquire additional genetic aberrations that launch them on the path to malignancy[90]; thus far, no light microscopic attributes have been elucidated that reliably identify which benign PTs harbor such ominous potential.

In the evaluation of fibroepithelial breast lesions on core biopsy, a balance must be struck between achieving maximal sensitivity of PT diagnosis, and the avoidance of assigning excessive weight to minor changes that might result in overzealous excisions of fibroadenomas. Although stromal Ki67 index ≥5% may be suggestive of PT on a core biopsy,[22,23] this is of potential use only when such immunoreactivity exists; low or absent Ki67 labeling does not distinguish between a fibroadenoma and PT.

In practice, when a constellation of features suggestive of PT is present, the diagnosis should be formulated such that excision with an adequate tissue rim, rather than simple enucleation or observation, is considered by the treating clinician. However, recent studies suggest that expectant management may be a reasonable policy to adopt in cases of benign PTs with positive surgical margins[91,92]; given the relatively low rates of recurrence in these tumors, repeat surgery to achieve pathologically negative margins would be unnecessary in most patients. A study of 90 patients with low-grade fibroepithelial lesions by Cowan and colleagues[93] revealed no statistically significant difference in local recurrence rates between patients with positive or negative surgical margins, and those with positive margins who did or did not undergo reexcision; neither did the extent of margin positivity predict recurrence. A holistic evaluation of clinical and radiological factors, such as lesional size and rate of growth, is useful in steering management.

Aside from the distinction of cellular fibroadenoma from PT as discussed previously, other considerations can arise in the setting of a limited core biopsy.

A relatively bland spindle cell proliferation may represent portions of a benign or borderline PT, mammary fibromatosis, or fibromatosis-like metaplastic carcinoma. Although routinely used as a confirmatory immunohistochemical marker of fibromatosis, aberrant nuclear expression of β-catenin has been reported in PT stroma, as well as in metaplastic carcinomas.[21,94–96] Sole reliance on β-catenin in the evaluation of mammary spindle cell lesions must therefore be cautioned against.

At the other extreme of the histologic spectrum, a malignant spindle cell proliferation raises the main differential diagnoses of malignant PT with stromal overgrowth, spindle cell metaplastic breast carcinoma, and sarcoma. The presence, even as a small component, of epithelium-lined clefts typical of a PT will strongly support that diagnosis. As mentioned, malignant heterologous stromal elements, such as liposarcoma, chondrosarcoma, osteosarcoma, or rhabdomyosarcoma may be present. Except in rare cases of coexistent epithelial malignancy, no in situ carcinoma is seen. Squamous differentiation is not a usual feature of the stromal component of PT. Cytokeratin and p63 immunohistochemistry should not, except in rare cases, stain the stromal cells of a PT to a significant degree.[97,98]

Significant cytokeratin or p63 immunoreactivity in malignant spindle cells, the presence of squamous differentiation, as well as adjacent DCIS, favor a diagnosis of metaplastic carcinoma. p40 has been found to be more specific but less sensitive than p63 in this setting.[98–100] As a note of caution, cytokeratin, p63, and p40 staining of PT stroma has been reported[97,98] (Fig. 13). Although CD34 is known to stain the stromal cells of PT, it is of limited utility in the diagnostic workup of a high-grade spindle cell breast lesion, as malignant PTs are less likely to express CD34 compared with their lower-grade counterparts.[20,23,24,101–103] Other markers, such as bcl-2[23,104,105] and CD117,[106,107] are not in routine use for this purpose.

In the absence of a known primary, breast sarcoma is a diagnosis arrived at after diligent exclusion of malignant PT and metaplastic carcinoma. Probes for sarcoma-specific molecular cytogenetic alterations can be an aid to rendering the diagnosis in individual cases.

Core Biopsy of Cellular Fibroepithelial Breast Lesions

Author	Key Findings Predicting Phyllodes Tumor
Jacobs et al,[22] 2005	• Marked stromal cellularity
	• Mitotic rate >2 per 10 HPFs in lesions with moderate cellularity
	• Elevated Ki67 and topoisomerase IIα indices
Lee et al,[33] 2007	• Stromal cellularity increased ≥50%
	• Stromal overgrowth
	• Core fragmentation
	• Adipose tissue is present within stroma
Jara-Lazaro et al,[23] 2010	• Marked stromal cellularity
	• Stromal atypia
	• Stromal overgrowth
	• Mitotic rate ≥2 per 10 HPFs
	• Ill-defined lesional borders
	• Ki67 and topoisomerase IIα indices ≥5%
	• Reduced or patchy CD34 staining
Resetkova et al,[83] 2010	• No clinical, radiological, or histologic parameters accurately predicted final histologic classification
Yasir et al,[84] 2014	• Mitotic rate ≥3 per 10 HPFs, and/or
	• 3 or more of the following features:
	○ Stromal overgrowth
	○ Increased stromal cellularity
	○ Stromal heterogeneity
	○ Subepithelial stromal condensation
	○ Stromal nuclear pleomorphism
	○ Core fragmentation
	○ Adipose tissue infiltration/fat entrapment

Fig. 13. Malignant phyllodes tumor. (*A*) Areas of hemorrhage are seen at low magnification. (*B*) Patchy nuclear reactivity for p63 is seen in stromal cells.

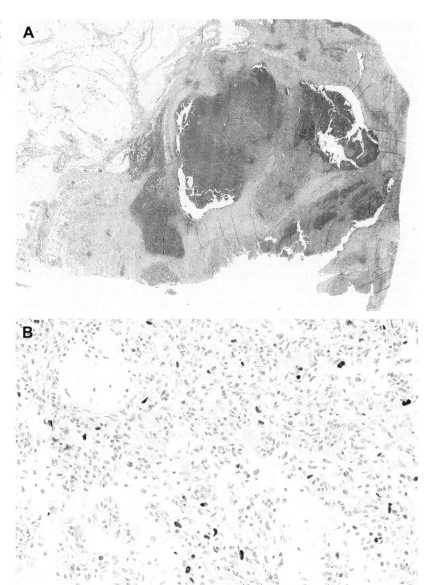

DISTINGUISHING FIBROADENOMA AND PHYLLODES TUMOR ON CYTOLOGY

Although largely superseded by core needle biopsy in many centers, fine needle aspiration cytology retains an important role in resource-limited settings. Cytologic distinction of fibroadenomas from PTs can be fraught with difficulty, owing to considerable cytomorphological overlap between the 2 entities.[48,49,108] Both may yield cellular stromal fragments. In numerous studies, the relative abundance of spindled stromal nuclei was a clue to a diagnosis of PT[50,52,109,110]; 1 study established a cutoff of more than 30% long spindled nuclei within background dispersed stromal cells as the threshold beyond which a PT diagnosis might be favored.[111] A high stromal-epithelial ratio, marked stromal cellularity, stromal cell pleomorphism and mitotic activity are cytologic attributes of malignant PTs.[112,113] Judicious cytologic interpretation should be accompanied by careful clinico-radiological correlation in all cases.

A NOTE ON FIBROEPITHELIAL BREAST LESIONS IN YOUNG PATIENTS

In a study of 54 fibroepithelial lesions from adolescent girls (age ≤18 years), Ross and colleagues[114] elucidated mean mitotic rates per 10 HPFs in various lesions as follows: 1.3 (range 0–6) in usual fibroadenomas, 1.8 in juvenile fibroadenomas, 3.1 in benign PTs, 10 in borderline PTs, and 17 in malignant PTs.

In another study of 68 fibroepithelial lesions from 53 pediatric subjects by Tay and colleagues,[115] 27 (39.7%) fibroadenomas, 32 (47.1%) juvenile fibroadenomas, 3 (4.4%) cellular fibroadenomas, and 3 (4.4%) benign PTs were found, with the remaining 3 (4.4%) cases comprising benign fibroepithelial neoplasms displaying focal infarction and hybrid features. Half of the lesions exhibited small leaflike fronds, whereas most (83.8%) demonstrated (at least) moderate stromal cellularity. In this study, 23.5% (16/68) of lesions showed ≥1 mitoses per 10 HPFs, whereas the remainder had no discernible mitotic activity. Faiz and colleagues[116] found stromal mitoses in all fibroadenoma subtypes (cellular, classic, and juvenile) in a study of 119 pediatric cases, with up to 5 mitoses per 10 HPFs documented in 2 cases. In a study of 379 pediatric fibroepithelial lesions by Ozerdem and Tavassoli,[117] epithelial atypia amounting to ADH was seen in 1.3% of the cases; other observations included the presence of usual ductal hyperplasia (8.4%), infarct (1.6%), PASH (1.3%), and fibrocystic changes (1.3%), as well as overlapping features of fibroadenoma and tubular adenoma (3.6%).

Recognition of unique morphologic features in pediatric fibroepithelial lesions should engender a measured evaluation of these tumors, with the aim of avoiding PT overdiagnosis, thereby averting unnecessary and cosmetically deleterious surgery.

Pitfalls
FIBROEPITHELIAL BREAST LESIONS

! Additional pathology, including in situ or invasive carcinoma, may be present

Fibroadenoma

! Juvenile fibroadenomas can exhibit rapid growth, increased stromal cellularity, and florid epithelial proliferation

Phyllodes Tumor

! Significant intratumoral heterogeneity may exist. Some PTs may harbor fibroadenomalike areas

! Due to marked overgrowth of stroma in some malignant PTs, extensive sampling may be required to reveal characteristic epithelium-lined architecture

MOLECULAR BIOLOGY OF FIBROEPITHELIAL BREAST LESIONS

Although PTs had historically been regarded as de novo lesions arising from mammary intralobular or periductal stroma, clonal analysis demonstrated findings suggestive of fibroadenoma-to-PT progression.[118] More recently, *MED12* exon 2 somatic mutations, reported in most uterine leiomyomas,[119–122] have been shown to occur with high prevalence in fibroadenomas, benign and borderline PTs,[123–125] while being significantly less common in malignant PTs.[124,126] *MED12* exon 2 mutations, which likely represent genomic drivers of breast fibroepithelial tumorigenesis, are restricted to the stromal elements of these tumors.[123] Further work has uncovered somatic mutations in *PIK3CA*, *RARA*, *FLNA*, *SETD2*, and *KMT2D* within PTs, with borderline and malignant lesions acquiring additional aberrations in cancer-associated genes, such as *TP53*, *RB1*, *EGFR*, and *NF1*.[124,127–130] Regions of intratumoral heterogeneity within malignant PT appear to exhibit increasing numbers of mutations in parallel with morphologic attributes of increasing cellularity and pleomorphism.[131] Fibroadenomas and PTs in patients with multiple fibroepithelial breast lesions have been found to harbor both identical and nonidentical *MED12* somatic mutations,[125] suggesting that although some malignant *MED12*-mutant PTs may indeed arise from fibroadenomas, other *MED12*–wild-type malignant PTs likely possess alternative driver mutations. Recent work has correlated prevalence of *TERT* promoter mutations with increasing malignancy in fibroepithelial breast lesions, suggesting a mechanistic role for *TERT* alterations in the progression of these tumors.[129,132,133] Elucidation of clinically actionable targets is an active area of research.[124,130,134,135]

A molecular assay for fibroepithelial breast lesions, comprising a 5-gene transcript set (ABCA8, APOD, CCL19, FN1, and PRAME), has been developed for use on formalin-fixed paraffin-embedded tissue samples.[136] This assay, which accurately classified 92.6% of fibroepithelial lesions in 230 preoperative core biopsies as either fibroadenomas or PTs, had a sensitivity of 82.9% and specificity of 94.7%. It is important to note that the study's investigators "do not advocate that the current diagnostic framework be replaced by the assay." However, if validated by prospective studies, the assay may assume a useful adjunctive role in histologically ambiguous cases.[136]

SUMMARY

"Gray-zone" lesions, such as cellular fibroepithelial breast lesions, often impose formidable demands on a pathologist's diagnostic skills. The World Health Organization Working Group has recognized the difficulty pathologists face in accurate classification of histologically indeterminate lesions, with a recommendation that in cases of histologic ambiguity, a diagnosis of fibroadenoma should be favored over that of a benign PT to avoid overtreatment.[137] However, the Working Group also acknowledged that in some circumstances, a circumspect diagnosis of "cellular fibroepithelial neoplasm" may be most appropriate. On the other hand, the accurate diagnosis of malignant PTs is emphasized. A recent multicenter consensus review offers several practical recommendations regarding the diagnostic approach to fibroepithelial breast lesions,[58] including the following recommendations of direct relevance to practicing pathologists:

1. Accuracy and consistency in PT grading should be strived for at the benign and malignant extremes of the histologic spectrum.
2. Definitive distinction between cellular fibroadenomas and benign PTs may not be critical, given similar reported recurrence rates. The term "benign fibroepithelial lesion/neoplasm" may be useful in cases in which diagnostic ambiguity exists, although this term should be used sparingly.
3. Malignant PTs are diagnosed in the presence of the following histologic features: marked stromal hypercellularity, stromal atypia, stromal mitoses ≥10 per 10 HPFs, stromal overgrowth, and permeative tumor borders. A malignant heterologous component classifies a PT as malignant without a requirement for other histologic features.
4. Accurate recognition of malignant PTs will allow timely institution of management for these lesions, which have a relatively infrequent but well-established risk of recurrence and metastasis.[34]

REFERENCES

1. Weinstein SP, Orel SG, Collazzo L, et al. Cyclosporin A-induced fibroadenomas of the breast: report of five cases. Radiology 2001;220(2):465–8.
2. Son EJ, Oh KK, Kim EK, et al. Characteristic imaging features of breast fibroadenomas in women given cyclosporin A after renal transplantation. J Clin Ultrasound 2004;32(2):69–77.
3. Iaria G, Pisani F, De Luca L, et al. Prospective study of switch from cyclosporine to tacrolimus for fibroadenomas of the breast in kidney transplantation. Transplant Proc 2010;42(4):1169–70.
4. Powell CM, Cranor ML, Rosen PP. Multinucleated stromal giant cells in mammary fibroepithelial neoplasms. A study of 11 patients. Arch Pathol Lab Med 1994;118(9):912–6.
5. Berean K, Tron VA, Churg A, et al. Mammary fibroadenoma with multinucleated stromal giant cells. Am J Surg Pathol 1986;10(11):823–7.
6. Heneghan HM, Martin ST, Casey M, et al. A diagnostic dilemma in breast pathology–benign fibroadenoma with multinucleated stromal giant cells. Diagn Pathol 2008;3:33.
7. Powell CM, Cranor ML, Rosen PP. Pseudoangiomatous stromal hyperplasia (PASH). A mammary stromal tumor with myofibroblastic differentiation. Am J Surg Pathol 1995;19(3):270–7.
8. Tan PH, Sahin A. Fibroepithelial lesions. In: Tan PH, Sahin AS, editors. Atlas of differential diagnosis in breast pathology. 1st edition. New York: Springer Science+Business Media LLC; 2017. p. 51–96.
9. Malberger E, Yerushalmi R, Tamir A, et al. Diagnosis of fibroadenoma in breast fine needle aspirates devoid of typical stroma. Acta Cytol 1997; 41(5):1483–8.
10. Bottles K, Chan JS, Holly EA, et al. Cytologic criteria for fibroadenoma. A step-wise logistic regression analysis. Am J Clin Pathol 1988;89(6): 707–13.
11. V S, R K, Murthy VS. Multinucleate giant cells in FNAC of benign breast lesions: its significance. J Clin Diagn Res 2014;8(12):FC01–4.
12. Huo L, Gilcrease MZ. Fibroepithelial lesions of the breast with pleomorphic stromal giant cells: a clinicopathologic study of 4 cases and review of the literature. Ann Diagn Pathol 2009;13(4):226–32.
13. Sklair-Levy M, Sella T, Alweiss T, et al. Incidence and management of complex fibroadenomas. Am J Roentgenol 2008;190(1):214–8.
14. Dupont WD, Page DL, Parl FF, et al. Long-term risk of breast cancer in women with fibroadenoma. N Engl J Med 1994;331(1):10–5.
15. McCague A, Davis JV. Giant fibroadenoma in a 22 year old patient: case report and literature review. Breast Dis 2010;31(1):49–52.
16. Alagaratnam TT, Ng WF, Leung EY. Giant fibroadenomas of the breast in an oriental community. J R Coll Surg Edinb 1995;40(3):161–2.
17. Ross DS, Giri DD, Akram MM, et al. Fibroepithelial lesions in the breast of adolescent females: a clinicopathological profile of 35 cases. Mod Pathol 2012;25(Suppl.2):64A.
18. Carney JA, Toorkey BC. Myxoid fibroadenoma and allied conditions (myxomatosis) of the breast. A heritable disorder with special associations including cardiac and cutaneous myxomas. Am J Surg Pathol 1991;15(8):713–21.
19. Chauhan H, Abraham A, Phillips JRA, et al. There is more than one kind of myofibroblast: analysis of CD34 expression in benign, in situ, and invasive breast lesions. J Clin Pathol 2003;56(4):271–6.
20. Moore T, Lee AH. Expression of CD34 and bcl-2 in phyllodes tumours, fibroadenomas and spindle cell

lesions of the breast. Histopathology 2001;38(1): 62–7.

21. Sawyer EJ, Hanby AM, Poulsom R, et al. Beta-catenin abnormalities and associated insulin-like growth factor overexpression are important in phyllodes tumours and fibroadenomas of the breast. J Pathol 2003;200(5):627–32.

22. Jacobs TW, Chen Y-Y, Guinee DG Jr, et al. Fibroepithelial lesions with cellular stroma on breast core needle biopsy: are there predictors of outcome on surgical excision? Am J Clin Pathol 2005;124(3): 342–54.

23. Jara-Lazaro AR, Akhilesh M, Thike AA, et al. Predictors of phyllodes tumours on core biopsy specimens of fibroepithelial neoplasms. Histopathology 2010;57(2):220–32.

24. Vilela MHT, de Almeida FM, de Paula GM, et al. Utility of Ki-67, CD10, CD34, p53, CD117, and mast cell content in the differential diagnosis of cellular fibroadenomas and in the classification of phyllodes tumors of the breast. Int J Surg Pathol 2014;22(6):485–91.

25. Branchini G, Schneider L, Cericatto R, et al. Progesterone receptors A and B and estrogen receptor alpha expression in normal breast tissue and fibroadenomas. Endocrine 2009;35(3):459–66.

26. Sapino A, Bosco M, Cassoni P, et al. Estrogen receptor-beta is expressed in stromal cells of fibroadenoma and phyllodes tumors of the breast. Mod Pathol 2006;19(4):599–606.

27. Umekita Y, Yoshida H. Immunohistochemical study of hormone receptor and hormone-regulated protein expression in phyllodes tumour: comparison with fibroadenoma. Virchows Arch 1998;433(4): 311–4.

28. Khanna AK, Tapodar JK, Khanna HD, et al. Behaviour of estrogen receptor, histological correlation, and clinical outcome in patients with benign breast disorders. Eur J Surg 2002;168(11):631–4.

29. Tochika N, Ogawa Y, Kumon M, et al. Rapid growing fibroadenoma in an adolescent. Breast Cancer 1998;5(3):321–4.

30. Mechtersheimer G, Krüger KH, Born IA, et al. Antigenic profile of mammary fibroadenoma and cystosarcoma phyllodes. A study using antibodies to estrogen- and progesterone receptors and to a panel of cell surface molecules. Pathol Res Pract 1990;186(4):427–38.

31. Shoker BS, Jarvis C, Clarke RB, et al. Abnormal regulation of the oestrogen receptor in benign breast lesions. J Clin Pathol 2000;53(10):778–83.

32. Pilichowska M, Kimura N, Fujiwara H, et al. Immunohistochemical study of TGF-alpha, TGF-beta1, EGFR, and IGF-1 expression in human breast carcinoma. Mod Pathol 1997;10(10):969–75.

33. Lee AHS, Hodi Z, Ellis IO, et al. Histological features useful in the distinction of phyllodes tumour

and fibroadenoma on needle core biopsy of the breast. Histopathology 2007;51(3):336–44.

34. Lakhani SR, Ellis IO, Schnitt SJ, et al. WHO classification of tumours of the breast. Lyon (France): IARC Press; 2012.

35. Chua CL, Thomas A, Ng BK. Cystosarcoma phyllodes–Asian variations. Aust N Z J Surg 1988; 58(4):301–5.

36. Tan P-H, Jayabaskar T, Chuah K-L, et al. Phyllodes tumors of the breast: the role of pathologic parameters. Am J Clin Pathol 2005;123(4):529–40.

37. Bernstein L, Deapen D, Ross RK. The descriptive epidemiology of malignant cystosarcoma phyllodes tumors of the breast. Cancer 1993;71(10):3020–4.

38. Pimiento JM, Gadgil PV, Santillan AA, et al. Phyllodes tumors: race-related differences. J Am Coll Surg 2011;213(4):537–42.

39. Barrio AV, Clark BD, Goldberg JI, et al. Clinicopathologic features and long-term outcomes of 293 phyllodes tumors of the breast. Ann Surg Oncol 2007;14(10):2961–70.

40. Mallory MA, Chikarmane SA, Raza S, et al. Bilateral synchronous benign phyllodes tumors. Am Surg 2015;81(5):E192–4.

41. Seal SK, Kuusk U, Lennox PA. Bilateral and multifocal phyllodes tumours of the breast: a case report. Can J Plast Surg 2010;18(4):145–6.

42. Tan PH, Thike AA, Tan WJ, et al. Predicting clinical behaviour of breast phyllodes tumours: a nomogram based on histological criteria and surgical margins. J Clin Pathol 2012;65(1):69–76.

43. Reisenbichler ES, Krontiras H, Hameed O. Beta-human chorionic gonadotropin production associated with phyllodes tumor of the breast: an unusual paraneoplastic phenomenon. Breast J 2009;15(5): 527–30.

44. Hino N, Nakagawa Y, Ikushima Y, et al. A case of a giant phyllodes tumor of the breast with hypoglycemia caused by high-molecular-weight insulin-like growth factor II. Breast Cancer 2010;17(2):142–5.

45. Bujanda DA, Vera JCR, Suárez MÁC, et al. Hypoglycemic coma secondary to big insulin-like growth factor II secretion by a giant phyllodes tumor of the breast. Breast J 2007;13(2):189–91.

46. Kataoka T, Haruta R, Goto T, et al. Malignant phyllodes tumor of the breast with hypoglycemia: report of a case. Jpn J Clin Oncol 1998;28(4):276–80.

47. Saito Y, Suzuki Y, Inomoto C, et al. A case of giant borderline phyllodes tumor of the breast associated with hypoglycemia. Tokai J Exp Clin Med 2016;41(3):118–22.

48. Tse GM, Tan P-H. Diagnosing breast lesions by fine needle aspiration cytology or core biopsy: which is better? Breast Cancer Res Treat 2010;123(1):1–8.

49. Deen SA, McKee GT, Kissin MW. Differential cytologic features of fibroepithelial lesions of the breast. Diagn Cytopathol 1999;20(2):53–6.

50. El Hag IA, Aodah A, Kollur SM, et al. Cytological clues in the distinction between phyllodes tumor and fibroadenoma. Cancer Cytopathol 2010; 118(1):33–40.

51. Scolyer RA, Mckenzie PR, Achmed D, et al. Can phyllodes tumours of the breast be distinguished from fibroadenomas using fine needle aspiration cytology? Pathology 2001;33(4):437–43.

52. Jayaram G, Sthaneshwar P. Fine-needle aspiration cytology of phyllodes tumors. Diagn Cytopathol 2002;26(4):222–7.

53. Stanley MW, Tani EM, Rutqvist LE, et al. Cystosarcoma phyllodes of the breast: a cytologic and clinicopathologic study of 23 cases. Diagn Cytopathol 1989;5(1):29–34.

54. Shimizu K, Masawa N, Yamada T, et al. Cytologic evaluation of phyllodes tumors as compared to fibroadenomas of the breast. Acta Cytol 1994; 38(6):891–7.

55. Vladescu T, Klijanienko J, Caillaud J-M, et al. Fine-needle sampling in malignant phyllodes tumors: clinicopathologic study of 22 cases seen at the Institut Curie. Diagn Cytopathol 2004;31(2):71–6.

56. Satou T, Matsunami N, Fujiki C, et al. Malignant phyllodes tumor with liposarcomatous components: a case report with cytological presentation. Diagn Cytopathol 2000;22(6):364–9.

57. Rao BR, Meyer JS, Fry CG. Most cystosarcoma phyllodes and fibroadenomas have progesterone receptor but lack estrogen receptor: stromal localization of progesterone receptor. Cancer 1981; 47(8):2016–21.

58. Tan BY, Acs G, Apple SK, et al. Phyllodes tumours of the breast: a consensus review. Histopathology 2016;68(1):5–21.

59. Tse GMK, Hoon Tan P, Rowan AJ, et al. Recent advances in the pathology of fibroepithelial tumours of the breast. Curr Diagn Pathol 2005;11(6):426–34.

60. Karim RZ, Gerega SK, Yang YH, et al. p16 and pRb immunohistochemical expression increases with increasing tumour grade in mammary phyllodes tumours. Histopathology 2010;56(7):868–75.

61. Dacic S, Kounelis S, Kouri E, et al. Immunohistochemical profile of cystosarcoma phyllodes of the breast: a study of 23 cases. Breast J 2002;8(6): 376–81.

62. Umekita Y, Yoshida H. Immunohistochemical study of MIB1 expression in phyllodes tumor and fibroadenoma. Pathol Int 1999;49(9):807–10.

63. Kočová L, Skálová A, Fakan F, et al. Phyllodes tumour of the breast: immunohistochemical study of 37 tumours using MIB1 antibody. Pathol Res Pract 1998;194(2):97–104.

64. Munawer NH, Md Zin R, Md Ali S-A, et al. ER, p53 and MIB-1 are significantly associated with malignant phyllodes tumor. Biomed J 2012;35(6): 486–92.

65. Abbasi SL, Namara KM, Absar MS, et al. Periductal stromal tumor of breast: a case report and a review of literature. Korean J Pathol 2014;48(6):442–4.

66. White SR, Auguste LJ, Guo H, et al. Periductal stromal sarcoma of the breast with liposarcomatous differentiation: a case report with 10-year follow-up and literature review. Int J Surg Pathol 2015;23(3):221–4.

67. Tomas D, Janković D, Marušić Z, et al. Low-grade periductal stromal sarcoma of the breast with myxoid features: immunohistochemistry. Pathol Int 2009;59(8):588–91.

68. Masbah O, Lalya I, Mellas N, et al. Periductal stromal sarcoma in a child: a case report. J Med Case Rep 2011;5:249.

69. Burga AM, Tavassoli FA. Periductal stromal tumor: a rare lesion with low-grade sarcomatous behavior. Am J Surg Pathol 2003;27(3):343–8.

70. Abdalla HM, Sakr MA. Predictive factors of local recurrence and survival following primary surgical treatment of phyllodes tumors of the breast. J Egypt Natl Canc Inst 2006;18(2):125–33.

71. Chaney AW, Pollack A, McNeese MD, et al. Primary treatment of cystosarcoma phyllodes of the breast. Cancer 2000;89(7):1502–11.

72. Tsubochi H, Sato N, Kaimori M, et al. Osteosarcomatous differentiation in lung metastases from a malignant phyllodes tumour of the breast. J Clin Pathol 2004;57(4):432–4.

73. West TL, Weiland LH, Clagett OT. Cystosarcoma phyllodes. Ann Surg 1971;173(4):520–8.

74. Kracht J, Sapino A, Bussolati G. Malignant phyllodes tumor of breast with lung metastases mimicking the primary. Am J Surg Pathol 1998; 22(10):1284–90.

75. Koh V, Thike AAT, Chng TW, et al. Predict metastases in malignant phyllodes tumors of the breast. Mod Pathol 2017;30(Suppl. 2. Abstracts: 106th Annual Meeting of the United States and Canadian Academy of Pathology (USCAP)):51A.

76. Chng TW, Lee JYH, Lee CS, et al. Validation of the Singapore nomogram for outcome prediction in breast phyllodes tumours: an Australian cohort. J Clin Pathol 2016;69(12):1124–6.

77. Nishimura R, Tan PH, Thike AA, et al. Utility of the Singapore nomogram for predicting recurrence-free survival in Japanese women with breast phyllodes tumours. J Clin Pathol 2014;67(8):748–50.

78. Cristando C, Li HH, Almekinders M, et al. Validation of the Singapore Nomogram for outcome prediction in a US-based population of women with breast phyllodes tumors (PT). Mod Pathol 2017;30(Suppl 2. Abstract: 106th Annual Meeting of the United States and Canadian Academy of Pathology (USCAP)):36A.

79. Chng TW, Gudi M, Li HL, et al. Validation of the Singapore Nomogram for outcome prediction in

breast phyllodes tumors in a large patient cohort. J Clin Pathol [Epub ahead of print].

80. Giri D. Recurrent challenges in the evaluation of fibroepithelial lesions. Arch Pathol Lab Med 2009; 133(5):713–21.

81. Lawton TJ, Acs G, Argani P, et al. Interobserver variability by pathologists in the distinction between cellular fibroadenomas and phyllodes tumors. Int J Surg Pathol 2014;22(8):695–8.

82. Bandyopadhyay S, Barak S, Hayek K, et al. Can problematic fibroepithelial lesions be accurately classified on core needle biopsies? Hum Pathol 2016;47(1):38–44.

83. Resetkova E, Khazai L, Albarracin CT, et al. Clinical and radiologic data and core needle biopsy findings should dictate management of cellular fibroepithelial tumors of the breast. Breast J 2010;16(6): 573–80.

84. Yasir S, Gamez R, Jenkins S, et al. Significant histologic features differentiating cellular fibroadenoma from phyllodes tumor on core needle biopsy specimens. Am J Clin Pathol 2014;142(3):362–9.

85. Tsang AK, Chan SK, Lam CC, et al. Phyllodes tumours of the breast – differentiating features in core needle biopsy Histopathology 2011;59(4): 600–8.

86. Grady I, Gorsuch H, Wilburn-Bailey S. Long-term outcome of benign fibroadenomas treated by ultrasound-guided percutaneous excision. Breast J 2008;14(3):275–8.

87. Nigro DM, Organ CH. Fibroadenoma of the female breast. Some epidemiologic surprises. Postgrad Med 1976;59(5):113–7.

88. Organ CH, Organ BC. Fibroadenoma of the female breast: a critical clinical assessment. J Natl Med Assoc 1983;75(7):701–4.

89. Barth RJ. Histologic features predict local recurrence after breast conserving therapy of phyllodes tumors. Breast Cancer Res Treat 1999;57(3):291–5.

90. Jones AM, Mitter R, Springall R, et al. A comprehensive genetic profile of phyllodes tumours of the breast detects important mutations, intra-tumoral genetic heterogeneity and new genetic changes on recurrence. J Pathol 2008; 214(5):533–44.

91. Cristando C, Almekinders M, Pareja F, et al. Is re-excision of benign and borderline phyllodes tumors with positive margins necessary? Mod Pathol 2017; 30(Suppl. 2. Abstracts: 106th Annual Meeting of the United States and Canadian Academy of Pathology (USCAP)):36A.

92. Tan EY, Tan PH, Hoon TP, et al. Recurrent phyllodes tumours of the breast: pathological features and clinical implications. ANZ J Surg 2006;76(6): 476–80.

93. Cowan ML, Argani P, Cimino-Mathews A. Benign and low-grade fibroepithelial neoplasms of the breast have low recurrence rate after positive surgical margins. Mod Pathol 2016;29(3):259–65.

94. Lacroix-Triki M, Geyer FC, Lambros MB, et al. β-catenin/Wnt signalling pathway in fibromatosis, metaplastic carcinomas and phyllodes tumours of the breast. Mod Pathol 2010;23(11):1438–48.

95. Sawyer EJ, Hanby AM, Rowan AJ, et al. The Wnt pathway, epithelial-stromal interactions, and malignant progression in phyllodes tumours. J Pathol 2002;196(4):437–44.

96. Tsang JYS, Mendoza P, Lam CCF, et al. Involvement of α- and β-catenins and E-cadherin in the development of mammary phyllodes tumours. Histopathology 2012;61(4):667–74.

97. Chia Y, Thike AA, Cheok PY, et al. Stromal keratin expression in phyllodes tumours of the breast: a comparison with other spindle cell breast lesions. J Clin Pathol 2012;65(4):339–47.

98. Cimino-Mathews A, Sharma R, Illei PB, et al. A subset of malignant phyllodes tumors express p63 and p40: a diagnostic pitfall in breast core needle biopsies. Am J Surg Pathol 2014;38(12):1689–96.

99. Kim SK, Jung WH, Koo JS. p40 (ΔNp63) expression in breast disease and its correlation with p63 immunohistochemistry. Int J Clin Exp Pathol 2014; 7(3):1032–41.

100. D'Alfonso TM, Ross DS, Liu Y-F, et al. Expression of p40 and laminin 332 in metaplastic spindle cell carcinoma of the breast compared with other malignant spindle cell tumours. J Clin Pathol 2015. https://doi.org/10.1136/jclinpath-2015-202923.

101. Noronha Y, Raza A, Hutchins B, et al. CD34, CD117, and Ki-67 expression in phyllodes tumor of the breast: an immunohistochemical study of 33 cases. Int J Surg Pathol 2011;19(2):152–8.

102. Cîmpean AM, Raica M, Narița D. Diagnostic significance of the immunoexpression of CD34 and smooth muscle cell actin in benign and malignant tumors of the breast. Rom J Morphol Embryol 2005;46(2):123–9.

103. Ho SK, Thike AA, Cheok PY, et al. Phyllodes tumours of the breast: the role of CD34, vascular endothelial growth factor and β-catenin in histological grading and clinical outcome. Histopathology 2013;63(3):393–406.

104. Dunne B, Lee AHS, Pinder SE, et al. An immunohistochemical study of metaplastic spindle cell carcinoma, phyllodes tumor and fibromatosis of the breast. Hum Pathol 2003;34(10):1009–15.

105. Lee AHS. Recent developments in the histological diagnosis of spindle cell carcinoma, fibromatosis and phyllodes tumour of the breast. Histopathology 2008;52(1):45–57.

106. Esposito NN, Mohan D, Brufsky A, et al. Phyllodes tumor: a clinicopathologic and immunohistochemical study of 30 cases. Arch Pathol Lab Med 2006;130(10):1516–21.

107. Tan P-H, Jayabaskar T, Yip G, et al. p53 and c-kit (CD117) protein expression as prognostic indicators in breast phyllodes tumors: a tissue microarray study. Mod Pathol 2005;18(12):1527–34.

108. Dusenbery D, Frable WJ. Fine needle aspiration cytology of phyllodes tumor. Potential diagnostic pitfalls. Acta Cytol 1992;36(2):215–21.

109. Veneti S, Manek S. Benign phyllodes tumour vs fibroadenoma: FNA cytological differentiation. Cytopathology 2001;12(5):321–8.

110. Pătraşcu A, Popescu CF, Pleşea IE, et al. Clinical and cytopathological aspects in phyllodes tumors of the breast. Rom J Morphol Embryol 2009; 50(4):605–11.

111. Krishnamurthy S, Ashfaq R, Shin HJ, et al. Distinction of phyllodes tumor from fibroadenoma: a reappraisal of an old problem. Cancer 2000;90(6): 342–9.

112. Bhattarai S, Kapila K, Verma K. Phyllodes tumor of the breast. A cytohistologic study of 80 cases. Acta Cytol 2000;44(5):790–6.

113. Tse GMK, Ma TKF, Pang LM, et al. Fine needle aspiration cytologic features of mammary phyllodes tumors. Acta Cytol 2002;46(5):855–63.

114. Ross DS, Giri DD, Akram MM, et al. Fibroepithelial lesions in the breast of adolescent females: a clinicopathological study of 54 cases. Breast J 2017; 23(2):182–92.

115. Tay TKY, Chang KTE, Thike AA, et al. Paediatric fibroepithelial lesions revisited: pathological insights. J Clin Pathol 2015;68(8):633–41.

116. Faiz S, Tudor V, Yasim G-P, et al. Fibroadenomatous lesions in pediatric age group. Mod Pathol 2013;26(Supp.2):39A.

117. Ozerdem U, Tavassoli F. Paucity of atypical epithelial proliferations in 379 pediatric fibroepithelial breast lesions. Mod Pathol 2017;30(Suppl 2. Abstract: 106th Annual Meeting of the United States and Canadian Academy of Pathology (USCAP)):62A.

118. Noguchi S, Yokouchi H, Aihara T, et al. Progression of fibroadenoma to phyllodes tumor demonstrated by clonal analysis. Cancer 1995;76(10):1779–85.

119. Makinen N, Mehine M, Tolvanen J, et al. MED12, the mediator complex subunit 12 gene, is mutated at high frequency in uterine leiomyomas. Science 2011;334(6053):252–5.

120. Je EM, Kim MR, Min KO, et al. Mutational analysis of MED12 exon 2 in uterine leiomyoma and other common tumors. Int J Cancer 2012;131(6): E1044–7.

121. Matsubara A, Sekine S, Yoshida M, et al. Prevalence of *MED12* mutations in uterine and extrauterine smooth muscle tumours. Histopathology 2013;62(4):657–61.

122. Markowski DN, Huhle S, Nimzyk R, et al. *MED12* mutations occurring in benign and malignant mammalian smooth muscle tumors. Genes Chromosomes Cancer 2013;52(3):297–304.

123. Lim WK, Ong CK, Tan J, et al. Exome sequencing identifies highly recurrent MED12 somatic mutations in breast fibroadenoma. Nat Genet 2014; 46(8):877–80.

124. Cani AK, Hovelson DH, McDaniel AS, et al. Next-gen sequencing exposes frequent MED12 mutations and actionable therapeutic targets in phyllodes tumors. Mol Cancer Res 2015;13(4): 613–9.

125. Piscuoglio S, Murray M, Fusco N, et al. MED12 somatic mutations in fibroadenomas and phyllodes tumours of the breast. Histopathology 2015. https://doi.org/10.1111/his.12712.

126. Laé M, Gardrat S, Rondeau S, et al. MED12 mutations in breast phyllodes tumors: evidence of temporal tumoral heterogeneity and identification of associated critical signaling pathways. Oncotarget 2016;7(51):84428–38.

127. Tan J, Ong CK, Lim WK, et al. Genomic landscapes of breast fibroepithelial tumors. Nat Genet 2015; 47(11):1341–5.

128. Nozad S, Sheehan CE, Gay LM, et al. Comprehensive genomic profiling of malignant phyllodes tumors of the breast. Breast Cancer Res Treat 2017;162(3):597–602.

129. Liu S-Y, Joseph NM, Ravindranathan A, et al. Genomic profiling of malignant phyllodes tumors reveals aberrations in FGFR1 and PI-3 kinase/RAS signaling pathways and provides insights into intratumoral heterogeneity. Mod Pathol 2016; 29(9):1012–27.

130. Tan PH, Nasir NDBM, Ng C, et al. Genomic alterations in breast fibroadenomas and phyllodes tumors – preliminary findings from the International Fibroepithelial Consortium. Mod Pathol 2017; 30(Suppl 2. Abstract: 106th Annual Meeting of the United States and Canadian Academy of Pathology (USCAP)):73A.

131. Tan BY, Ng CCY, Nasir ND, et al. Morphological and genomic heterogeneity in a malignant phyllodes tumor. Mod Pathol 2017;30(Suppl 2. Abstract: 106th Annual Meeting of the United States and Canadian Academy of Pathology (USCAP)):72A–3A.

132. Yoshida M, Ogawa R, Yoshida H, et al. TERT promoter mutations are frequent and show association with MED12 mutations in phyllodes tumors of the breast. Br J Cancer 2015;113(8): 1244–8.

133. Piscuoglio S, Ng CK, Murray M, et al. Massively parallel sequencing of phyllodes tumours of the breast reveals actionable mutations, and TERT promoter hotspot mutations and TERT gene amplification as likely drivers of progression. J Pathol 2016; 238(4):508–18.

134. Jardim D, Conley A, Subbiah V. Comprehensive characterization of malignant phyllodes tumor by whole genomic and proteomic analysis: biological implications for targeted therapy opportunities. Orphanet J Rare Dis 2013;8(1):112.

135. Gatalica Z, Vranic S, Ghazalpour A, et al. Multiplatform molecular profiling identifies potentially targetable biomarkers in malignant phyllodes tumors of the breast. Oncotarget 2016;7(2):1707–16.

136. Tan WJ, Cima I, Choudhury Y, et al. A five-gene reverse transcription-PCR assay for pre-operative classification of breast fibroepithelial lesions. Breast Cancer Res 2016;18(1):31.

137. Tan PH, Ellis IO. Myoepithelial and epithelial-myoepithelial, mesenchymal and fibroepithelial breast lesions: updates from the WHO Classification of Tumours of the Breast 2012. J Clin Pathol 2013;66(6):465–70.

Axillary Lymph Node Inclusions

Ashley Cimino-Mathews, MD

KEYWORDS

- Axillary lymph node • Lymph node inclusions • Endosalpingiosis • Nodal nevi

---

Key points

- Lymph node inclusions include both epithelial inclusions and nonepithelial inclusions.

- Epithelial lymph node inclusions include mammary-type glandular inclusions, Mullerian-type glandular inclusions, squamous inclusions, and mixed glandular-squamous inclusions.

- The primary diagnostic pitfall with glandular lymph node inclusions is metastatic mammary carcinoma, or metastatic adenocarcinoma of another site, such as the gynecologic tract.

- Nonepithelial inclusions include nodal nevi, and the primary diagnostic pitfall with nodal nevi is metastatic melanoma or less commonly metastatic spindle cell (sarcomatoid) mammary carcinoma.

- Examining the histologic features of the nodal inclusions, comparing the inclusion with the primary mammary carcinoma, and performing a targeted immunohistochemical panel can resolve the diagnosis.

ABSTRACT

Lymph node inclusions can occur in axillary lymph nodes, where they can mimic metastatic breast carcinoma. This article provides an overview of epithelial and nonepithelial lymph node inclusions, including mammary-type glandular inclusions, Mullerian-type glandular inclusions, squamous inclusions, mixed glandular-squamous inclusions, and nodal nevi. The discussion emphasizes the histologic and immunophenotypic features and differential diagnoses of each entity.

OVERVIEW

Benign lymph node inclusions can occur in any anatomic location, including the axilla, where they pose a potential diagnostic pitfall in the evaluation of sentinel lymph nodes in patients with breast carcinoma. Lymph node inclusions fall into 2 broad categories: epithelial, and nonepithelial (**Box 1**).[1] Epithelial inclusions include those that consist of mammary-type glandular epithelium, Mullerian-type glandular epithelium, squamous epithelium, and mixed glandular-squamous epithelium. Nonepithelial inclusions include benign nodal nevi.

The potential for misdiagnosis of a benign lymph node inclusion as metastatic breast carcinoma is greatest on frozen section evaluation of sentinel lymph nodes,[2] where frozen section artifact can obscure cytologic detail, sections of the primary tumor are often not available for histologic comparison, and the intraoperative nature generally precludes the use of supplemental immunohistochemistry. Fortunately, in this regard, the frequency of frozen section analysis of sentinel lymph nodes has in general decreased with the results of the ACOSOG Z0011 trial indicating that axillary radiation can supplant surgical axillary nodal dissection for a subset of patients with axillary nodal disease.[3,4] However, diagnostic pitfalls of nodal inclusions still remain in permanent histologic sections of lymph node evaluation (**Box 2, Table 1**).[2,5,6]

Disclosure Statement: The author declares no financial disclosures or conflicts of interest.
Department of Pathology, Johns Hopkins Hospital, 401 North Broadway Street, Weinberg 2242, Baltimore, MD 21287, USA
E-mail address: acimino1@jhmi.edu

Surgical Pathology 11 (2018) 43–59
https://doi.org/10.1016/j.path.2017.09.004

surgpath.theclinics.com

EPITHELIAL INCLUSIONS

MAMMARY-TYPE GLANDULAR INCLUSIONS (HETEROTOPIC BREAST PARENCHYMA)

Mammary-type glandular inclusions (heterotopic breast parenchyma) have been described in axillary lymph nodes.[1,7–14] As most axillary lymph node sampling occurs in patients with primary breast carcinoma, the main diagnostic pitfall of benign mammary-type glandular inclusions is of course metastatic breast carcinoma (see Box 2, Table 1). Postulated mechanisms to explain the pathogenesis of mammary-type glandular inclusions include benign displacement or mechanical transport (eg, due to prior biopsy),[15–19] as well as the presence of ectopic mammary tissue or embryogenic malformation during development.[1]

Pathologic Features

Microscopic foci of mammary-type glandular inclusions lack gross pathologic changes. Large, proliferative or cystic inclusions may be grossly visible as cystic spaces or solid, firm, tan and well-circumscribed nodules. Microscopically, mammary-type glandular inclusions are most commonly located within the lymph node capsule, but can occur in the node parenchyma (Fig. 1).[1] The inclusions can be solitary or multiple. Mammary-type glandular inclusions display a range of histologic appearances, from simple glands with low-cuboidal epithelium to those with apocrine metaplasia and microcysts, and to those containing architectural complexity including florid epithelial hyperplasia (Fig. 2),[20] adenosis,[21] and papillary proliferations.[1,22] The luminal epithelial cells are typically bland, with hypochromatic nuclei, inconspicuous nucleoli, and minimal mitotic activity. Mammary-type glandular inclusions have an associated myoepithelial cell layer (see Box 1),[7] which can be visible on hematoxylin-eosin (H&E) inspection alone, but also confirmed by immunohistochemistry (see Fig. 2; Figs. 3–5).

Atypical epithelial proliferations can involve, and most likely arise from, underlying mammary-type glandular inclusions. Ductal carcinoma in situ[14,23] and papillary carcinoma[23] have been reported within axillary nodal inclusions.

Differential Diagnosis

The primary differential diagnosis of mammary-type glandular inclusions in axillary lymph nodes is metastatic ductal carcinoma. Metastatic carcinoma typically involves the lymph node sinuses, in contrast to inclusions, which are most commonly located in the node capsule. However, as indicated previously, glandular inclusions can also occur in the node parenchyma. The differential diagnosis also includes other benign inclusions, specifically Mullerian-type glandular inclusions discussed later in this article, or metastatic well-differentiated adenocarcinoma of another primary site, such as lung or upper gastrointestinal tract.

Diagnosis

By immunohistochemistry, mammary-type glandular inclusions label like benign mammary glands. They are immunoreactive for pancytokeratin and CK7 and thus present a potential diagnostic pitfall if a cytokeratin is performed on a sentinel lymph node excision for breast carcinoma (see Fig. 3). The luminal epithelial cells are also immunoreactive for gross cystic disease fluid protein (GCDFP),

Table 1
Differential diagnosis of nodal inclusions

Diagnosis	Histologic Features	Immunohistochemical Features	Differential Diagnosis
Mammary-type glandular inclusions	Bland mammary glands with associated myoepithelial layer	+ ER, GATA3, GCDFP, mammaglobin +/− S100 + p63, SMMHC (myoepithelial cells) - PAX8, WT1	Metastatic mammary carcinoma
Mullerian-type glandular inclusions	Bland glands with ciliated cells admixed with intercalated (peg) cells	+ ER, PAX8, WT1 - GATA3, GCDFP, mammaglobin, S100 - p63, SMMHC (myoepithelial cells)	Metastatic mammary or gynecologic carcinoma
Squamous inclusions	Bland squamous nests or squamous-lined cysts	+ p63, CK5/6 +/− GATA3 - ER, GCDFP, mammaglobin, PAX8, WT1, S100, SMMHC	Metastatic squamous cell carcinoma, or metastatic metaplastic/sarcomatoid mammary carcinoma
Nodal nevi	Bland, spindled nevocytes located within lymph node capsule	+ Melan A, SOX10, S100, MITF - HMB45, cytokeratins, ER, GATA3, GCDFP, mammaglobin, PAX8, WT1	Metastatic melanoma, or metastatic spindle cell (sarcomatoid) carcinoma

mammaglobin, and GATA binding protein 3 (GATA3), with mosaic pattern reactivity for estrogen receptor (ER). The associated myoepithelial cell layer can be highlighted by immunostains for p63, smooth muscle myosin heavy chain (SMMHC), and calponin (see **Fig. 4**). In contrast, metastatic mammary carcinoma lacks myoepithelial cells; in addition, low-grade ductal carcinomas are typically strongly and diffusely positive for ER. Immunohistochemistry can also distinguish between mammary-type glandular inclusions and Mullerian-type glandular inclusions. Unlike, Mullerian-type

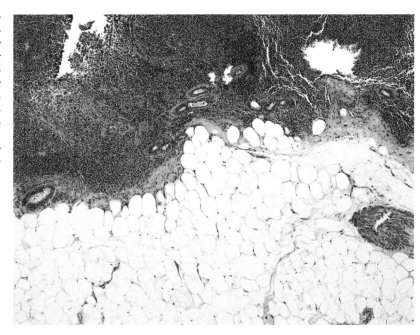

Fig. 1. Mammary-type glandular inclusion. Multiple glands lined by bland, simple columnar epithelial cells are present in this axillary sentinel lymph node in a patient with breast carcinoma. The glands are located both in the nodal capsule and immediately beneath the subcapsular sinus space (H&E, original magnification ×40).

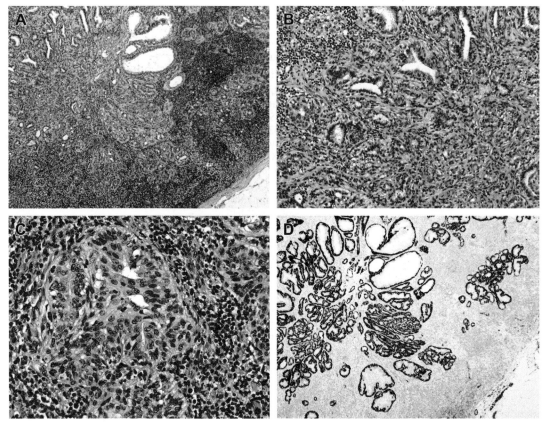

Fig. 2. Mammary-type glandular inclusion with hyperplasia. (*A*) This axillary sentinel lymph node contains a complex glandular proliferation (H&E, ×40). (*B*) Areas consist of sclerosing adenosis (H&E, original magnification ×100). (*C*) Areas contain florid epithelial hyperplasia of bland cells with punctate nucleoli, overlapping and elongated nuclei, nuclear variability, and slitlike spaces. An outer, second cell layer is visible (H&E, original magnification ×200). (*D*) A smooth-muscle myosin heavy chain immunostain is positive in the myoepithelial cell layer (original magnification ×40).

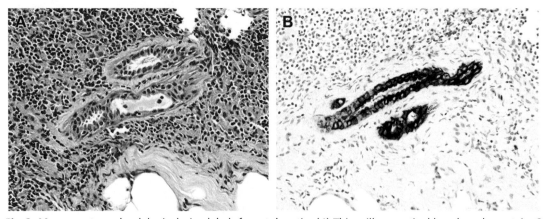

Fig. 3. Mammary-type glandular inclusion labels for cytokeratin. (*A*) This axillary sentinel lymph node contains 2 bland glands in the subcapsular space, each composed of 2 cell layers (H&E, original magnification ×200). (*B*) A cytokeratin AE/1/AE3 immunostain is positive, mimicking metastatic mammary carcinoma (original magnification ×200).

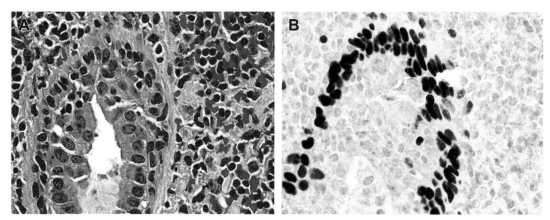

Fig. 4. Mammary-type glandular inclusion has myoepithelial cells. (*A*) A double cell layer is clearly visible in this glandular inclusion; the inner, luminal cell layer is composed of bland cuboidal cells, and the outer myoepithelial cells layer is composed of bland uniform cells with minimal cytoplasm (H&E, original magnification ×400). (*B*) A p63 immunostain highlights myoepithelial cells (original magnification ×400).

glandular inclusions, mammary-type glandular inclusions are negative for PAX8 and WT1 (see Fig. 5),[24–26] although PAX8 is preferred in this setting because WT1 labeling has rarely been reported in breast carcinomas.[27]

In addition to the use of immunohistochemistry, histologic comparison of the primary mammary carcinoma to the glandular nodal inclusion can be a useful diagnostic tool (Figs. 6 and 7). The discordance between a primary ductal

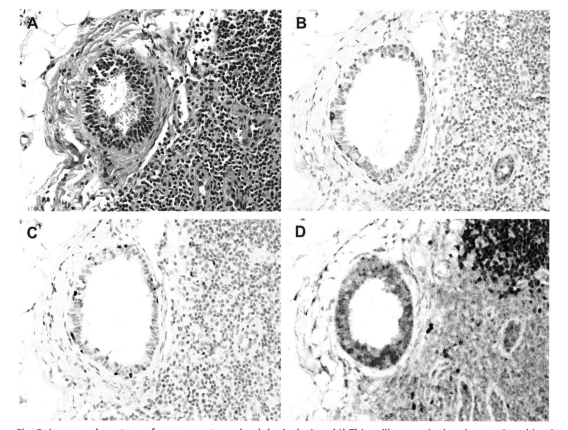

Fig. 5. Immunophenotype of mammary-type glandular inclusion. (*A*) This axillary sentinel node contains a bland gland in the capsule (H&E, original magnification ×200). Immunostains for smooth (*B*) SMMHC and (*C*) p63 highlight intact myoepithelial cells (original magnification ×200). (*D*) The gland is negative for PAX8 (original magnification ×200).

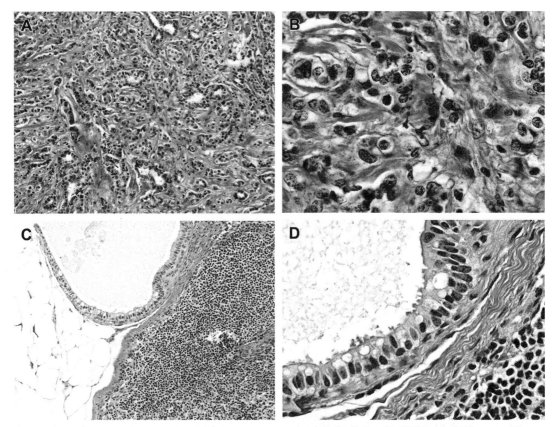

Fig. 6. Primary breast carcinoma and a nodal mammary-type glandular inclusion. (*A, B*) This primary breast carcinoma consists of irregular, poorly formed glands with nuclear size variability, high nuclear-to-cytoplasmic ratio, and frequent mitoses (H&E, original magnification ×100 and ×400). (*C, D*) The axillary sentinel lymph node contains a single, cystically dilated gland in the capsule. The gland is lined by bland columnar epithelium with uniform nuclei, supranuclear vacuoles, luminal secretions, and an outer myoepithelial cell layer (H&E, original magnification ×100 and ×400).

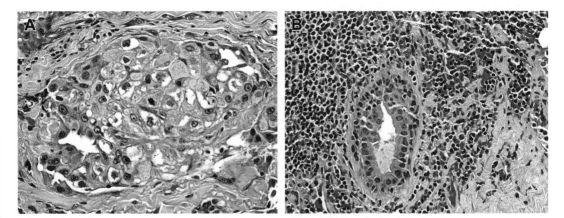

Fig. 7. Primary breast carcinoma and a nodal mammary-type glandular inclusion. (*A*) This primary breast carcinoma is composed of large polygonal cells with eosinophilic cytoplasm, round nuclei with prominent central nucleoli, and frequent mitoses (H&E, original magnification ×200). (*B*) The axillary sentinel lymph node contains a bland gland within the subcapsular space; the lining cells are bland and simple cuboidal, and there is a distinct outer myoepithelial cell layer (H&E, original magnification ×200).

carcinoma with minimal gland formation or marked atypia and the presence of bland, well-differentiated glands in the lymph node should raise the possibility of a glandular inclusion (see Figs. 6 and 7).

Prognosis

Mammary-type glandular inclusions are benign, incidental findings. In the absence of associated atypia, no additional therapy is indicated.

MULLERIAN-TYPE GLANDULAR INCLUSIONS

Mullerian-type glandular inclusions resemble the gynecologic tract Mullerian epithelium and most commonly consist of endosalpingiosis. Nodal endosalpingiosis is well recognized in abdominal and pelvic sites, but has also been rarely described in supra-diaphragmatic locations including axillary and intramammary lymph nodes.[1,2,5,28-35] Mullerian-type glandular inclusions mimic metastatic carcinoma of the breast or gynecologic tract (see Box 2, Table 1). The pathogenesis of supra-diaphragmatic endosalpingiosis is unclear. Subdiaphragmatic nodal endosalpingiosis has been linked to salpingitis[36] and metastases from unsampled serous borderline tumors.[37] Postulated mechanisms include precursor lesions or metastasis from an unsampled primary gynecologic malignancy.[1]

Pathologic Features

Microscopic Mullerian-type glandular inclusions lack gross findings. Microscopically, Mullerian-type glandular inclusions are typically located within the lymph node capsule (Fig. 8), but may also extend into the lymph node parenchyma. Endosalpingiosis glands are typically lined by bland columnar cells with cilia, with admixed intercalated cells consisting of smaller round cells with more prominent cytoplasm (Fig. 9) (see Box 1).[1,2] The cells are bland and lack nuclear atypia or mitotic figures. Occasionally, Mullerian-type glandular inclusions can lack the ciliated cells and/or intercalated cells (Fig. 10)[30,32]; however, the immunophenotype aids in the correct identification. There is one case report of atypical endosalpingiosis in an axillary lymph node.[38]

Mullerian-type glandular inclusions can have the histology of endocervicosis or endometriosis. Endocervicosis has been reported in axillary lymph nodes[39] and consists of glands lined by low-cuboidal epithelium. Endometriosis consists of glands lined by columnar epithelium with associated endometrial-type stroma, as well as foci of hemorrhage or hemosiderin-laden macrophages.

Differential Diagnosis

The primary differential diagnoses of axillary node Mullerian-type glandular inclusions are benign mammary-type glandular inclusions, metastatic mammary carcinoma, and metastatic gynecologic tract adenocarcinoma.[40] As with mammary-type glandular inclusions, Mullerian-type glandular inclusions most commonly (but not always) involve the lymph node capsule, whereas metastatic carcinomas most commonly involve subcapsular sinus. The differential diagnosis also includes metastatic adenocarcinoma of other sites, such as lung or upper gastrointestinal tract.

Diagnosis

By immunohistochemistry, Mullerian-type glandular inclusions label like the glandular epithelium of the gynecologic tract, and this distinct immunoprofile can readily verify the diagnosis. However, they do have some overlapping immunophenotypic features with mammary epithelium. Mullerian-type glandular inclusions are immunoreactive for CK7, PAX8, WT1, and ER (see Box 1, Fig. 10; Fig. 11),[1,2] and they are negative for GATA3 (see Fig. 11D),[41] GCDFP, and mammaglobin. Low-grade ductal carcinoma is also immunoreactive for CK7 and ER (Fig. 12A-C), but in contrast is positive for GATA3 (see Fig. 12C),[42] GCDFP, and mammaglobin, and is negative for PAX8 (Fig. 12D).[24,25] Most mammary carcinomas are also negative for WT1,[26] but WT1 labeling has rarely been reported in breast carcinomas[27]; hence PAX8 is the preferred immunostain in this setting. Mullerian-type glandular inclusions also lack associated myoepithelial cells (Fig. 13),[2] and in this way they also mimic metastatic breast carcinoma. However, the histologic features of the ciliated cells along with immunoreactivity for PAX8 and WT1 can confirm the diagnosis.

Both immunophenotypic and histologic comparison of a patient's primary breast carcinoma with the Mullerian-type nodal inclusion can be a useful diagnostic tool.[1] The presence of a poorly differentiated, ER-negative primary breast carcinoma with a bland ER + gland in the axillary node capsule should raise suspicion of a benign nodal inclusion. Careful histologic examination for the presence of cilia or intercalated cells, along with immunostains for PAX8 and

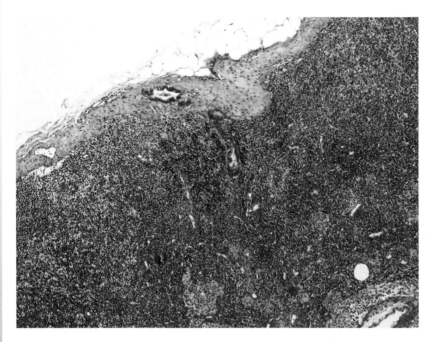

Fig. 8. Mullerian-type glandular inclusion (endosalpingiosis). This axillary lymph node contains bland individual glands in the capsule and extending into the lymph node parenchyma along the septa (H&E, original magnification ×4).

GATA3 as necessary, can then confirm the diagnosis.

Prognosis

Mullerian-type glandular inclusions are benign and are incidentally discovered in nodal excisions performed for other reasons. However, some observers have recommended clinical workup for an occult gynecologic primary malignancy.[1]

SQUAMOUS INCLUSIONS

Benign squamous inclusions occur throughout the body, including in the axillary[1,43,44] and intramammary[45] lymph nodes. Squamous inclusions

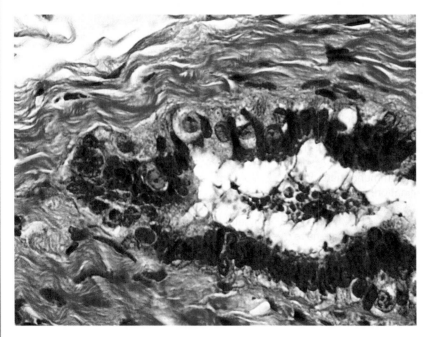

Fig. 9. Histology of Mullerian-type glandular inclusion (endosalpingiosis). This bland single gland within an axillary lymph node capsule is lined by ciliated columnar cells with elongated nuclei, interspersed with round cells with round nuclei and pale cytoplasm (H&E, original magnification ×400).

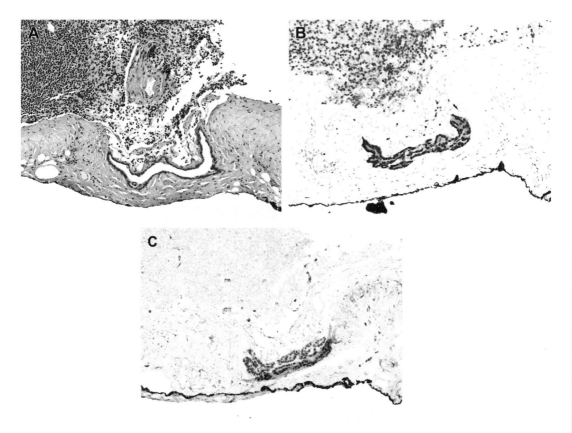

Fig. 10. Immunophenotype of Mullerian-type glandular inclusion that lacks intercalated cells. (*A*) This axillary sentinel lymph node excised in a patient with breast ductal carcinoma contains a single bland gland in the lymph node capsule; no obvious intercalated cells are identified (H&E, original magnification ×100). Immunostains for (*B*) PAX8 and (*C*) WT1 are diffusely positive (original magnification ×100).

can also present as isolated axillary masses in the absence of any breast lesion.[1] Axillary nodal squamous inclusions can mimic metastatic squamous cell carcinoma and metastatic sarcomatoid (metaplastic) breast carcinoma (see **Box 2**, **Table 1**). The mechanisms of development are unclear.

Pathologic Features

Microscopic squamous inclusions lack gross pathologic findings. Larger squamous inclusions may display grossly apparently cystic structures with central keratinaceous debris. Microscopically, squamous inclusions can be located within the lymph node parenchyma (**Fig. 14**)[1] or capsule, and can be multiple (see **Fig. 14**) or individual. Squamous inclusions can be squamous-lined cysts with central keratinaceous debris (**Fig. 15**),[1] or individual squamous nests (**Fig. 16**). The cells lining squamous inclusions are keratinocytes that mature from a basal layer through a spinous cell layer and finally to a granular cell layer (see **Box 1**, **Fig. 16**). The cells lack

atypia or mitotic activity. There have been no reports of malignancy arising from in axillary nodal squamous inclusion.

Differential Diagnosis

The differential diagnosis of nodal squamous inclusions includes metastatic squamous cell carcinoma and sarcomatoid (metaplastic) breast carcinoma with a squamous component. Metastatic squamous cell carcinoma of any site can be cystic, but should also display some degree of atypia. The differential diagnosis may also include dermal-based epidermal inclusion cysts with a brisk lymphocytic response; however, the presence of a capsule and subcapsular sinus aids in identifying an underlying lymph node architecture.

Diagnosis

The diagnosis of benign nodal squamous inclusions is made on the basis of histology and clinical history. Benign squamous inclusions lack nuclear atypia and mitotic figures, in contrast to metastatic squamous cell carcinomas, which

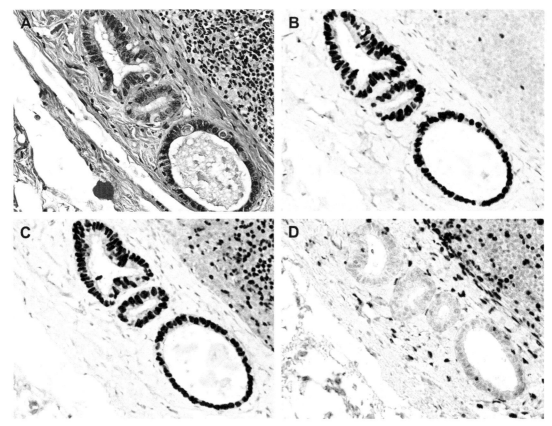

Fig. 11. Immunophenotype of Mullerian-type glandular inclusion (endosalpingiosis). (*A*) This axillary lymph node in a patient with a primary breast carcinoma (see Fig. 12) contains multiple bland glands with ciliated columnar cells admixed with intercalated cells (H&E, original magnification ×200). The bland glands are positive for (*B*) ER and (*C*) PAX8, and are negative for (*D*) GATA3 (original magnification ×200).

will display some degree of atypia and lack of maturation. In addition, the absence of a clinical history of squamous cell carcinoma is helpful. Axillary lymph nodes would be an uncommon first site of presentation of metastatic squamous cell carcinoma of head and neck or lung origin. A cutaneous squamous cell carcinoma of the upper extremities or truck could metastasize to the axillary lymph nodes, but is unlikely to be an occult primary.

In general, immunohistochemistry is not helpful in differentiating between a benign squamous inclusion and a metastatic squamous cell carcinoma, as both label for p63 (Fig. 17), p40, and CK5/6 and lack myoepithelial cells. However, if the patient has a primary human papilloma virus (HPV)-related squamous cell carcinoma of the head and neck or anogenital region, these tumors are diffusely immunoreactive for p16 and are positive for high-risk HPV by RNA or DNA in situ hybridization. In contrast, benign squamous inclusions (as well as squamous cell carcinomas of other sites such as the skin) are not HPV-related.

Prognosis

Lymph node squamous inclusions are benign. No additional treatment is required.

MIXED GLANDULAR-SQUAMOUS INCLUSIONS

In addition to pure glandular or squamous inclusions, some nodal inclusions display mixed glandular and squamous components.[1]

Pathologic Features

Microscopic foci of mixed glandular-squamous inclusions lack gross findings. If either the glandular or the squamous component is particularly florid or cystic, this component may be visible on gross examination. Microscopically, mixed glandular-squamous inclusions consist of varying degrees of benign glands with benign squamous nests or squamous-lined cysts. The epithelial cells lack atypia or mitotic activity. There have been no reported instances of malignancy arising from a nodal mixed glandular-squamous inclusions.

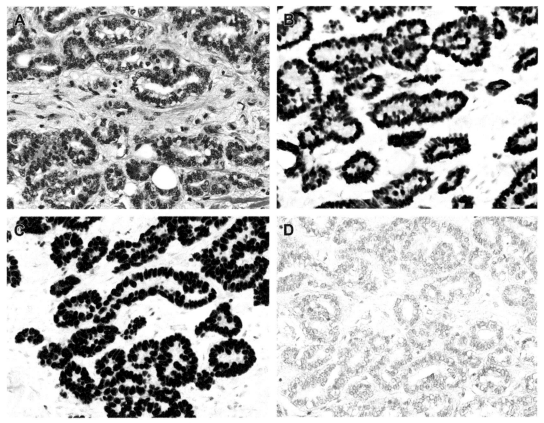

Fig. 12. Immunophenotype of well-differentiated infiltrating ductal carcinoma of the breast. (*A*) The primary breast carcinoma in the patient with a Mullerian-type glandular inclusion (see Fig. 11) is shown here. The carcinoma is composed of well-formed glands lined by uniform cuboidal cells with minimal cytologic atypia, eliciting a stromal desmoplastic response (H&E, original magnification ×200). The glands are diffusely immunoreactive for (*B*) ER and (*C*) GATA3, and are negative for (*D*) PAX8 (original magnification ×200).

Differential Diagnosis

One differential diagnosis of mixed glandular-squamous inclusions is metastatic breast adenosquamous carcinoma. However, most mixed glandular-squamous inclusions have distinct, separate but adjacent components of glandular and squamous elements[1]; in contrast, adenosquamous carcinomas have intimately associated glandular

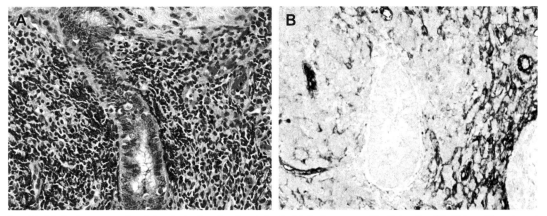

Fig. 13. Mullerian-type glandular inclusion (endosalpingiosis) lacks myoepithelial cells. (*A*) This axillary lymph node contains a bland gland lined by ciliated columnar cells with interspersed intercalated cells (H&E, original magnification ×200). (*B*) The gland lacks myoepithelial cells by SMMHC, mimicking metastatic mammary carcinoma (original magnification ×200).

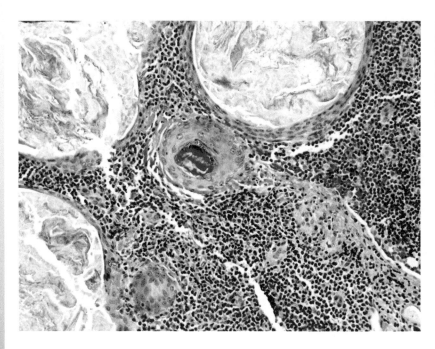

Fig. 14. Multiple squamous inclusions. Multiple squamous-lined cysts and squamoid nests involve this axillary sentinel lymph node (H&E, original magnification ×100).

and squamous elements. Furthermore, breast adenosquamous carcinomas have a very low risk of metastatic spread.[46]

Diagnosis

The presence of mixed glandular and squamous elements on microscopic examination favors the diagnosis of a benign mixed glandular-squamous inclusion over metastatic ductal carcinoma or squamous cell carcinoma.

The histologic and immunophenotypic feature of a myoepithelial cell layer in the glandular component excludes the diagnosis of metastatic adenocarcinoma.

Prognosis

Mixed glandular-squamous inclusions are benign and are typically incidental findings in lymph nodes excised for other reasons. No additional treatment is necessary.

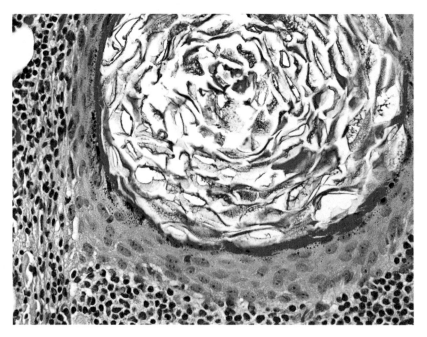

Fig. 15. Cystic squamous inclusion. This axillary sentinel lymph node contains a squamous-lined cyst with central keratinaceous debris (H&E, original magnification ×200).

Fig. 16. Solid squamous inclusion. This squamous inclusion displays a solid next of squamous cells with epithelial maturation from a basal cell layer through a spinous cell layer, a granular cell layer, and central keratin (H&E, original magnification ×400).

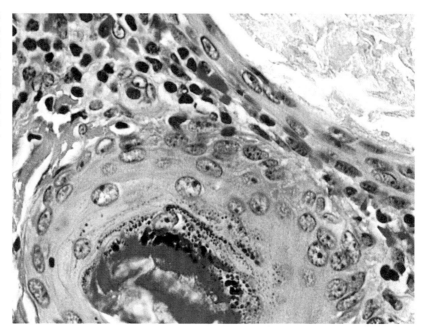

NONEPITHELIAL INCLUSIONS

NODAL NEVI

Nodal nevi have frequently been described in axillary lymph nodes,[47] including sentinel nodes excised for a workup of melanoma[48,49] and of breast carcinoma.[1,11,50–52] Nodal nevi are composed of bland nevocytes located in the lymph node capsule. The primary potential diagnostic pitfall of nodal nevi is metastatic melanoma (see **Box 2, Table 1**). Postulated mechanisms for the pathogenesis of nodal nevi includes benign mechanical transport of nevocytes, lymphatic drainage of nevocytes from the skin, and aberrant embryogenesis.[53]

Pathologic Features

There are no gross pathologic features associated with microscopic nodal nevi. Microscopically, nodal nevi consist of bland, spindled nevocytes with no nuclear atypia, indistinct nucleoli and no mitotic activity (see **Box 1**; **Fig. 18**A,B). Nodal nevi are located in the lymph node capsule and may extend into the lymph node fibrous trabeculae.

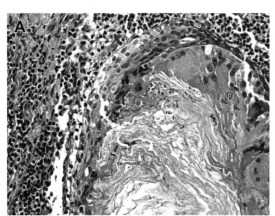
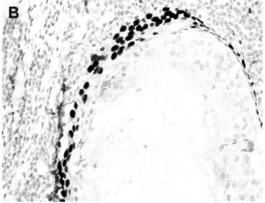

Fig. 17. Immunophenotype of squamous inclusion. (*A*) This axillary sentinel lymph node contains a bland squamous-lined cystic space with central keratinaceous debris and associated histiocytes (H&E, original magnification ×200). (*B*) An immunostain for p63 highlights the keratinocytes (original magnification ×200).

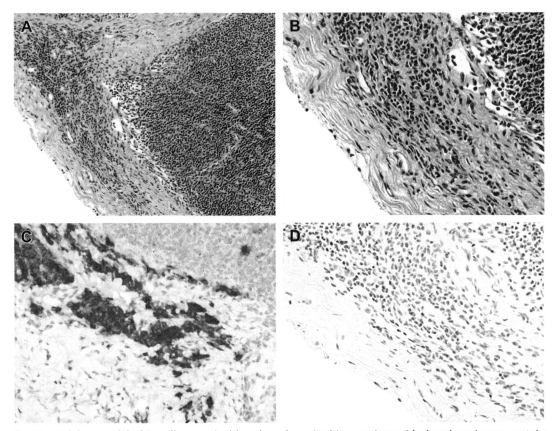

Fig. 18. Nodal nevus. (*A*) This axillary sentinel lymph node excised in a patient with ductal carcinoma contains bland spindled to epithelioid cells within the capsule (H&E, original magnification ×100). (*B*) The cells lack nuclear atypia, have minimal cytoplasm, and show no gland formation or mitotic activity (H&E, original magnification ×200). The cells are immunoreactive for (*C*) Melan A and are negative for (*D*) cytokeratin AE1/AE3 (original magnification ×200).

Differential Diagnosis

The primary differential diagnosis of nodal nevi is metastatic melanoma. This is particularly an issue because nodal nevi can occur in the sentinel nodes or regional lymph nodes excised as part of a melanoma staging procedure. The secondary differential diagnosis of nodal nevi is metastatic carcinoma, and in the setting of an axillary node excised in a patient with breast carcinoma, the differential diagnosis may specifically be metastatic spindle cell (sarcomatoid) carcinoma. Nodal nevi are typically located within the node capsule, whereas both metastatic melanoma and carcinoma preferentially involve the subcapsular sinus.

Diagnosis

The diagnosis of nodal nevi is made on the basis of histologic and immunophenotypic features. Nodal nevi are bland and located in the lymph node capsule. In contrast, most cases of metastatic melanoma show nuclear atypia in the form of increased nuclear-to-cytoplasmic ratio and prominent nucleoli, and typically involve the subcapsular space. Comparison of the nodal melanocytic proliferation with the primary melanoma can be helpful, as the primary will often display marked cytologic atypia. However, if the primary melanoma is a nevoid melanoma, the malignant cells may be smaller and display less atypia than other subtypes. In this setting, immunostains can be essential. Nodal nevi are immunoreactive for Melan A (**Fig. 18**C),[54] SOX10, and S100,[55,56] but are negative for HMB45.[54] In contrast, metastatic melanomas are typically immunoreactive for Melan A, SOX10, S100, and HMB45. Desmoplastic melanomas are an exception to this staining pattern, as they may label only for S100 and SOX10. Nodal nevi and melanomas are negative for cytokeratin (**Fig. 18**D).

In differentiating nodal nevi from metastatic breast carcinoma, histologic comparison of the nodal nevus to the primary carcinoma is helpful. The presence of a primary high-grade ductal carcinoma would be incongruous to a metastasis consisting of bland spindled cells in a lymph node capsule. Immunohistochemistry can easily resolve this differential, as nodal nevi are negative for cytokeratin (see **Fig. 18**D). Caution should be used in interpreting positive labeling for S100 protein and SOX10 without an accompanying cytokeratin immunostain, however, as mammary carcinomas can label for S100[57] as well as SOX10.[58]

Prognosis

Nodal nevi are benign incidental findings in lymph nodes excised for other reasons, such as staging for primary melanoma or breast carcinoma. No additional treatment is necessary.

In summary, benign lymph node inclusions pose a potential for misdiagnosis as metastatic breast carcinoma. However, with careful attention to cytologic features and the location in the lymph node, comparison with the breast primary, and judicious use of adjunctive immunostains, most inclusions can be readily recognized.

ACKNOWLEDGMENTS

Special thanks to Dr Pedram Argani for providing the original cases used in this review.

REFERENCES

1. Fellegara G, Carcangiu ML, Rosai J. Benign epithelial inclusions in axillary lymph nodes: report of 18 cases and review of the literature. Am J Surg Pathol 2011;35(8):1123–33.
2. Corben AD, Nehhozina T, Garg K, et al. Endosalpingiosis in axillary lymph nodes: a possible pitfall in the staging of patients with breast carcinoma. Am J Surg Pathol 2010;34(8):1211–6.
3. Yi M, Kuerer HM, Mittendorf EA, et al. Impact of the American College of Surgeons oncology group Z0011 criteria applied to a contemporary patient population. J Am Coll Surg 2013;216(1):105–13.
4. Giuliano AE, Hunt KK, Ballman KV, et al. Axillary dissection vs no axillary dissection in women with invasive breast cancer and sentinel node metastasis: a randomized clinical trial. JAMA 2011; 305(6):569–75.
5. Norton LE, Komenaka IK, Emerson RE, et al. Benign glandular inclusions a rare cause of a false positive sentinel node. J Surg Oncol 2007;95(7): 593–6.
6. Peng Y, Ashfaq R, Ewing G, et al. False-positive sentinel lymph nodes in breast cancer patients caused by benign glandular inclusions: report of three cases and review of the literature. Am J Clin Pathol 2008;130(1):21–7, [quiz: 146].
7. Maiorano E, Mazzarol GM, Pruneri G, et al. Ectopic breast tissue as a possible cause of false-positive axillary sentinel lymph node biopsies. Am J Surg Pathol 2003;27(4):513–8.
8. Kadowaki M, Nagashima T, Sakata H, et al. Ectopic breast tissue in axillary lymph node. Breast Cancer 2007;14(4):425–8.
9. Holdsworth PJ, Hopkinson JM, Leveson SH. Benign axillary epithelial lymph node inclusions–a histological pitfall. Histopathology 1988;13(2):226–8.
10. Turner DR, Millis RR. Breast tissue inclusions in axillary lymph nodes. Histopathology 1980;4(6):631–6.
11. Fisher CJ, Hill S, Millis RR. Benign lymph node inclusions mimicking metastatic carcinoma. J Clin Pathol 1994;47(3):245–7.
12. Resetkova E, Hoda SA, Clarke JL, et al. Benign heterotopic epithelial inclusions in axillary lymph nodes. Histological and immunohistochemical patterns. Arch Pathol Lab Med 2003;127(1):e25–27.
13. Chuang C, Hicks DG, Berenson M, et al. Benign inclusion of axillary lymph nodes: report of two cases and literature review. Breast J 2009;15(6):664–5.
14. Fitzpatrick-Swallow VL, Helin H, Cane P, et al. Synchronous ductal carcinoma in situ of the breast and within epithelial inclusions in an ipsilateral sentinel lymph node. Hum Pathol 2013;44(1):142–4.
15. Carter BA, Jensen RA, Simpson JF, et al. Benign transport of breast epithelium into axillary lymph nodes after biopsy. Am J Clin Pathol 2000;113(2): 259–65.
16. Bleiweiss IJ, Nagi CS, Jaffer S. Axillary sentinel lymph nodes can be falsely positive due to iatrogenic displacement and transport of benign epithelial cells in patients with breast carcinoma. J Clin Oncol 2006;24(13):2013–8.
17. Diaz NM, Cox CE, Ebert M, et al. Benign mechanical transport of breast epithelial cells to sentinel lymph nodes. Am J Surg Pathol 2004;28(12):1641–5.
18. Diaz NM, Mayes JR, Vrcel V. Breast epithelial cells in dermal angiolymphatic spaces: a manifestation of benign mechanical transport. Hum Pathol 2005; 36(3):310–3.
19. Diaz NM, Vrcel V, Centeno BA, et al. Modes of benign mechanical transport of breast epithelial cells to axillary lymph nodes. Adv Anat Pathol 2005;12(1):7–9.
20. Migliorini L. Proliferative intraductal lesion arising in ectopic breast tissue within axillary lymph node. Histopathology 2006;48(3):316–7.
21. Chen YB, Magpayo J, Rosen PP. Sclerosing adenosis in sentinel axillary lymph nodes from a patient with invasive ductal carcinoma: an unusual variant of benign glandular inclusions. Arch Pathol Lab Med 2008;132(9):1439–41.
22. Dzodic R, Stanojevic B, Saenko V, et al. Intraductal papilloma of ectopic breast tissue in axillary lymph node of a patient with a previous

intraductal papilloma of ipsilateral breast: a case report and review of the literature. Diagn Pathol 2010;5:17.

23. Boulos FI, Granja NM, Simpson JF, et al. Intranodal papillary epithelial proliferations: a local process with a spectrum of morphologies and frequent association with papillomas in the breast. Am J Surg Pathol 2014;38(3):383–8.

24. Nonaka D, Chiriboga L, Soslow RA. Expression of pax8 as a useful marker in distinguishing ovarian carcinomas from mammary carcinomas. Am J Surg Pathol 2008;32(10):1566–71.

25. Laury AR, Perets R, Piao H, et al. A comprehensive analysis of PAX8 expression in human epithelial tumors. Am J Surg Pathol 2011;35(6):816–26.

26. Tornos C, Soslow R, Chen S, et al. Expression of WT1, CA 125, and GCDFP-15 as useful markers in the differential diagnosis of primary ovarian carcinomas versus metastatic breast cancer to the ovary. Am J Surg Pathol 2005;29(11):1482–9.

27. Domfeh AB, Carley AL, Striebel JM, et al. WT1 immunoreactivity in breast carcinoma: selective expression in pure and mixed mucinous subtypes. Mod Pathol 2008;21(10):1217–23.

28. Henley JD, Michael HB, English GW, et al. Benign Mullerian lymph node inclusions. An unusual case with implications for pathogenesis and review of the literature. Arch Pathol Lab Med 1995;119(9): 841–4.

29. Piana S, Asioli S, Cavazza A. Benign Mullerian inclusions coexisting with breast metastatic carcinoma in an axillary lymph node. Virchows Arch 2005;446(4): 467–9.

30. Stolnicu S, Preda O, Kinga S, et al. Florid, papillary endosalpingiosis of the axillary lymph nodes. Breast J 2011;17(3):268–72.

31. Salehi AH, Omeroglu G, Kanber Y, et al. Endosalpingiosis in axillary lymph nodes simulating metastatic breast carcinoma: a potential diagnostic pitfall. Int J Surg Pathol 2013;21(6):610–2.

32. Carney E, Cimino-Mathews A, Argani C, et al. A subset of nondescript axillary lymph node inclusions have the immunophenotype of endosalpingiosis. Am J Surg Pathol 2014;38(12):1612–7.

33. Consensus conference on the classification of ductal carcinoma in situ. The Consensus Conference Committee. Cancer 1997;80(9):1798–802.

34. Nomani L, Calhoun BC, Biscotti CV, et al. Endosalpingiosis of axillary lymph nodes: a rare histopathologic pitfall with clinical relevance for breast cancer staging. Case Rep Pathol 2016;2016:2856358.

35. Groth JV, Prabhu S, Wiley E. Coexistent isolated tumor cell clusters of infiltrating lobular carcinoma and benign glandular inclusions of Mullerian (endosalpingiosis) type in an axillary sentinel node: case report and review of the literature. Appl Immunohistochem Mol Morphol 2016;24(2):144–8.

36. Kheir SM, Mann WJ, Wilkerson JA. Glandular inclusions in lymph nodes. The problem of extensive involvement and relationship to salpingitis. Am J Surg Pathol 1981;5(4):353–9.

37. Moore WF, Bentley RC, Berchuck A, et al. Some Mullerian inclusion cysts in lymph nodes may sometimes be metastases from serous borderline tumors of the ovary. Am J Surg Pathol 2000;24(5):710–8.

38. Sarode VR, Euhus D, Thompson M, et al. Atypical endosalpingiosis in axillary sentinel lymph node: a potential source of false-positive diagnosis of metastasis. Breast J 2011;17(6):672–3.

39. Mukonoweshuro P, McCluggage WG. Endocervicosis involving axillary lymph nodes: first case report. Int J Gynecol Pathol 2014;33(6):620–3.

40. Recine MA, Deavers MT, Middleton LP, et al. Serous carcinoma of the ovary and peritoneum with metastases to the breast and axillary lymph nodes: a potential pitfall. Am J Surg Pathol 2004;28(12):1646–51.

41. White M, Vang R, Sharma R, et al. GATA3 is negative in endosalpingiosis: a useful marker in distinguishing metastatic breast carcinoma from a benign mimicker. Mod Pathol 2016;30(S2):78A.

42. Asch-Kendrick R, Cimino-Mathews A. The role of GATA3 in breast carcinomas: a review. Hum Pathol 2016;48:37–47.

43. Garret R, Ada AE. Epithelial inclusion cysts in an axillary lymph node; report of a case simulating metastatic adenocarcinoma. Cancer 1957;10(1):173–8.

44. Fraggetta F, Vasquez E. Epithelial inclusion in axillary lymph node associated with a breast carcinoma: report of a case with a review of the literature. Pathol Res Pract 1999;195(4):263–6.

45. Layfield LJ, Mooney E. Heterotopic epithelium in an intramammary lymph node. Breast J 2000;6(1): 63–7.

46. Rosen PP, Ernsberger D. Low-grade adenosquamous carcinoma. A variant of metaplastic mammary carcinoma. Am J Surg Pathol 1987;11(5):351–8.

47. Bautista NC, Cohen S, Anders KH. Benign melanocytic nevus cells in axillary lymph nodes. A prospective incidence and immunohistochemical study with literature review. Am J Clin Pathol 1994;102(1):102–8.

48. Carson KF, Wen DR, Li PX, et al. Nodal nevi and cutaneous melanomas. Am J Surg Pathol 1996; 20(7):834–40.

49. Holt JB, Sangueza OP, Levine EA, et al. Nodal melanocytic nevi in sentinel lymph nodes. Correlation with melanoma-associated cutaneous nevi. Am J Clin Pathol 2004;121(1):58–63.

50. Ridolfi RL, Rosen PP, Thaler H. Nevus cell aggregates associated with lymph nodes: estimated frequency and clinical significance. Cancer 1977; 39(1):164–71.

51. Andreola S, Clemente C. Nevus cells in axillary lymph nodes from radical mastectomy specimens. Pathol Res Pract 1985;179(6):616–8.

52. Subramony C, Lewin JR. Nevus cells within lymph nodes. Possible metastases from a benign intradermal nevus. Am J Clin Pathol 1985;84(2):220–3.

53. Johnson WT, Helwig EB. Benign nevus cells in the capsule of lymph nodes. Cancer 1969;23(3):747–53.

54. Biddle DA, Evans HL, Kemp BL, et al. Intraparenchymal nevus cell aggregates in lymph nodes: a possible diagnostic pitfall with malignant melanoma and carcinoma. Am J Surg Pathol 2003;27(5):673–81.

55. Bichel P, Ornsholt J. Benign nevus cells in the lymph nodes. An immunohistochemical study. APMIS 1988;96(2):117–22.

56. Yazdi HM. Nevus cell aggregates associated with lymph nodes. Immunohistochemical observations. Arch Pathol Lab Med 1985;109(11):1044–6.

57. Dwarakanath S, Lee AK, Delellis RA, et al. S-100 protein positivity in breast carcinomas: a potential pitfall in diagnostic immunohistochemistry. Hum Pathol 1987;18(11):1144–8.

58. Cimino-Mathews A, Subhawong AP, Elwood H, et al. Neural crest transcription factor Sox10 is preferentially expressed in triple-negative and metaplastic breast carcinomas. Hum Pathol 2013; 44(6):959–65.

An Update of Mucinous Lesions of the Breast

Beth T. Harrison, MD*, Deborah A. Dillon, MD

KEYWORDS

- Breast • Mucinous carcinoma • Mucocele-like lesion • Solid papillary carcinoma

---

Key points

- A diverse group of entities in the breast are associated with extracellular mucin production.
- The most important differential diagnosis is between mass-forming mucocelelike lesions and mucinous carcinoma.
- Mucocelelike lesions may be associated with benign proliferative and nonproliferative changes, atypia, and neoplasia, and inadequate sampling at biopsy is a concern.
- Mucinous carcinoma may be pure or mixed with other histologic subtypes and in its pure form is associated with a good prognosis.
- Solid papillary carcinoma often exhibits neuroendocrine and mucinous features and in some cases, may be a precursor to mucinous carcinoma.

ABSTRACT

Mucinous lesions of the breast include a variety of benign and malignant epithelial processes that display intracytoplasmic or extracellular mucin, including mucocelelike lesions, mucinous carcinoma, solid papillary carcinoma, and other rare subtypes of mucin-producing carcinoma. The most important diagnostic challenge is the finding of free-floating or stromal mucin accumulations for which the significance depends on the clinical, radiologic, and pathologic context. This article emphasizes the differential diagnosis between mucocelelike lesions and mucinous carcinoma, with a brief consideration of potential mimics, such as biphasic and mesenchymal lesions with myxoid stroma ("stromal mucin") and foreign material.

OVERVIEW

Mucins are a family of high molecular weight, heavily glycosylated proteins that are classified into 2 groups: membrane-bound mucins (eg, MUC1, MUC3, and MUC4) involved in signal transduction and gel-forming secreted mucins released into the extracellular space (eg, MUC2, MUC5AC, MUC5B and MUC6).[1] At least 18 mucin genes have been cloned to date.[2] The classic mucin genes are primarily expressed by epithelial cells.[3] A membrane-bound mucin, MUC1, is found at the apical surface of most normal breast epithelium, whereas its polarity is lost and its expression increased in neoplastic epithelium.[4] Secreted mucins are produced by various benign and malignant lesions of the breast. Mucinous carcinoma characteristically produces MUC2 (gel-forming intestinal-type secretory mucin) and MUC6 (pyloric gland–type secretory mucin), a finding uncommon in other mammary adenocarcinomas.[1] Secreted mucins are neutral or acidic and the chemical composition determines reactivity on special stains, such as periodic acid-Schiff, Alcian blue, and mucicarmine.[5,6]

In the older literature, proteoglycan-rich extracellular matrix secreted by connective tissue cells was referred to as "connective tissue mucin" or

Disclosure Statement: The authors have no disclosures.

Department of Pathology, Brigham and Women's Hospital, 75 Francis Street, Amory 3, Boston, MA 02115, USA

* Corresponding author.

E-mail address: bharrison3@bwh.harvard.edu

surgpath.theclinics.com

"stromal mucin," but this is a misnomer, as there are biochemical differences between the 2 families of glycoproteins. Nevertheless, prominent "myxoid" stromal change is morphologically similar to extracellular mucin on a macroscopic and microscopic level, related in large part to the hydrophilic, gel-forming properties of proteoglycans.[6]

This review is focused on mammary epithelial lesions with extracellular mucin production, especially mucocelelike lesions (MLLs) and mucinous carcinoma, with a brief consideration of biphasic and mesenchymal lesions with myxoid stroma and other mucin mimics as they relate to the differential diagnosis.

MUCOCELELIKE LESIONS

Key Points
MUCOCELELIKE LESIONS

- MLLs consist of ruptured mucinous cysts and extravasated mucin.

- The cysts may be lined by flat-to-columnar epithelium or involved by usual, atypical or neoplastic epithelial proliferations. Large, granular calcifications are often present within the mucin.

- Mucinous carcinoma is the most important consideration in the differential diagnosis of an MLL, especially if the lesion is associated with intraductal neoplasia, abundant stromal mucin, and/or floating epithelium.

- MLLs without evidence of atypia on core needle biopsy have a rate of upgrade to malignancy on excision of less than 5%.

- Excision has been traditionally recommended; however, conservative management may be possible in selected incidental or small benign lesions.

Pitfalls
MUCOCELELIKE LESIONS

! The presence of strips or clusters of epithelium floating within the mucin of an MLL involved by atypical ductal hyperplasia or ductal carcinoma in situ may raise consideration for mucinous carcinoma. Epithelial displacement is favored if the floating epithelium is scant, associated with myoepithelial cells, or contiguous with the cyst lining.

MLL was first described by Rosen[7] in 1986 as a benign lesion analogous to mucocele of the minor salivary glands. Rosen[7] defined this lesion as benign mucin-filled cysts lined by flat or cuboidal epithelium frequently associated with rupture and mucin extravasation. It is now appreciated that MLLs arise in the setting of various pathologic processes, including benign proliferative and nonproliferative changes, atypical ductal hyperplasia (ADH), and in situ or invasive carcinoma. The biology of the lesions depends on the nature of the lining epithelium, which may be hyperplastic, atypical, or neoplastic.[8,9] Therefore, "mucocelelike lesion" is best considered a descriptive term, insufficient on its own as a diagnosis without further classification of the underlying process.

GROSS FEATURES

An MLL may present as a palpable breast mass, a mammographic abnormality, or an incidental finding. The most common presentation is indeterminate microcalcifications on screening mammography.[10–12] The microcalcifications are typically described as clustered and pleomorphic, but also may be coarse and eggshell-shaped or fine and linear or granular. If a mass lesion is present, it is usually a single round or lobulated mass with circumscribed or indistinct borders or possibly multiple masses with a "rosarylike" appearance.[11]

Grossly, there may be well-defined multiloculated cystic nodules or ill-defined shiny areas with a gelatinous cut surface. Yellow flecks or gritty texture are found in lesions with prominent calcifications. Most lesions measure between 0.5 and 1.0 cm.[8]

MICROSCOPIC FEATURES

MLLs consist of cysts with mucinous contents and extravasated mucin within the surrounding stroma. In benign lesions, the cysts are lined by attenuated, flat-to-cuboidal epithelium (**Figs. 1** and **2**). With rupture, strips of epithelium detach from the cyst wall and float within the mucin. Mucin collects as pools within the stroma. Large, granular calcifications are often present within the mucin and are characteristic (**Figs. 3** and **4**). Some lesions are associated with chronic inflammation and stromal fibrosis (see **Fig. 2**). The epithelium commonly exhibits areas of columnar cell change or proliferative change ranging from usual ductal hyperplasia to ADH (see **Fig. 2**; **Figs. 5–9**).

MLLs may be associated with neoplastic proliferations that warrant a diagnosis of in situ or invasive carcinoma. Ductal carcinoma in situ (DCIS)

Fig. 1. Ruptured mucinous cyst with extruded contents (H&E, original magnification ×20).

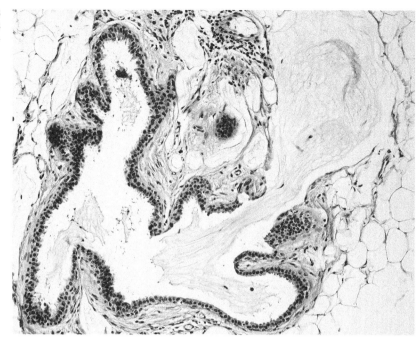

involving MLLs usually displays micropapillary, papillary, or cribriform growth patterns. A diagnosis of DCIS should be rendered only when at least 2 duct profiles are completely involved. The extent criterion (>0.2 cm) must be applied with caution, as the true extent of the lesion may be difficult to assess due to significant cystic dilatation of the involved ducts (see Fig. 9; Figs. 10 and 11). A focus of invasive carcinoma arising in the background of an MLL is diagnosed when there are detached clusters of cytologically malignant epithelial cells within stromal mucin pools

Fig. 2. Small benign MLL in a background of columnar cell change and hyperplasia, fibrosis, and inflammation on core biopsy for calcifications (H&E, original magnification ×10).

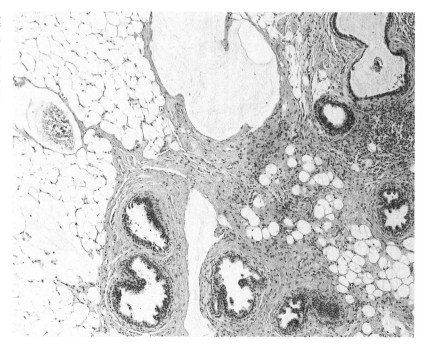

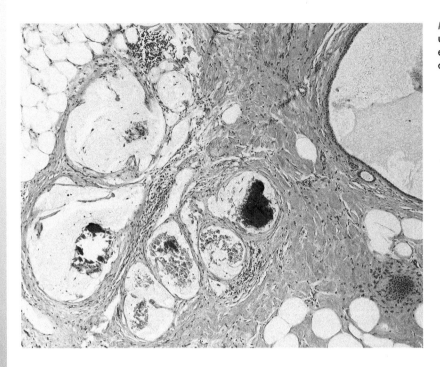

Fig. 3. Characteristic granular calcifications within extravasated mucin (H&E, original magnification ×10).

(see **Fig. 10**) (see later in this article for further discussion).

DIFFERENTIAL DIAGNOSIS

Benign cysts, atypical and neoplastic intraductal proliferations, and invasive carcinoma may be associated with extracellular mucin production, and in our opinion, should be considered an MLL only in the presence of cyst formation with at least focal mucin extravasation.

Invasive mucinous carcinoma is the most important consideration in the differential diagnosis of MLLs. Mucinous carcinoma features tumor cells

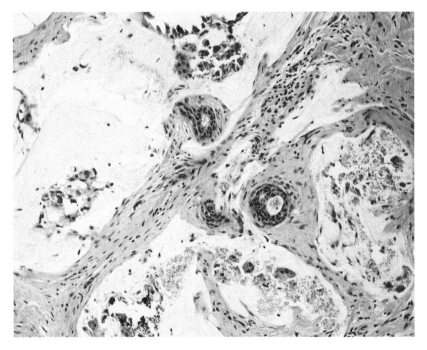

Fig. 4. Free-floating benign epithelium within extravasated mucin should not be mistaken for mucinous carcinoma (H&E, original magnification ×20).

Fig. 5. A large MLL corresponding to a radiologic mass lesion measuring larger than 2 cm (H&E, original magnification ×4).

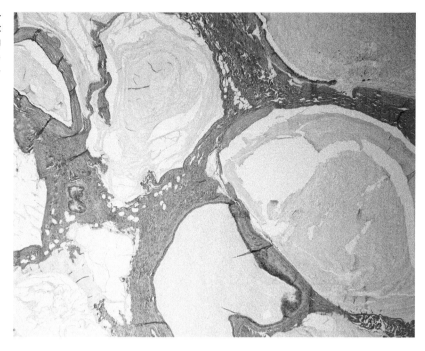

arranged in clusters, solid nests, micropapillae, or cribriform structures within pools of extracellular mucin. Cytologic atypia is conspicuous. Paucicellular tumors and foci of microinvasive mucinous carcinoma may be particularly challenging to distinguish from MLLs, although the presence of a subtle network of arborizing fibrovascular septae should raise suspicion for carcinoma.

Conversely, MLLs in which small fragments of epithelium have dislodged into the extracellular mucin may be worrisome for mucinous carcinoma. If an MLL is free of significant atypia, it is unlikely

Fig. 6. The cyst lining ranges from columnar cell change to flat epithelial atypia (H&E, original magnification ×20).

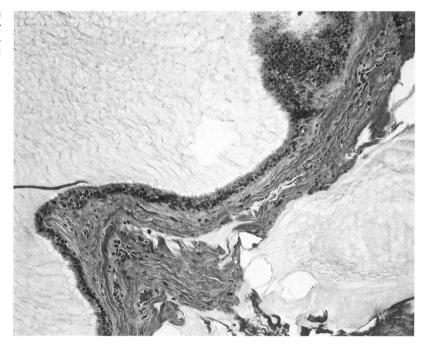

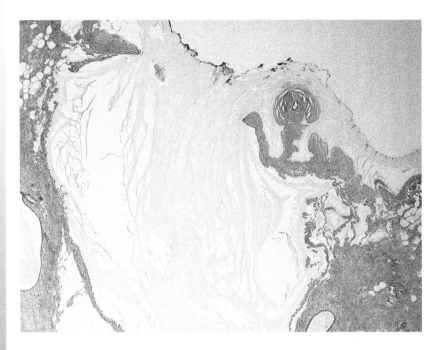

Fig. 7. A mucin lake extends to the inked margin of the excision and should prompt consideration of reexcision (H&E, original magnification ×4).

that small epithelial fragments floating within the mucin represent a malignant process. It is more difficult to determine the significance of free-floating epithelial clusters in cases of MLL associated with DCIS. It would be prudent to favor epithelial displacement when the floating clusters of neoplastic cells are scant, associated with myoepithelial cells, or contiguous with the cyst lining. Deeper levels and immunohistochemistry (IHC) for myoepithelial cell markers (eg, p63, smooth muscle myosin heavy chain, calponin) assist in the diagnosis,[13] although IHC is helpful

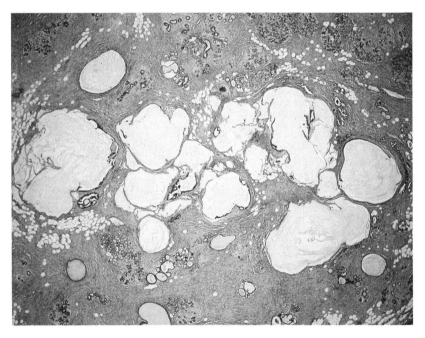

Fig. 8. ADH bordering on DCIS involving a large MLL. This lesion is difficult to classify by quantitative and qualitative criteria due to cystic dilatation and distortion of involved ducts (H&E, original magnification ×2).

Fig. 9. ADH adjacent to a ruptured mucinous cyst and extravasated mucin (H&E, original magnification ×20).

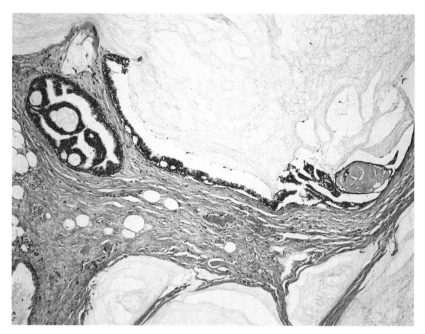

only when positive; an absence of myoepithelial cells is not necessarily confirmatory of invasion in this setting.

Cystic hypersecretory lesions (change, hyperplasia, and intraductal carcinoma) may bear superficial resemblance to MLLs because they are also composed of cysts with prominent secretions. Like MLLs, the cyst lining encompasses a variety of morphologies, including flat or cuboidal (change), columnar with apical blebs (hyperplasia), or micropapillary (intraductal carcinoma). The secretions are colloidlike, dense, and eosinophilic, with fracture lines and scalloped contours, and stand in contrast to the pale blue-gray, translucent mucin of MLLs (**Fig. 12**).[14]

Breast lesions that contain stromal mucin, such as nodular mucinosis, myxoma and myxoid fibroepithelial lesions, are other entities that may resemble the extravasated mucin of an MLL, especially in limited core needle biopsies (see discussion later in this article).

PROGNOSIS

The management of MLLs diagnosed on core needle biopsy is a topic of debate. Historically, it has been common practice to excise all MLLs regardless of the presence of epithelial atypia due to concern for inadequate sampling of mucinous carcinoma. Studies have reported widely variable upgrade rates (0%–43%),[12,15–28]

but many have been limited by small numbers, insufficient radiologic-pathologic correlation, varying inclusion criteria (MLLs with and without atypia), and varying definitions of what constitutes an upgrade (ADH vs in situ and invasive carcinoma).

Rakha and colleagues[29] recently published one of the largest studies on MLLs without atypia diagnosed on core biopsy as well as a comprehensive review of the literature. The investigators found a 4% rate of upgrade to in situ or invasive carcinoma in their cohort (2 of 54 cases) and in previous studies (4 of 106 cases), which just exceeds the upgrade rate ($\geq$3%) used in the radiologic literature to define a high-risk lesion requiring excision.[30] Three subsequent studies, by Sutton and colleagues,[27] Ha and colleagues,[28] and Park and Kim,[10] have not identified any additional examples of in situ or invasive carcinoma in 45 excisions of MLLs without atypia, suggesting that the contemporary upgrade rate is even lower and likely less than the 3% threshold (6 of 205 cases to date).

Surgical excision of atypical or malignant MLLs is clearly recommended, as the upgrade rate is more than 20%.[29] The management of MLLs without atypia is subject to institutional practice patterns. We recommend discussion of these cases at radiology-pathology correlation conferences when possible. Also, in our opinion, it appears reasonable to recommend excision for all cases that present as a radiologic

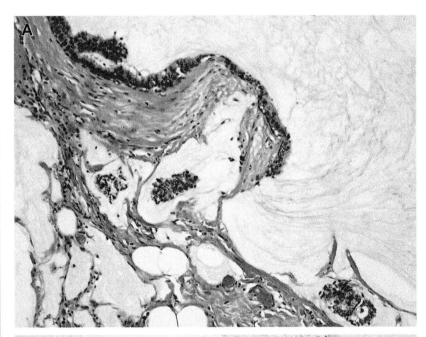

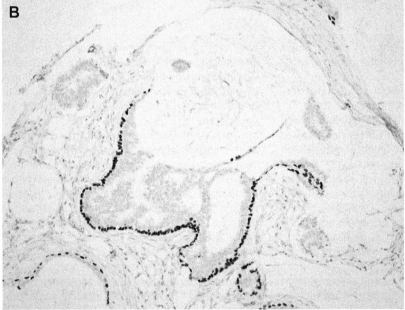

Fig. 10. A focus suspicious for microinvasion associated with a ruptured mucinous cyst with atypia (H&E, original magnification ×20) (*A*). The clusters of neoplastic cells lack myoepithelial cells (p63 immunoperoxidase stain, original magnification ×20) (*B*).

mass lesion to exclude the possibility of sampling error. Conservative management may be appropriate for small or incidental MLLs in the absence of atypia.

The prognosis of MLLs is likely related to the accompanying pathologic process, and in the absence of malignancy, is excellent. Few recurrences have been documented, including an MLL with ADH that recurred as an MLL with DCIS[31] as well as an MLL with usual ductal hyperplasia that recurred as an MLL with lobular carcinoma

in situ.[8] Moreover, Meares and colleagues[32] recently reported long-term clinical outcomes of 102 MLLs identified from the benign breast disease cohort at Mayo Clinic with an average follow-up of 14.8 years. One-quarter of the lesions was associated with atypical hyperplasia. Breast cancer developed in 13 (12.7%) patients. This frequency is only slightly higher than expected population rates and not significantly different from that in women with proliferative breast disease in the cohort.

MUCINOUS CARCINOMA

Key Points
MUCINOUS CARCINOMA

- Mucinous carcinoma presents as a gelatinous mass with pushing borders.

- A diagnosis of pure mucinous carcinoma requires that at least 90% of the tumor contains extracellular mucin.

- Capella type A is the paucicellular subtype, with ribbonlike, annular, or cribriform growth patterns, whereas Capella type B is the highly cellular subtype with a sheetlike growth pattern and endocrine differentiation.

- Mucinous carcinoma is typically hormone receptor positive and human epidermal growth factor receptor 2 (HER2) negative and most exhibit a luminal A phenotype on gene expression analysis.

- Mucinous carcinoma has a more favorable prognosis than invasive carcinoma of no special type.

Pitfalls
MUCINOUS CARCINOMA

! In the neoadjuvant setting, acellular mucin remaining in the breast or lymph nodes does not preclude a pathologic complete response. If scant residual neoplastic epithelium can be identified within the mucin, the tumor is staged according to the size of the largest discrete area of involved mucin.

Mucinous carcinoma is a special subtype of invasive breast cancer generally associated with a favorable prognosis. Previously known as colloid carcinoma, the reported incidence varies somewhat according to histologic criteria. However, most studies show that fewer than 5% of all invasive breast cancers have a mucinous component and only approximately 2% represent pure mucinous carcinoma.[33–36]

GROSS FEATURES

Patients with mucinous carcinoma generally present at an older age than patients with breast carcinoma of no special type, in the sixth through early eighth decade in most studies. Although many patients present with palpable tumors, a substantial proportion present with nonpalpable mammographic abnormalities, including poorly defined or lobulated mass lesions that are rarely associated with calcification.[37–40] Approximately 20% of mucinous carcinomas are mammographically occult.[41]

On gross examination, mucinous carcinomas have a distinctive appearance. They are generally circumscribed, with a soft, gelatinous consistency and a glistening cut surface. Mucinous carcinomas with larger amounts of fibrous stroma may present with a firmer consistency. A wide range of sizes has been reported in the literature, with an average of approximately 3 cm.[42]

MICROSCOPIC FEATURES

Mucinous carcinomas are characterized by the presence of abundant extracellular mucin, varying somewhat in extent from tumor to tumor, separated by fibrous septae containing capillaries. The typical histologic appearance shows tumor cells in small clusters, solid nests, or cribriform structures present within extracellular mucin pools (Figs. 13–17). Nuclear features are generally low or intermediate-grade with a low mitotic rate. Tumors showing extracellular mucin production in conjunction with other nonmucinous histologic features are classified as "mixed" mucinous tumors. A DCIS component may accompany these cancers and may show papillary, micropapillary, cribriform, or solid patterns with or without prominent extracellular mucin production (Fig. 18).[42]

Capella and colleagues[43] divided mucinous carcinomas according to their cellularity, with paucicellular tumors having ribbon, annular, and cribriform growth patterns called "type A" and highly cellular tumors with clumped and sheetlike growth patterns and less extracellular mucin called "type B." Type B mucinous carcinomas typically show endocrine differentiation, including immunoreactivity for chromogranin or synaptophysin or cytoplasmic argyrophilic granules (see Fig. 18).

Recently, a histologic variant of mucinous carcinoma has been described with intermediate to high-grade nuclei, a hobnail pattern and micropapillary architecture (see Fig. 13B). These cases have been called pure mucinous carcinoma with micropapillary pattern[44,45] or mucinous micropapillary carcinoma.[46] In one study, 20% of these cases were HER2 positive.[46] Although the clinical significance of these findings has not been studied extensively, preliminary data, including an

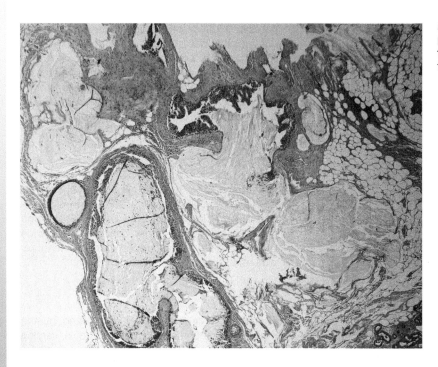

Fig. 11. DCIS with mucin production and extra-vasation (H&E, original magnification ×4).

association with lymphovascular invasion and positive lymph nodes, suggest aggressive behavior in these cases.[46–48]

DIAGNOSIS

The diagnosis of mucinous carcinoma is usually straightforward in the setting of prominent extracellular mucin. At least 90% of the tumor (or 100% according to some)[41] should show the characteristic histology to qualify for the diagnosis of mucinous carcinoma. Care should be taken to note any areas that are not purely mucinous, as mixed mucinous tumors have a less favorable prognosis than pure mucinous carcinomas.

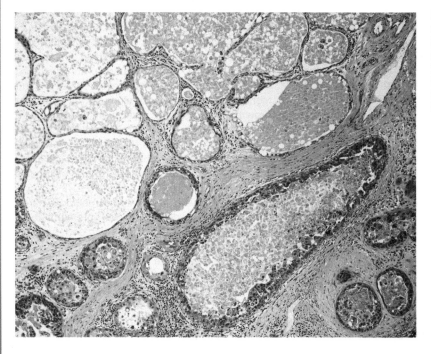

Fig. 12. Cystic hypersecretory carcinoma with colloid-like eosinophilic secretions should be distinguished from malignant mucocele-like lesions and mucinous DCIS (H&E, original magnification ×10).

Fig. 13. Capella type A mucinous carcinoma with low cellularity and micropapillary features (H&E, original magnification ×4) (*A*). The micropapillary clusters exhibit characteristic inverted architecture (H&E, original magnification ×20) (*B*).

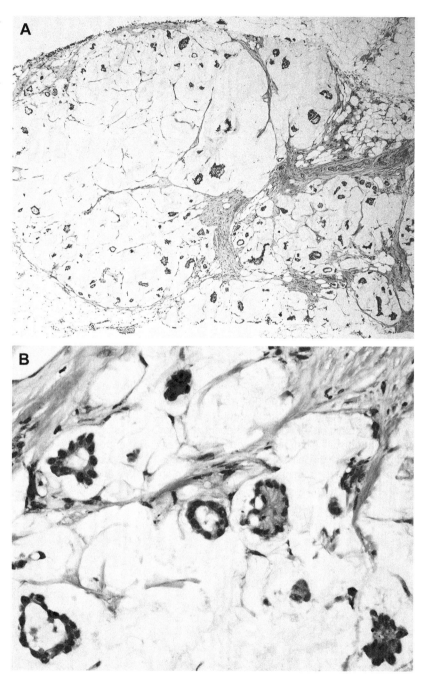

Most mucinous carcinomas are estrogen receptor (ER) positive and approximately 70% are also progesterone receptor (PR) positive. Overexpression of the HER2 protein or presence of HER2 gene amplification is rare.[49–52] Mucinous carcinomas show a relatively stable genome, with fewer chromosomal gains and losses than invasive carcinomas of no special type.[53] Mucinous carcinomas generally cluster within the luminal A subtype in gene expression studies. Type B mucinous carcinomas are distinct from type A mucinous carcinomas and cluster with other breast cancers showing neuroendocrine differentiation.[54]

DIFFERENTIAL DIAGNOSIS

Paucicellular mucinous carcinoma (Type A) may easily be mistaken for MLL in a small biopsy or insufficiently sampled lesion. Deeper levels or

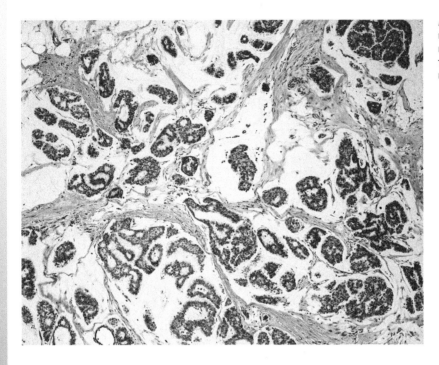

Fig. 14. Mucinous carcinoma composed of small nests, micropapillae, and festoons (H&E, original magnification ×10).

more extensive sampling may reveal nests of floating tumor cells required for a diagnosis of mucinous carcinoma. Small core biopsies showing prominent extracellular mucin without definite tumor cell clusters may represent under-sampling of a paucicellular mucinous carcinoma if a mass lesion is present on clinical examination and imaging. Excision is advised in such cases to exclude a mucinous carcinoma.

Conversely, fragments of detached benign, atypical, or DCIS epithelium in an MLL may raise the possibility of mucinous carcinoma. Careful attention to associated myoepithelium in the floating epithelial cell clusters, with IHC for

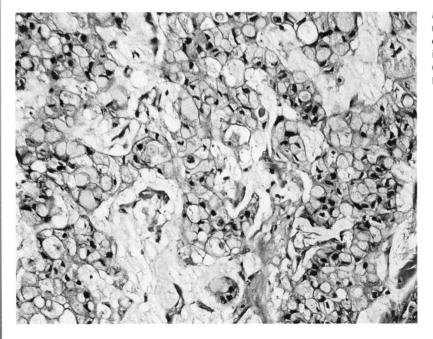

Fig. 15. Mucinous carcinoma with signet ring cell features (H&E, original magnification ×40). (Courtesy of Dr Susan Lester, Boston, MA.)

Fig. 16. Mucinous carcinoma with a cribriform growth pattern associated with DCIS (H&E, original magnification ×10).

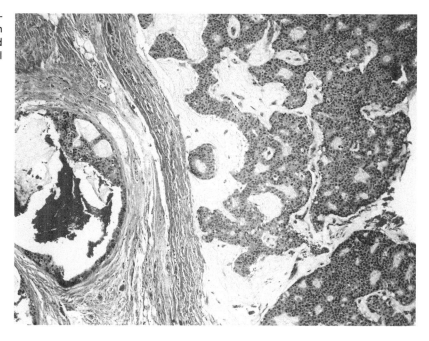

p63, smooth muscle myosin heavy chain, or other myoepithelial markers, may be helpful in resolving this dilemma. In some cases, deeper levels may reveal continuity between the suspicious cell clusters and epithelium lining adjacent ducts, supporting an artifact of duct rupture with mucin extravasation.

Mucin pools may be seen in the breast and lymph nodes following neoadjuvant chemotherapy and should not be considered residual carcinoma unless there are tumor cells floating in the mucin (**Figs. 19–21**). Submission of additional tissue and evaluation of levels may be required to confirm the absence of residual carcinoma.

In the absence of an associated in situ component, the differential diagnosis may sometimes include mucinous carcinoma metastatic from another site. In this case, stains for ER/PR,

Fig. 17. Mucinous DCIS with an unusual micropapillary growth pattern (H&E, original magnification ×4).

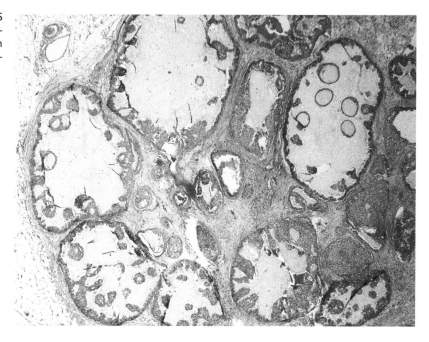

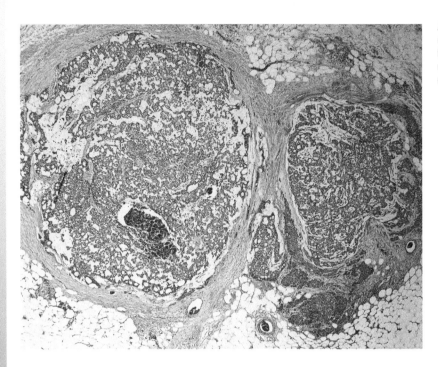

Fig. 18. Capella type B mucinous carcinoma with high cellularity and scant mucin (H&E, original magnification ×4).

CK7/20, GATA3, CDX2, PAX8, and others may be helpful, as well as additional clinical history and imaging studies.[55]

PROGNOSIS

Using the Surveillance, Epidemiology, and End Results (SEER) database, Di Saverio and colleagues[36] compared 20-year survival data from more than 11,000 patients with mucinous carcinoma and patients with invasive ductal carcinoma diagnosed between 1973 and 2002. In this report, there were no significant differences in overall survival; however, survival at 10 and 20 years for mucinous carcinoma was 89% and 81%, respectively, compared with 72% and 62% for invasive ductal carcinoma. In multivariate analyses, the most significant prognostic factors were nodal status, then age, tumor size, PR status, and nuclear grade. In the SEER database, patients with mucinous carcinoma most often presented with localized disease (86%). Only 12% had regional lymph node involvement and only 2% had distant metastases at the time of diagnosis. This is significantly less than the incidence of node positivity rate seen in mixed mucinous tumors or invasive breast cancers of no special type. Lymph node involvement is related to tumor size and is extremely rare in mucinous carcinomas measuring smaller than 1 cm,[52] prompting some groups to consider deferral of lymph node sampling in patients with very small tumors.[56]

There were 38 patients with mucinous carcinoma enrolled in the NSABP-B06 trial. Overall, these patients experienced better survival, as did patients with tubular carcinoma, especially in the node-negative group.[57] Ellis and coworkers[58] reported similar results in their retrospective series. In 2 additional series, one looking at patients with node-negative early-stage breast cancer treated with mastectomy (20-year follow-up), and the other looking at early-stage patients treated with breast-conserving therapy (10-year follow-up), patients with mucinous carcinoma had significantly lower rates of distant recurrence compared with patients with invasive ductal carcinoma.[59,60] Several studies have also noted late recurrences in patients with mucinous carcinoma, with 1 report documenting a recurrence 30 years after initial treatment.[61]

There are no significant differences in local recurrence rates following conservative surgery and radiation for mucinous carcinoma compared with invasive ductal carcinoma.[60,62,63] Given the favorable prognosis for most patients with mucinous carcinoma, some investigators have questioned whether radiation therapy might be safely omitted after breast-conserving surgery; however, data are insufficient at the current time to inform such a recommendation.

Unusual complications of metastatic disease have occasionally been seen in mucinous carcinomas, including mucin embolism resulting in cerebral infarct and pseudomyxoma peritonei.[64]

Fig. 19. Acellular mucin in the primary tumor bed (*A*) and lymph node (H&E, original magnification, [*A, B*] ×4) (*B*) is considered a pathologic complete response following neoadjuvant chemotherapy. Care should be taken to exclude residual tumor.

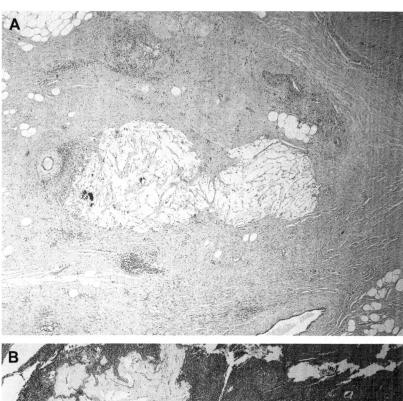

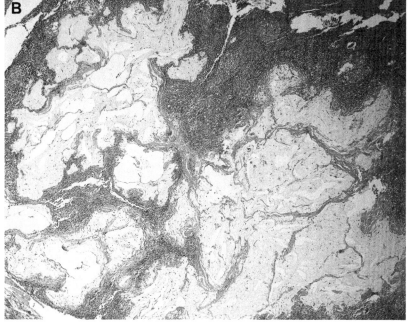

MUCINOUS CYSTADENOCARCINOMA

This cystic type of papillary mucinous carcinoma is a rare variant of mucin-producing carcinoma, characterized by multiple mucin-containing cysts lined by micropapillary, papillary, or cribriform carcinoma without evidence of a peripheral myoepithelial cell layer. It is negative for ERs and PRs, which sets it apart from other cystic papillary tumors of the breast. In the absence of ER-positivity and an in situ component, careful clinical correlation is required to exclude the possibility of metastatic ovarian or colorectal carcinoma. The prognosis of this rare form of triple-negative breast cancer is relatively favorable.[65]

SOLID PAPILLARY CARCINOMA

> ### *Key Points*
> #### SOLID PAPILLARY CARCINOMA
>
> - Solid papillary carcinoma (SPC) is an indolent breast cancer found in elderly women.
>
> - The tumor is characterized by circumscribed expansile, cellular nodules with delicate fibrovascular cores.
>
> - Mucinous and neuroendocrine features are characteristic.
>
> - SPC is considered a form of in situ carcinoma for staging purposes in the absence of an irregular, geographic, or "jigsawlike" growth pattern or a conventional invasive component.
>
> - A conventional invasive component is present in 50% of cases and is most commonly type B mucinous, neuroendocrinelike, or ductal in type.
>
> - Metastasis to axillary lymph nodes or distant sites is rare and generally seen only in SPC with a conventional invasive component.

SPC is a term that was originally coined by Maluf and Koerner[66] in 1995 to refer to a distinctive form of intraductal carcinoma with endocrine differentiation frequently associated with mucinous carcinoma. More recently, SPC has been defined by the World Health Organization Classification of Tumors of the Breast 2012[67] as a "distinctive form of papillary carcinoma characterized by closely apposed expansile, cellular nodules." The tumor nodules that define solid papillary carcinoma are circumscribed and resemble intraductal carcinoma, but they completely lack myoepithelial cells and likely represent a form of expansile invasion.[68] SPC frequently arises in a background of solid papillary and other patterns of DCIS and is associated with a frankly infiltrative component in half of cases.[69,70] SPC is thought in some cases to be a precursor of the Capella type B pattern of mucinous carcinoma.[69]

Although appropriate staging has been a matter of controversy, the World Health Organization recommends that SPC be classified as in situ disease in the absence of jagged borders or a conventional invasive component.[68]

GROSS FEATURES

SPC is primarily found in elderly women.[66,69–71] Most tumors arise in the central region of the

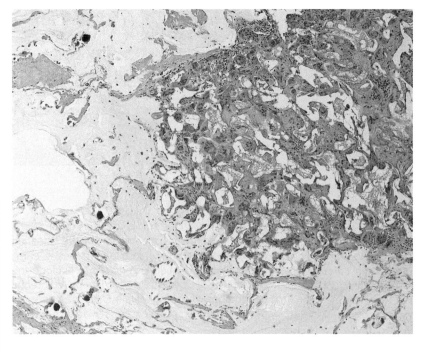

Fig. 20. A core biopsy site with foreign body giant cells is present within mucin and should not be mistaken for tumor (H&E, original magnification ×10).

Fig. 21. Scant mucin with calcifications in a core biopsy of a 1-cm mass detected in a patient with a history of ipsilateral mucinous carcinoma (*A*). On excision, only a single small cluster of neoplastic cells in present within neovascularized mucin (*B*), consistent with recurrent mucinous carcinoma. The tumor is staged according to the size of the involved mucin (eg, rpT1b) (H&E, original magnification [*A*] ×10; [*B*] ×20).

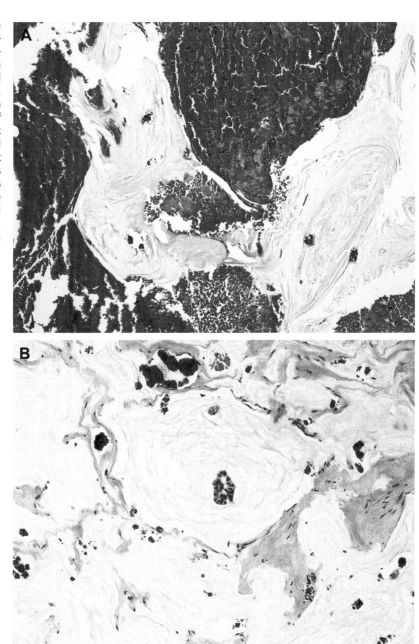

breast.[66] Patients present with a palpable mass, nipple discharge, or a density on screening mammogram. On gross examination, the tumor consists of a single nodule or multiple circumscribed nodules with a fleshy to firm consistency.[66,69] A gelatinous appearance is associated with mucinous differentiation.[66,69]

MICROSCOPIC FEATURES

SPC is characterized by circumscribed solid nodules that are variably sized, ranging from small and DCIS-like to expansive, with delicate, hyalinized fibrovascular cores (**Fig. 22**). The neoplastic proliferation is low to intermediate grade and commonly displays a streaming appearance resembling florid usual ductal hyperplasia. The tumor cells may be ovoid, spindled with nuclear grooves, or plasmacytoid with eosinophilic cytoplasm and eccentric nuclei, reflecting the neuroendocrine differentiation present in many of these tumors. The tumor cells may contain intracytoplasmic mucin vacuoles or signet ring cell morphology and

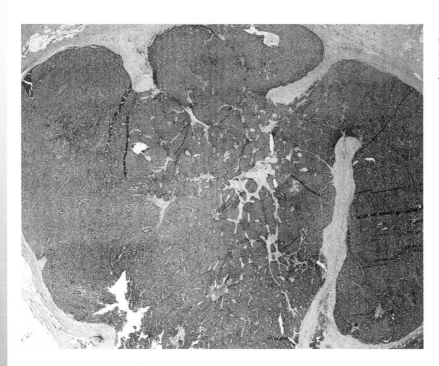

Fig. 22. SPC is present as a single nodule with an expansile growth pattern (H&E, original magnification ×2).

extracellular mucin may be present (**Figs. 23–26**). A type of SPC with extravasated mucin has been described in which the circumscribed tumor nodule is present within a clefted space containing mucin.[69]

SPC is considered invasive if it consists of tumor nodules with an irregular, geographic, or "jigsawlike" pattern and associated stromal desmoplasia. A conventional invasive carcinoma is found in approximately half of the cases and may be pure or mixed

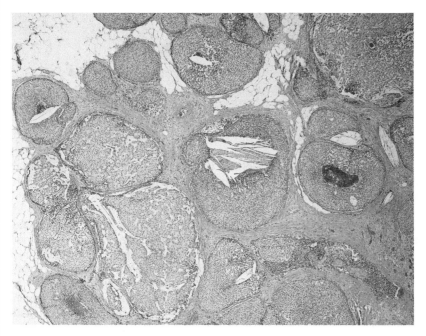

Fig. 23. SPC is present as several DCIS-like nodules with mucinous features (H&E, original magnification ×4).

Fig. 24. In situ SPC with mucin production. Note the delicate fibrovascular cores within the tumor nodule (H&E, original magnification ×10).

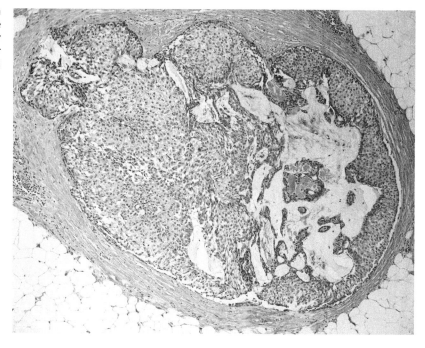

mucinous, neuroendocrinelike, ductal, and less commonly, lobular or tubular.[69,72] The associated mucinous carcinoma has type B morphology and is characterized by crowded or confluent clusters of tumor cells in relatively scant pools of mucin (**Fig. 27**).[69] Pathologic staging is based on the size of the frankly invasive component.[68]

DIAGNOSIS

Immunohistochemical studies for myoepithelial markers aid in the diagnosis of SPC and its distinction from other papillary lesions. In SPC, the myoepithelial cell layer is absent within the fibrovascular cores, but may or may not be

Fig. 25. The neoplastic cells of this SPC have a plasmacytoid morphology with abundant eosinophilic cytoplasm and eccentric nuclei. Intercellular mucin is present (H&E, original magnification ×40).

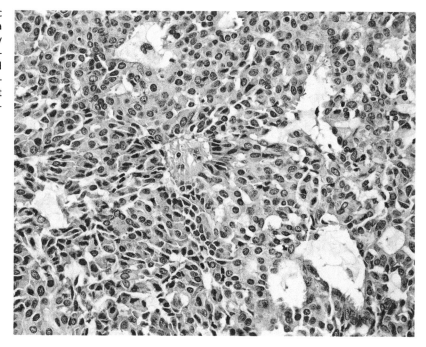

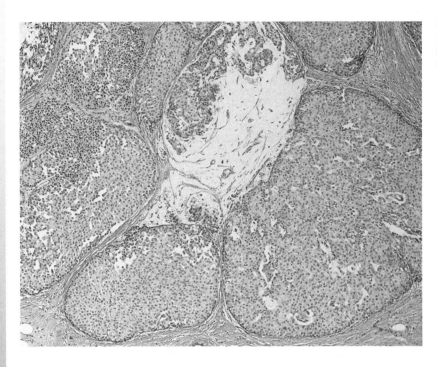

Fig. 26. SPC with at least microinvasive mucinous carcinoma (H&E, original magnification ×10).

present at the periphery of the tumor nodules.[73] As a low-grade neoplastic proliferation, SPC is almost always strongly and diffusely positive for ERs and negative for HER2[69] and typically lacks expression of cytokeratin (CK) 5/6. Most cases show IHC staining for neuroendocrine markers (synaptophysin, chromogranin, CD56,

or neuron-specific enolase).[66,69] SPCs associated with extracellular mucin production or mucinous carcinoma are more likely to express higher levels of WT-1 and MUC2 than those without.[74]

SPC has a luminal phenotype on gene expression array analysis and is closely related to

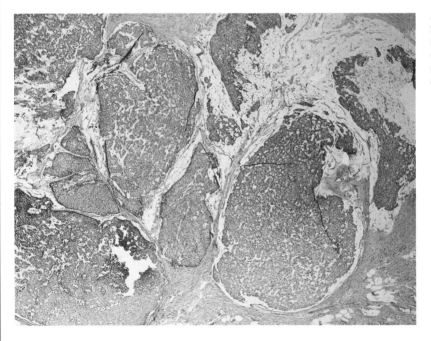

Fig. 27. Fragmentation of SPC within extravasated mucin and transition to Capella type B cellular mucinous carcinoma (H&E, original magnification ×4).

type B mucinous carcinomas at the transcriptomic level.[54,75]

DIFFERENTIAL DIAGNOSIS

SPC must be distinguished from hyperplastic and neoplastic proliferations involving an intraductal papilloma. SPC is composed of low-grade spindle cells with nuclear grooves and a streaming growth pattern closely resembles florid usual ductal hyperplasia. It is differentiated from florid hyperplasia by greater cellular monotony, readily identifiable mitotic activity, and hyalinized fibrovascular cores surrounded by nuclear palisading. Intracellular or extracellular mucin is a clue to the diagnosis of SPC, as this is not seen in florid hyperplasia. In challenging cases, an IHC panel of ER, CK 5/6, and myoepithelial markers is helpful. In contrast to SPC, a papilloma involved by florid hyperplasia shows heterogeneous ER and mosaic CK 5/6 expression in the epithelial proliferation and an intact myoepithelial cell layer within fibrovascular cores and at the periphery of the benign papilloma.

SPC containing low-grade to intermediate-grade monotonous epithelial tumor cells often raises consideration for DCIS or lobular carcinoma in situ superimposed on an underlying papilloma. Again, assessing the pattern of staining for myoepithelial cell markers is essential to the diagnosis of SPC versus papilloma. If plasmacytoid or signet ring cell morphology is especially prominent, the demonstration of normal membranous expression of E-cadherin and p120 catenin is helpful in excluding lobular neoplasia (see discussion later in this article).

PROGNOSIS

SPC has an indolent clinical course. Pure cases without extravasated mucin or invasive carcinoma rarely metastasize.[66,69,70] Axillary lymph node metastasis and distant metastasis are rare and are generally seen only in SPC with a conventional invasive component. A recent review of the literature revealed that 11 patients developed a local recurrence, 7 patients developed distant metastases, and 3 patients died of breast carcinoma of 253 patients.[70] A case of SPC with extravasated mucin with distant metastasis at 10 years after diagnosis has been reported and highlights the difficulties in differentiating it from mucinous carcinoma.[69] Metastases may retain the solid papillary morphology.[66,69]

Given the low incidence of recurrence, metastasis, and breast cancer–related death,

management with adequate local therapy is likely sufficient. This approach includes at least lumpectomy and sentinel lymph node biopsy. Hormonal therapy may be administered in the adjuvant setting.[76]

INVASIVE LOBULAR CARCINOMA WITH EXTRACELLULAR MUCIN PRODUCTION

> ### Key Points
> #### INVASIVE LOBULAR CARCINOMA WITH EXTRACELLULAR MUCIN PRODUCTION
>
> - Invasive lobular carcinoma with extracellular mucin production (ILCEMP) is a recently recognized, rare variant.
> - Invasive lobular carcinoma, most commonly classic type, is associated with a mucinous component composed of single cells, clusters or single file arrays floating in mucin.
> - Membranous E-cadherin is absent and p120 catenin is aberrantly cytoplasmic.
> - Limited data preclude comparison of outcomes with classic lobular carcinoma and other forms of mammary carcinoma.

ILCEMP is a rare variant that was first described by Rosa and colleagues[77] in 2009 and subsequently characterized further in a few case reports[78–81] and a small case series[82] (13 reported cases in total). Although intracellular mucin often in the form of "targetoid" intracytoplasmic vacuoles is characteristic of classic and variant forms of lobular carcinoma, extracellular mucin secretion has been traditionally considered a feature of ductal carcinoma.[77] This tumor is characterized by invasive lobular carcinoma, most commonly classic type, which features a mucinous component composed of single cells, clusters, or single file arrays floating within variably sized pools of mucin (**Figs. 28 and 29**). Like other forms of lobular neoplasia, E-cadherin staining is absent and p120 catenin staining is cytoplasmic. The tumors are ER and PR positive and HER2 negative,[82] except for 2 reported cases classified as HER2 positive.[81,82]

Given the previous assumptions about the origin of extracellular mucin, this tumor is likely underrecognized and rather reported as

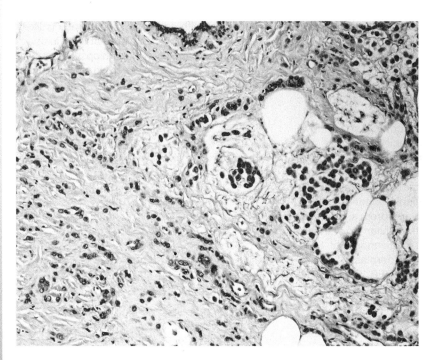

Fig. 28. ILCEMP with classic morphology in the nonmucinous component (H&E, original magnification ×20). (*Courtesy of* Dr Stuart Schnitt, Boston, MA.)

ductal or mucinous carcinoma. Of note, examples of mucinous carcinoma with significantly reduced E-cadherin staining have been reported, but these cases do not show redistribution of p120 into the cytoplasm.[81] The differential diagnosis also includes matrix-producing mammary carcinoma, a type of metaplastic carcinoma in which nests, cords, and single tumor cells are suspended in an abundant myxoid matrix (**Fig. 30**). Unlike ILCEMP, it is almost always negative for ER, PR, and HER2.[83]

Of 7 cases with follow-up ranging from 2 to 68 months, there are 3 cases with documented recurrences, including an ipsilateral breast recurrence; local recurrence and distant metastases to bone, liver, and brain; and a distant peritoneal metastasis.[82]

SALIVARY GLAND–TYPE TUMORS OF THE BREAST WITH MUCINOUS FEATURES

MUCOEPIDERMOID CARCINOMA

Mucoepidermoid carcinoma (MEC) is a very rare malignant epithelial salivary gland–type tumor of the breast.[84–86] Low-grade MEC is composed of varying proportions of distinctive mucinous, intermediate, epidermoid, and basaloid cells arranged in solid nests and cystic spaces. The cystic spaces are lined by flat-to-columnar mucinous epithelium and contain extracellular mucin (**Fig. 31**). High-grade MEC is an infiltrative, solid tumor with a higher degree of cytologic atypia, mitotic activity, necrosis, and inconspicuous mucinous elements. The differential diagnosis includes mucinous cystic lesions and squamous and adenosquamous carcinoma of the breast. MEC does not exhibit true keratinization. Limited evidence suggests that low-grade MEC can be included in the group of triple-negative breast cancers with a good prognosis.[85,86]

ADENOID CYSTIC CARCINOMA

Adenoid cystic carcinoma (AdCC) of the breast is a rare (<1%), special histologic type of triple-negative breast cancer analogous to the tumor of the salivary gland.[87] Classic AdCC features a dual population of epithelial (luminal) cells and myoepithelial (basal) cells arranged in glandular, cribriform (cylindromatous), and/or solid growth patterns. This tumor is notable for distinctive pseudolumina of the cylindromatous pattern that represent basal lamina material between myoepithelial cells. The basal lamina material consists of type IV collagen, laminin, fibronectin, and proteoglycans.[88] Depending on the composition, the appearance may be eosinophilic or

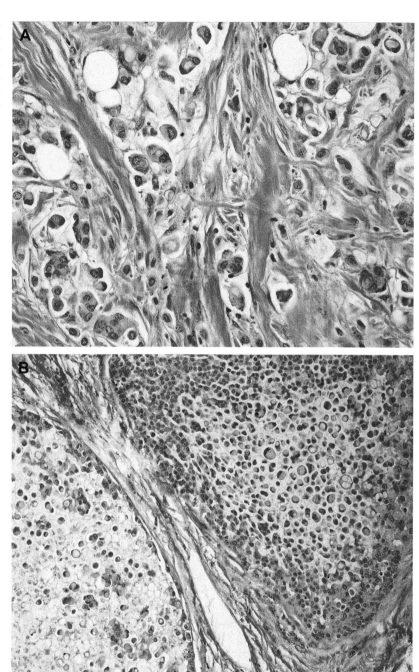

Fig. 29. ILCEMP with unusual pleomorphic and signet ring cell morphology (H&E, original magnification ×40) (*A*). Lobular carcinoma in situ with the same features (H&E, original magnification ×20) (*B*). (*Courtesy of* Dr Stuart Schnitt, Boston, MA.)

basophilic, the latter resembling epithelial mucin (Fig. 32). The differential diagnosis of AdCC includes collagenous or "mucinous" spherulosis, the spherules of which have a similar composition (Fig. 33).[89] Classic AdCC of the breast is a relatively indolent tumor with an excellent prognosis.[90]

BREAST LESIONS WITH MUCIN MIMICS

Several other mesenchymal or biphasic lesions of the breast may contain stromal ground substance that mimics extracellular mucin production. Nodular mucinosis is a very rare nonneoplastic lesion found in the subareolar region of young women. It consists of multiple nodules

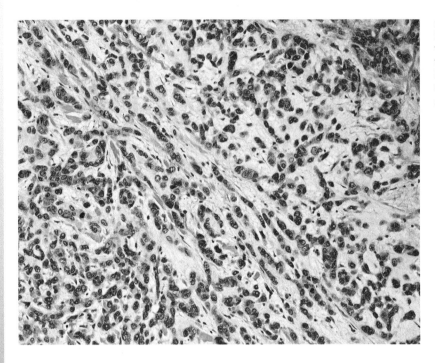

Fig. 30. Matrix-producing mammary carcinoma with cords and single cells within blue-gray extracellular matrix resembles IL-CEMP (H&E, original magnification ×20).

of basophilic myxoid material and sparse bland spindle cells. The myxoid material is strongly positive on Alcian blue and colloidal iron special stains. A lack of epithelial elements distinguishes nodular mucinosis from MLLs and mucinous carcinoma. It has been noted that the spindle cells have an immunophenotype similar to myofibroblasts and may be related to myxoid myofibroblastoma.[91] Additional mesenchymal neoplasms with a myxoid stroma include nodular

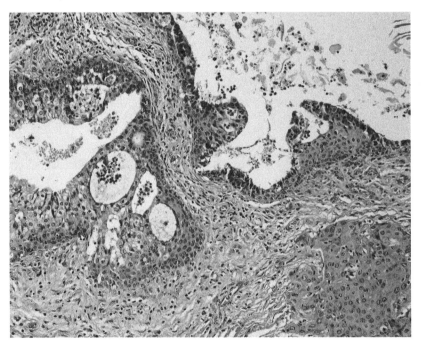

Fig. 31. Mucoepidermoid carcinoma with cysts lined by mucinous epithelium surrounded by epidermoid and intermediate cells (H&E, original magnification ×10). (courtesy of Dr Stuart Schnitt, Boston, MA.)

Fig. 32. AdCC with basophilic proteoglycan-containing basal lamina material in the pseudolumina of the cylindromatous pattern (H&E, original magnification ×4).

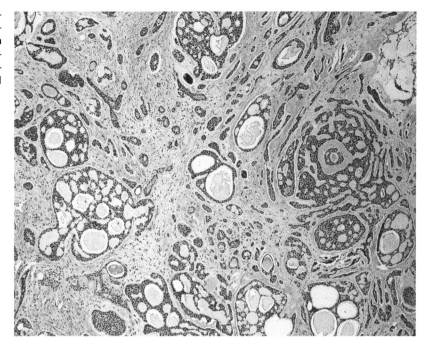

fasciitis, myxoma, superficial angiomyxoma, and myxoid sarcomas. Biphasic neoplasms with myxoid stromal change, such as myxoid fibroepithelial lesions, pleomorphic adenomas, and metaplastic carcinomas with matrix production, also may be considered in the differential diagnosis of mucinous lesions of the breast, especially when present as small fragments in

Fig. 33. Mucinous (collagenous) spherulosis involved by lobular carcinoma in situ. The spherules contain material similar to that seen in AdCC (H&E, original magnification ×20).

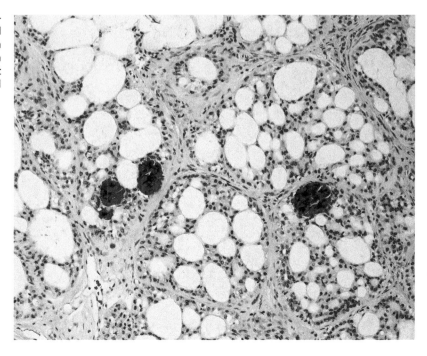

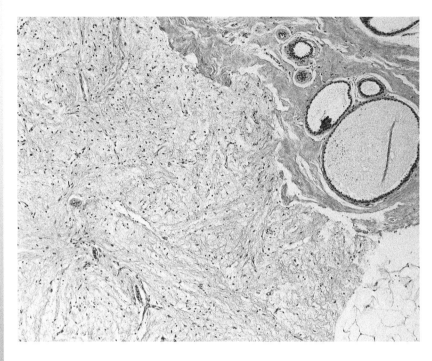

Fig. 34. Benign myxoid neoplasm, myxoid fibroadenoma versus myxoma, adjacent to a mucinous cyst on core biopsy. Prominent myxoid stroma superficially resembles extracellular mucin (H&E, original magnification ×10).

limited biopsy specimens (**Fig. 34**).[92] A complete discussion of these entities is beyond the scope of this review.

Miscellaneous mimics of extracellular mucin include the foreign material marking a core needle biopsy site, leakage from a silicone implant (**Fig. 35**), or injected for breast augmentation. The foreign material is almost always accompanied by multinucleated giant cells, other inflammatory changes, and fibrosis.[93]

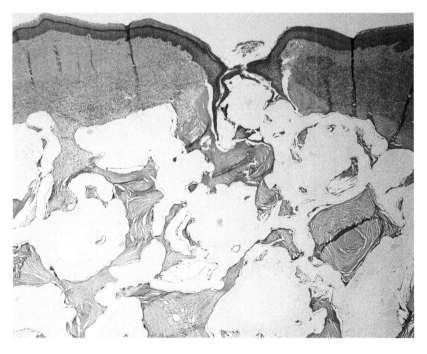

Fig. 35. Silicone leakage from implant in reconstructed breast after mastectomy. It is distinguished from mucin by a foreign body giant cell reaction to polarizable material (H&E, original magnification ×2).

SUMMARY

In summary, mucinous lesions of the breast represent a variety of lesions, most of which feature extracellular mucin production. Of these lesions, MLLs and mucinous carcinomas are among the most commonly encountered, and their distinction from one another perhaps the most challenging issue in the differential diagnosis.

REFERENCES

1. Mukhopadhyay P, Chakraborty S, Ponnusamy MP, et al. Mucins in the pathogenesis of breast cancer: implications in diagnosis, prognosis and therapy. Biochim Biophys Acta 2011;1815(2):224–40.
2. Voynow JA, Rubin BK. Mucins, mucus, and sputum. Chest 2009;135(2):505–12.
3. Foschini MP, Fulcheri E, Baracchini P, et al. Squamous cell carcinoma with prominent myxoid stroma. Hum Pathol 1990;21(8):859–65.
4. Adsay NV, Merati K, Nassar H, et al. Pathogenesis of colloid (pure mucinous) carcinoma of exocrine organs: coupling of gel-forming mucin (MUC2) production with altered cell polarity and abnormal cell-stroma interaction may be the key factor in the morphogenesis and indolent behavior of colloid carcinoma in the breast and pancreas. Am J Surg Pathol 2003;27(5):571–8.
5. Hanna WM, Corkill M. Mucins in breast carcinoma. Hum Pathol 1988;19(1):11–4.
6. Myers RB, Fredenburgh JL, Grizzle WE. Carbohydrates. In: Bancroft JD, editor. Theory and practice of histochemical techniques. 6th edition. London: Churchill Livingstone; 2008. p. 161–86.
7. Rosen PP. Mucocele-like tumors of the breast. Am J Surg Pathol 1986;10(7):464–9.
8. Hamele-Bena D, Cranor ML, Rosen PP. Mammary mucocele-like lesions. Benign and malignant. Am J Surg Pathol 1996;20(9):1081–5.
9. Weaver MG, Abdul-Karim FW, al-Kaisi N. Mucinous lesions of the breast. A pathological continuum. Pathol Res Pract 1993;189(8):873–6.
10. Park YJ, Kim EK. A pure mucocele-like lesion of the breast diagnosed on ultrasonography-guided core-needle biopsy: is imaging follow-up sufficient? Ultrasonography 2015;34(2):133–8.
11. Kim JY, Han BK, Choe YH, et al. Benign and malignant mucocele-like tumors of the breast: mammographic and sonographic appearances. AJR Am J Roentgenol 2005;185(5):1310–6.
12. Carkaci S, Lane DL, Gilcrease MZ, et al. Do all mucocele-like lesions of the breast require surgery? Clin Imaging 2011;35(2):94–101.
13. Tan PH, Tse GM, Bay BH. Mucinous breast lesions: diagnostic challenges. J Clin Pathol 2008;61(1):11–9.
14. Brogi E. Cystic hypersecretory carcinoma and cystic hypersecretory hyperplasia. In: Hoda SA, Brogi E, Koerner FC, et al, editors. Rosen's breast pathology. 4th edition. Philadelphia: Lippincott Williams & Wilkins; 2014. p. 715–24.
15. Deschryver K, Radford DM, Schuh ME. Pathology of large-caliber stereotactic biopsies in nonpalpable breast lesions. Semin Diagn Pathol 1999;16(3):224–34.
16. Renshaw AA. Can mucinous lesions of the breast be reliably diagnosed by core needle biopsy? Am J Clin Pathol 2002;118(1):82–4.
17. Glazebrook K, Reynolds C. Original report. Mucocele-like tumors of the breast: mammographic and sonographic appearances. AJR Am J Roentgenol 2003;180(4):949–54.
18. Carder PJ, Murphy CE, Liston JC. Surgical excision is warranted following a core biopsy diagnosis of mucocoele-like lesion of the breast. Histopathology 2004;45(2):148–54.
19. Ramsaroop R, Greenberg D, Tracey N, et al. Mucocele-like lesions of the breast: an audit of 2 years at BreastScreen Auckland (New Zealand). Breast J 2005;11(5):321–5.
20. Wang J, Simsir A, Mercado C, et al. Can core biopsy reliably diagnose mucinous lesions of the breast? Am J Clin Pathol 2007;127(1):124–7.
21. El-Sayed ME, Rakha EA, Reed J, et al. Predictive value of needle core biopsy diagnoses of lesions of uncertain malignant potential (B3) in abnormalities detected by mammographic screening. Histopathology 2008;53(6):650–7.
22. Begum SM, Jara-Lazaro AR, Thike AA, et al. Mucin extravasation in breast core biopsies–clinical significance and outcome correlation. Histopathology 2009;55(5):609–17.
23. Ouldamer L, Body G, Arbion F, et al. Mucocele-like lesions of the breast: management after diagnosis on ultrasound guided core biopsy or stereotactic vacuum-assisted biopsy. Gynecol Obstet Fertil 2010;38(7–8):455–9, [in French].
24. Flegg KM, Flaherty JJ, Bicknell AM, et al. Surgical outcomes of borderline breast lesions detected by needle biopsy in a breast screening program. World J Surg Oncol 2010;8:78.
25. Jaffer S, Bleiweiss IJ, Nagi CS. Benign mucocele-like lesions of the breast: revisited. Mod Pathol 2011;24(5):683–7.
26. Weigel S, Decker T, Korsching E, et al. Minimal invasive biopsy results of "uncertain malignant potential" in digital mammography screening: high prevalence but also high predictive value for malignancy. Rofo 2011;183(8):743–8.
27. Sutton B, Davion S, Feldman M, et al. Mucocele-like lesions diagnosed on breast core biopsy: assessment of upgrade rate and need for surgical excision. Am J Clin Pathol 2012;138(6):783–8.

28. Ha D, Dialani V, Mehta TS, et al. Mucocele-like lesions in the breast diagnosed with percutaneous biopsy: is surgical excision necessary? AJR Am J Roentgenol 2015;204(1):204–10.

29. Rakha EA, Shaaban AM, Haider SA, et al. Outcome of pure mucocele-like lesions diagnosed on breast core biopsy. Histopathology 2013;62(6):894–8.

30. Calhoun BC, Collins LC. Recommendations for excision following core needle biopsy of the breast: a contemporary evaluation of the literature. Histopathology 2016;68(1):138–51.

31. Ohi Y, Umekita Y, Rai Y, et al. Mucocele-like lesions of the breast: a long-term follow-up study. Diagn Pathol 2011;6:29.

32. Meares AL, Frank RD, Degnim AC, et al. Mucocele-like lesions of the breast: a clinical outcome and histologic analysis of 102 cases. Hum Pathol 2016;49: 33–8.

33. Norris HJ, Taylor HB. Prognosis of mucinous (gelatinous) carcinoma of the breast. Cancer 1965;18:879.

34. Silverberg SG, Kay S, Chitale AR, et al. Colloid carcinoma of the breast. Am J Clin Pathol 1971;55(3): 355–63.

35. Rasmussen BB. Human mucinous breast carcinomas and their lymph node metastases. A histological review of 247 cases. Pathol Res Pract 1985; 180(4):377–82.

36. Di Saverio S, Gutierrez J, Avisar E. A retrospective review with long term follow up of 11,400 cases of pure mucinous breast carcinoma. Breast Cancer Res Treat 2008;111(3):541–7.

37. Wilson TE, Helvie MA, Oberman HA, et al. Pure and mixed mucinous carcinoma of the breast: pathologic basis for differences in mammographic appearance. AJR Am J Roentgenol 1995;165(2): 285–9.

38. Cardenosa G, Doudna C, Eklund GW. Mucinous (colloid) breast cancer: clinical and mammographic findings in 10 patients. AJR Am J Roentgenol 1994; 162(5):1077–9.

39. Goodman DN, Boutross-Tadross O, Jong RA. Mammographic features of pure mucinous carcinoma of the breast with pathological correlation. Can Assoc Radiol J 1995;46(4):296–301.

40. Chopra S, Evans AJ, Pinder SE, et al. Pure mucinous breast cancer—mammographic and ultrasound findings. Clin Radiol 1996;51(6):421–4.

41. Lam WW, Chu WC, Tse GM, et al. Sonographic appearance of mucinous carcinoma of the breast. AJR Am J Roentgenol 2004;182(4):1069–74.

42. Rosen PP, Oberman HA. In: Tumors of the mammary gland, vol. 7. Washington, DC: Armed Forces Institute of Pathology; 1993.

43. Capella C, Eusebi V, Mann B, et al. Endocrine differentiation in mucoid carcinoma of the breast. Histopathology 1980;4(6):613–30.

44. Shet T, Chinoy R. Presence of a micropapillary pattern in mucinous carcinomas of the breast and its impact on the clinical behavior. Breast J 2008; 14(5):412–20.

45. Ranade A, Batra R, Sandhu G, et al. Clinicopathological evaluation of 100 cases of mucinous carcinoma of breast with emphasis on axillary staging and special reference to a micropapillary pattern. J Clin Pathol 2010;63(12):1043–7.

46. Barbashina V, Corben AD, Akram M, et al. Mucinous micropapillary carcinoma of the breast: an aggressive counterpart to conventional pure mucinous tumors. Hum Pathol 2013;44(8): 1577–85.

47. Kim HJ, Park K, Kim JY, et al. Prognostic significance of a micropapillary pattern in pure mucinous carcinoma of the breast: comparative analysis with micropapillary carcinoma. J Pathol Transl Med 2017;51(4):403–9.

48. Liu F, Yang M, Li Z, et al. Invasive micropapillary mucinous carcinoma of the breast is associated with poor prognosis. Breast Cancer Res Treat 2015;151(2):443–51.

49. Soomro S, Shousha S, Taylor P, et al. c-erbB-2 expression in different histological types of invasive breast carcinoma. J Clin Pathol 1991;44(3): 211–4.

50. Somerville JE, Clarke LA, Biggart JD. c-erbB-2 overexpression and histological type of in situ and invasive breast carcinoma. J Clin Pathol 1992;45(1): 16–20.

51. Rosen PP, Lesser ML, Arroyo CD, et al. p53 in node-negative breast carcinoma: an immunohistochemical study of epidemiologic risk factors, histologic features, and prognosis. J Clin Oncol 1995;13(4): 821–30.

52. Diab SG, Clark GM, Osborne CK, et al. Tumor characteristics and clinical outcome of tubular and mucinous breast carcinomas. J Clin Oncol 1999; 17(5):1442–8.

53. Fujii H, Anbazhagan R, Bornman DM, et al. Mucinous cancers have fewer genomic alterations than more common classes of breast cancer. Breast Cancer Res Treat 2002;76(3):255–60.

54. Weigelt B, Geyer FC, Horlings HM, et al. Mucinous and neuroendocrine breast carcinomas are transcriptionally distinct from invasive ductal carcinomas of no special type. Mod Pathol 2009;22(11): 1401–14.

55. O'Connell FP, Wang HH, Odze RD. Utility of immunohistochemistry in distinguishing primary adenocarcinomas from metastatic breast carcinomas in the gastrointestinal tract. Arch Pathol Lab Med 2005; 129(3):338–47.

56. Barkley CR, Ligibel JA, Wong JS, et al. Mucinous breast carcinoma: a large contemporary series. Am J Surg 2008;196(4):549–51.

57. Fisher ER, Anderson S, Redmond C, et al. Pathologic findings from the National Surgical Adjuvant Breast Project protocol B-06. 10-year pathologic and clinical prognostic discriminants. Cancer 1993;71(8):2507–14.

58. Ellis IO, Galea M, Broughton N, et al. Pathological prognostic factors in breast cancer. II. Histological type. Relationship with survival in a large study with long-term follow-up. Histopathology 1992; 20(6):479–89.

59. Rosen PP, Groshen S, Kinne DW, et al. Factors influencing prognosis in node-negative breast carcinoma: analysis of 767 T1N0M0/T2N0M0 patients with long-term follow-up. J Clin Oncol 1993;11(11): 2090–100.

60. Haffty BG, Perrotta PL, Ward BE, et al. Conservatively treated breast cancer: outcome by histologic subtype. Breast J 1997;3:7.

61. Sharnhorst D, Huntrakoon M. Mucinous carcinoma of the breast: recurrence 30 years after mastectomy. South Med J 1988;81:656–7.

62. Weiss MC, Fowble BL, Solin LJ, et al. Outcome of conservative therapy for invasive breast cancer by histologic subtype. Int J Radiat Oncol Biol Phys 1992;23(5):941–7.

63. Kurtz JM, Jacquemier J, Torhorst J, et al. Conservation therapy for breast cancers other than infiltrating ductal carcinoma. Cancer 1989;63(8):1630–5.

64. Hawes D, Robinson R, Wira R. Pseudomyxoma peritonei from metastatic colloid carcinoma of the breast. Gastrointest Radiol 1991;16(1):80–2.

65. Corben A, Brogi E. Mucinous carcinoma. In: Hoda SA, Brogi E, Koerner FC, et al, editors. Rosen's breast pathology. 4th edition. Philadelphia: Lippincott Williams & Wilkins; 2014. p. 611–44.

66. Maluf HM, Koerner FC. Solid papillary carcinoma of the breast. A form of intraductal carcinoma with endocrine differentiation frequently associated with mucinous carcinoma. Am J Surg Pathol 1995; 19(11):1237–44.

67. Lakhani SR, Ellis IO, Schnitt SJ, et al, editors. WHO classification of tumors of the breast. Lyon (France): IARC; 2012.

68. Tan PH, Schnitt SJ, van de Vijver MJ, et al. Papillary and neuroendocrine breast lesions: the WHO stance. Histopathology 2015;66(6):761–70.

69. Nassar H, Qureshi H, Adsay NV, et al. Clinicopathologic analysis of solid papillary carcinoma of the breast and associated invasive carcinomas. Am J Surg Pathol 2006;30(4):501–7.

70. Guo S, Wang Y, Rohr J, et al. Solid papillary carcinoma of the breast: a special entity needs to be distinguished from conventional invasive carcinoma avoiding over-treatment. Breast 2016;26:67–72.

71. Otsuki Y, Yamada M, Shimizu S, et al. Solid-papillary carcinoma of the breast: clinicopathological study of 20 cases. Pathol Int 2007;57(7):421–9.

72. Tan BY, Thike AA, Ellis IO, et al. Clinicopathologic characteristics of solid papillary carcinoma of the breast. Am J Surg Pathol 2016;40(10):1334–42.

73. Moritani S, Ichihara S, Kushima R, et al. Myoepithelial cells in solid variant of intraductal papillary carcinoma of the breast: a potential diagnostic pitfall and a proposal of an immunohistochemical panel in the differential diagnosis with intraductal papilloma with usual ductal hyperplasia. Virchows Arch 2007; 450(5):539–47.

74. Oh EJ, Koo JS, Kim JY, et al. Correlation between solid papillary carcinoma and associated invasive carcinoma according to expression of WT1 and several MUCs. Pathol Res Pract 2014;210(12):953–8.

75. Weigelt B, Horlings HM, Kreike B, et al. Refinement of breast cancer classification by molecular characterization of histological special types. J Pathol 2008;216(2):141–50.

76. Saremian J, Rosa M. Solid papillary carcinoma of the breast: a pathologically and clinically distinct breast tumor. Arch Pathol Lab Med 2012;136(10): 1308–11.

77. Rosa M, Mohammadi A, Masood S. Lobular carcinoma of the breast with extracellular mucin: new variant of mucin-producing carcinomas? Pathol Int 2009;59(6):405–9.

78. Bari VB, Bholay SU, Sane KC. Invasive lobular carcinoma of the breast with extracellular mucin—a new rare variant. J Clin Diagn Res 2015;9(4): ED05–06.

79. Gomez Macias GS, Perez Saucedo JE, Cardona Huerta S, et al. Invasive lobular carcinoma of the breast with extracellular mucin: a case report. Int J Surg case Rep 2016;25:33–6.

80. Haltas H, Bayrak R, Yenidunya S, et al. Invasive lobular carcinoma with extracellular mucin as a distinct variant of lobular carcinoma: a case report. Diagn Pathol 2012;7:91.

81. Yu J, Bhargava R, Dabbs DJ. Invasive lobular carcinoma with extracellular mucin production and HER-2 overexpression: a case report and further case studies. Diagn Pathol 2010;5:36.

82. Cserni G, Floris G, Koufopoulos N, et al. Invasive lobular carcinoma with extracellular mucin production—a novel pattern of lobular carcinomas of the breast. Clinico-pathological description of eight cases. Virchows Arch 2017;471(1):3–12.

83. Downs-Kelly E, Nayeemuddin KM, Albarracin C, et al. Matrix-producing carcinoma of the breast: an aggressive subtype of metaplastic carcinoma. Am J Surg Pathol 2009;33(4):534–41.

84. Patchefsky AS, Frauenhoffer CM, Krall RA, et al. Low-grade mucoepidermoid carcinoma of the breast. Arch Pathol Lab Med 1979;103(4):196–8.

85. Di Tommaso L, Foschini MP, Ragazzini T, et al. Mucoepidermoid carcinoma of the breast. Virchows Arch 2004;444(1):13–9.

86. Camelo-Piragua SI, Habib C, Kanumuri P, et al. Mucoepidermoid carcinoma of the breast shares cytogenetic abnormality with mucoepidermoid carcinoma of the salivary gland: a case report with molecular analysis and review of the literature. Hum Pathol 2009;40(6):887–92.

87. Bennett AK, Mills SE, Wick MR. Salivary-type neoplasms of the breast and lung. Semin Diagn Pathol 2003;20(4):279–304.

88. Cheng J, Saku T, Okabe H, et al. Basement membranes in adenoid cystic carcinoma. An immunohistochemical study. Cancer 1992;69(11):2631–40.

89. Grignon DJ, Ro JY, Mackay BN, et al. Collagenous spherulosis of the breast. Immunohistochemical and ultrastructural studies. Am J Clin Pathol 1989; 91(4):386–92.

90. Foschini MP, Krausz T. Salivary gland-type tumors of the breast: a spectrum of benign and malignant tumors including "triple negative carcinomas" of low malignant potential. Semin Diagn Pathol 2010; 27(1):77–90.

91. Sanati S, Leonard M, Khamapirad T, et al. Nodular mucinosis of the breast: a case report with pathologic, ultrasonographic, and clinical findings and review of the literature. Arch Pathol Lab Med 2005; 129(3):e58–61.

92. Magro G, Cavanaugh B, Palazzo J. Clinico-pathological features of breast myxoma: report of a case with histogenetic considerations. Virchows Arch 2010;456(5):581–6.

93. Shim JY, Sahin AA. Mucinous lesions of the breast. Surg Pathol Clin 2009;2(2):413–40.

Differential Diagnosis of Benign Spindle Cell Lesions

Gaetano Magro, MD, PhD

KEYWORDS

• Breast • Benign tumors • Spindle cells • Differential diagnosis • Immunohistochemistry

ABSTRACT

Spindle cell lesions of the breast cover a wide spectrum of diseases ranging from reactive tumor-like lesions to high-grade malignant tumors. The recognition of the benign spindle cell tumor-like lesions (nodular fasciitis; reactive spindle cell nodule after biopsy, inflammatory pseudotumor/inflammatory myofibroblastic tumor; fascicular variant of pseudoangiomatous stromal hyperplasia) and tumors (myofibroblastoma, benign fibroblastic spindle cell tumor, leiomyoma, schwannoma, spindle cell lipoma, solitary fibrous tumor, myxoma) is crucial to avoid confusion with morphologically similar but more aggressive bland-appearing spindle cell tumors, such as desmoid-type fibromatosis, low-grade (fibromatosis-like) spindle cell carcinoma, low-grade fibrosarcoma/myofibroblastic sarcoma and dermatofibrosarcoma protuberans.

OVERVIEW

Spindle cell lesions of the breast cover a wide spectrum of diseases ranging from reactive tumor-like lesions to high-grade malignant tumors.[1–6] Although most of the lesions are mesenchymal in nature, there is the possibility that some *carcinomas* may be composed exclusively/predominantly of neoplastic cells that adopt spindled rather than epithelioid morphology. A subset of potentially malignant lesions, consisting of bland-looking spindle cells, are closely reminiscent of several benign entities. In this regard it should be emphasized that benign spindle cells lesions are usually underrecognized and can represent potential pitfalls of malignancy, particularly on a small biopsy. The lack of strict diagnostic criteria and expertise in soft tissue pathology are likely the main reasons that, in the past, have led some investigators to use different names for the same lesion or, conversely, to collect different lesions under the same term.

Benign spindle cell lesions of the breast encompass a wide and heterogeneous spectrum of fibroblastic and myofibroblastic tumor-like or tumor entities.[7,8] By definition, they should be composed exclusively of spindle cells (pure spindle cell lesions), with no mixed epithelial component.[7,8] However, pathologists should be aware of the possibility that normal epithelial mammary structures can be entrapped or displaced within some lesions, particularly in pseudoangiomatous stromal hyperplasia and reactive spindle cell nodule/exuberant scar. Similarly, mature adipose tissue admixed with the proliferating spindle cell component may be part of the lesion (see lipomatous myofibroblastoma and benign fibroblastic spindle cell tumor) and should not be confused with entrapped fat tissue from the adjacent breast parenchyma as seen in desmoid-type fibromatosis, low-grade (fibromatosis-like)

I state I have no conflicts of interests with any commercial or financial company that has a direct financial interest in subject matter or materials discussed in article or with a company making a competing product.
Department of Medical and Surgical Sciences and Advanced Technologies, G.F. Ingrassia, Anatomic Pathology, University of Catania, Via S. Sofia 87, Catania 95123, Italy
E-mail address: g.magro@unict.it

spindle cell carcinoma and dermatofibrosarcoma protuberans.

To better understand the different morphologies of the lesions, pathologists should keep in mind that myofibroblasts are modified fibroblasts with the capability to contract, and that play a crucial role in both wound healing and tissue remodeling. Myofibroblasts, plumper than fibroblasts, show more abundant pale to slightly eosinophilic cytoplasm, and ovoid nuclei with evident small nucleoli. Although myofibroblasts are usually spindle-shaped cells, their morphology is highly variable, ranging from round, stellate, epithelioid to ganglion-like cells. Immunohistochemically they are variably stained with α-smooth muscle actin, desmin, and calponin. The distinction of each single entity among the benign spindle cell lesions of the breast may be challenging, especially in core needle biopsies. This is mainly because there is overlap among all these mesenchymal proliferations, as they are composed of relatively bland-looking spindle cells with the morphologic features of myofibroblasts, arranged haphazardly, or in short fascicles or with a storiform growth pattern. Similarly, the stroma is usually fibrotic but myxoid changes are not uncommon. Although immunohistochemistry is helpful in revealing the myofibroblastic nature of the cells, it cannot distinguish with certainty the different lesions, as they frequently stain with α-smooth muscle actin and stain variably with desmin. Although there has been progress in cytogenetics and molecular biology, the difficulty in defining, at least in some lesions, the boundaries between a reactive versus a neoplastic process (see inflammatory pseudotumor/inflammatory myofibroblastic tumor) still remains. The differential diagnosis between benign spindle cell lesions and the bland-looking spindle cell tumors with potentially aggressive behavior is crucial to avoid overtreatment of patients. Although immunohistochemistry is mandatory in ruling out low-grade (fibromatosis-like) spindle cell carcinoma (absence of epithelial markers and p63), its role is limited when dealing with desmoid-type fibromatosis and low-grade myofibroblastic sarcoma.

For a practical diagnostic approach, benign spindle cell lesions of the breast parenchyma can be divided into 2 main categories: reactive and neoplastic lesions (Table 1). The former is represented by nodular fasciitis, reactive spindle cell nodule/exuberant scar following biopsy/fine-needle aspiration, inflammatory pseudotumor/inflammatory myofibroblastic tumor, and pseudoangiomatous stromal hyperplasia. Among the

Table 1	
Benign spindle cell lesions of the breast	
Classification	**Differential Diagnosis**
Tumor-like lesions	• Desmoid-type fibromatosis
• Nodular fasciitis	
• Reactive spindle cell nodule/exuberant scar	• Low-grade (fibromatosis-like) spindle cell carcinoma
• Inflammatory pseudotumor/inflammatory myofibroblastic tumor	• Low-grade myofibroblastic sarcoma
• Pseudoangiomatous stromal hyperplasia (fascicular variant)	• Low-grade fibrosarcoma
Tumor lesions	• Dermatofibrosar coma protuberans
Specific to mammary stroma	
• Myofibroblastoma	
• Benign fibroblastic spindle cell tumor	
Not specific to mammary stroma	
• Leiomyoma	
• Schwannoma/neurofibroma	
• Solitary fibrous tumor	
• Spindle cell lipoma	
• Myxoma	

tumors, the most common is myofibroblastoma, followed by benign fibroblastic spindle cell tumor, leiomyoma, schwannoma/neurofibroma, solitary fibrous tumor, spindle cell lipoma, and myxoma. Both reactive and neoplastic benign lesions need to be distinguished from locally aggressive or potentially metastatic bland-looking spindle cell tumors, including desmoid-type fibromatosis, low-grade (fibromatosis-like) spindle cell carcinoma, low-grade myofibroblastic sarcoma, low-grade fibrosarcoma, and dermatofibrosarcoma protuberans (see Table 1).

This review focuses on the key diagnostic features of the most common benign spindle cell lesions of the breast to achieve a nosologically correct classification. The main clinicopathologic features, highlighting the differences between the various entities, are summarized in tables (See Tables 1–3). Representative illustrations of the most common lesions are also provided. Awareness by pathologists of the diversity of morphologic and immunohistochemical features exhibited by the most common benign spindle cell lesions of the breast, including their uncommon features/variants, is the first step toward accurate diagnosis. Correlation with clinical and imaging findings is often crucial to avoid confusion with aggressive monomorphic bland-looking malignant spindle cell tumors.

BENIGN SPINDLE CELL TUMOR-LIKE LESIONS

This group comprises biologically different lesions that can be generally viewed as exuberant, reactive myofibroblastic proliferations in response to unknown stimuli. This is the case for nodular fasciitis[9–16] and inflammatory pseudotumor/inflammatory myofibroblastic tumor,[17–33] which apparently seem to arise spontaneously in most cases. Conversely a history of a previous biopsy or fine-needle aspiration (FNA) is the rule in the so-called "reactive spindle cell nodule/exuberant scar."[34–38] Similarly pseudoangiomatous stromal hyperplasia, nodular variant, is usually considered a hormone-dependent proliferation of the specialized mammary stroma.[39–55] Although relatively rare, all the previously mentioned entities can pose serious differential diagnostic problems, particularly in core biopsy, with bland-looking aggressive spindle cell tumors. The clinicopathologic features of each entity are summarized in tables.

Benign spindle cell tumor-like lesions are often identified as incidental findings on mammography/sonography or may present as painless, less frequently painful, masses with fairly circumscribed borders. However some lesions, especially nodular fasciitis and inflammatory pseudotumor/inflammatory myofibroblastic tumor, may exhibit irregular margins raising the suspicion of malignancy.[9,10,12–14,23,26,28–30] The differential diagnosis may be challenging, especially when evaluating small biopsies or material from FNAs.[11,15,19,20] Rendering the correct diagnosis requires awareness on the part of pathologists that nodular fasciitis (Box 1) (Fig. 1), reactive spindle cell nodule/exuberant scar (Box 2) (Fig. 2), and inflammatory pseudotumor/inflammatory myofibroblastic tumor (Box 3) (Fig. 3) do occur in the breast parenchyma, with morphologic and immunohistochemical features similar, if not identical, to those seen elsewhere. Although reactive spindle cell nodule/exuberant scar and nodular fasciitis have overlapping morphologic and immunohistochemical features, clinical information of a previous biopsy or FNA cytology (FNAC) is extremely helpful for diagnosis of reactive spindle cell nodule/exuberant scar.[34–38] The presence of entrapped/displaced epithelial mammary structures,

stromal hemosiderin deposition, foamy and hemosiderin-laden macrophages, lymphocytes and plasma cells, fat necrosis, and foreign body giant cell reaction, are all features that strongly favor the diagnosis of the former lesion[34–38] (see Fig. 2). Notably, a pseudotumor composed of histiocytes with spindle cell morphology has been reported in the breast as the result of an exaggerated reaction to fat necrosis.[38] Conversely, the identification of irregular margins, at least focally, more abundant myxoid extracellular matrix, tissue culture/granulation-like appearance, numerous typical mitoses, and entrapped ducts/lobules at the periphery of the lesion are features consistent with the diagnosis of nodular fasciitis[14] (see Fig. 1).

Inflammatory pseudotumor/inflammatory myofibroblastic tumor is also considered to be a reactive lesion to unknown local stimuli. Only rarely is it the result of an exaggerated myofibroblastic proliferation to mechanical trauma.[27] A clear-cut distinction between inflammatory pseudotumor and a "true" inflammatory myofibroblastic tumor is still arbitrary, especially in the absence of a proven immunohistochemical expression of ALK-1 or rearrangements of ALK gene by means of fluorescence in situ hybridization. Some investigators are reluctant to make the diagnosis of inflammatory myofibroblastic tumor when dealing with ALK-negative lesions arising at unusual sites, including the adult breast.[27,56] Review of the literature on the topic shows that most lesions, regardless of ALK-1 expression, have a benign clinical course after follow-up of 6 to 85 months,[19,23,29] with only a few cases with local recurrence, or more rarely, distant metastases that cannot be predicted by ALK-1 expression.[17–33] However, at least in 1 case labeled as "inflammatory myofibroblastic tumor with brain metastases," the illustrations provided by the investigators could be more consistent with a low-intermediate–grade myofibroblastic sarcoma rather than inflammatory myofibroblastic tumor.[32] Based on these data, the combined diagnosis of "*inflammatory pseudotumor/inflammatory myofibroblastic tumor of the breast*," specifying the presence or not of ALK-1 expression, seems to be more appropriate for these lesions. As inflammatory pseudotumor/inflammatory myofibroblastic tumor has a low rate of local recurrence and a very low risk of metastatic potential, it needs to be distinguished from both nodular fasciitis and reactive spindle cell nodule/exuberant scar. Although nodular fasciitis may contain scattered lymphocytes admixed with spindle cells, the inflammatory component, namely lymphocytes and

---

Box 1
Key features of nodular fasciitis

Definition

- Reactive lesion of spindle cells with the morphologic and immunohistochemical features of myofibroblasts, arising spontaneously; similar to its counterpart occurring more frequently in soft tissues

Clinical and radiographic

- Female patients; rarely male patients

- Age (15–84 years)

- Painless breast mass (0.5–5.0 cm in diameter)

- Mammography and sonography: mass with irregular borders, often suspicious of malignancy; occasionally well-defined borders

Gross pathology

- Soft to firm in consistency

- Grayish-white in color

- Fairly circumscribed margins

Histopathology

- Partially circumscribed margins

- Spindle to stellate cells with the features of myofibroblasts

- Mild nuclear atypia can be seen

- Variable cellularity (more cellular in the early lesions)

- Variable mitotic activity; sometimes brisk

- Short, not well-formed, fascicles; whorls; focal storiform pattern

- Loose edematous stroma with microcystic changes (tissue culture–like appearance); areas of collagenous stroma are usually seen

- Extravasated erythrocytes and scattered lymphocytes

- Mammary ducts/lobules are entrapped, mainly at the periphery of the lesion.

Immunohistochemistry/molecular diagnostic features

- Positive markers: α-smooth muscle actin

- Negative markers: cytokeratins, desmin, h-caldesmon, CD34, S-100 protein, beta-catenin, STAT6

- Fluorescence in situ hybridization (FISH): *USP6* rearrangement

Diagnostic key features

- Proliferation of mitotically active, α-smooth muscle actin–positive spindle cells with the features of myofibroblasts, embedded in a myxoid to fibrous stroma usually containing extravasated red blood cells and lymphocytic infiltrates (tissue culture–like appearance)

Treatment/Prognosis

- Complete surgical excision is curative; rare local recurrence; occasionally spontaneous regression

---

plasma cells, is more abundant in inflammatory pseudotumor/inflammatory myofibroblastic tumor (see **Fig. 3**). In addition, the typical tissue culture/granulation-like appearance seen in nodular fasciitis is lacking in inflammatory pseudotumor/inflammatory myofibroblastic tumor. Reactive spindle cell nodule should be excluded based on clinical information of a previous biopsy/FNAC.

The diagnosis of pseudoangiomatous stromal hyperplasia is usually straightforward[39] (**Box 4**) (**Fig. 4** A, B); however some diagnostic problems may arise when dealing with its fascicular variant, which consists of a proliferation of

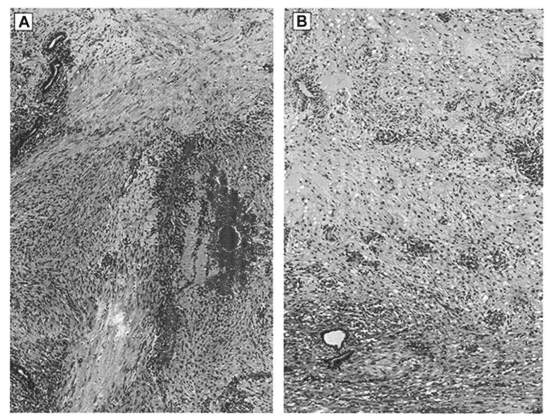

Fig. 1. Nodular fasciitis. (*A*) Spindle cell proliferation involving breast parenchyma (mammary ducts are at the periphery). Stroma is edematous and contains inflammatory cells and extravasated erythrocytes. (*B*) The typical tissue culture–like appearance is evident (H&E, original magnification [*A,B*] ×80).

spindle cells arranged in fascicles with interspersed keloid-like collagen fibers without any evidence of pseudovascular spaces[40,41] (**Fig. 4** C, D). In most cases, fascicular pseudoangiomatous stromal hyperplasia is closely reminiscent of classic-type myofibroblastoma[40] (see **Fig. 4** D). Unlike the other spindle cell tumor-like lesions, pseudoangiomatous stromal hyperplasia usually lacks myxoid stromal changes, an inflammatory infiltrate, and is consistently CD34 positive.[39,42]

BENIGN SPINDLE CELL TUMORS

For a practical diagnostic approach, it is helpful to separate benign spindle cell tumors into lesions that are relatively specific to mammary stroma and lesions typically occurring in soft tissues, but that can be occasionally encountered in the breast (see **Table 1**). The tumors that belong to the first group are closely related lesions within a continuous morphologic spectrum, variably composed of cells ranging from spindly fibroblast-like cells to plump myofibroblasts.[7,8] It has been postulated that these tumors arise from a common precursor stromal cell.[7,8] Over time, several names have been used for such tumors, including "benign spindle cell tumor," "fibroma," "myogenic stromal tumor," and "spindle cell lipoma."[7,8] Currently the prototypic benign spindle cell tumors of the mammary stroma are myofibroblastoma and benign fibroblastic spindle cell tumor.

Classic-type myofibroblastoma is a tumor composed of bland-looking spindle cells with the morphologic and immunohistochemical features of myofibroblasts.[57–60] The diagnosis is relatively straightforward if strict morphologic criteria are applied. Myofibroblastoma should be suspected when dealing with a pure spindle cell lesion with pushing borders, composed of cells with relatively abundant pale to slightly eosinophilic cytoplasm, arranged in short, haphazardly intersecting fascicles with interspersed thick,

---

Box 2
Key features of reactive spindle cell nodule/exuberant scar

Definition

- Reactive, tumor-like lesion of spindle cells with the morphologic and immunohistochemical features of myofibroblasts, following biopsy or fine-needle aspiration

Clinical and radiographic

- Nodule arising postoperatively or after biopsy (usually 2 weeks later) of any breast lesion
- Painless breast nodule (1.5–9.0 mm in greatest diameter)
- Age (36–70 years)
- Mammography and sonography: mass with circumscribed borders; parenchymal distortion

Gross pathology

- Firm in consistency
- Whitish in color
- Often circumscribed margins, sometimes focally infiltrative

Histopathology

- Well-circumscribed margins
- Plump spindle to epithelioid cells with the features of myofibroblasts
- Mild to focally moderate nuclear atypia can be seen
- Variable cellularity
- Intersecting short fascicles; focal storiform pattern
- Low mitotic count (1–4 mitoses per 10 high power fields [HPFs])
- Delicate collagen fibers can be seen among proliferating cells
- Entrapment/displacement of normal glands and/or epithelial structures of the preexisting lesion
- Capillary-like blood vessels
- Interspersed foamy and hemosiderin-laden macrophages, lymphocytes and plasma cells
- Hemosiderin deposition, fat necrosis, and foreign body giant cell reaction
- A needle tract can be identified in the center of the nodule

Immunohistochemistry

- Positive markers: α-smooth muscle actin, desmin focally positive
- Negative markers: cytokeratins, S-100 protein, CD34, beta-catenin, STAT6

Diagnostic key features

- Fairly circumscribed nodule, arising after biopsy or FNA, of α-smooth muscle actin–positive spindle cells with the features of myofibroblasts, set in a myxoid to fibrous stroma containing acute/chronic inflammation and often hemosiderin-laden macrophages

Treatment and prognosis

- Complete surgical excision; spontaneous regression can be seen

---

brightly eosinophilic keloid-like collagen fibers[58–60] (Box 5) (Fig. 5). Marked nuclear pleomorphism, high mitotic count (>3 mitoses per 10 high power fields [HPFs]), atypical mitoses, necrosis, and extensive infiltrating margins are not features of myofibroblastoma. Although the differential diagnosis with all bland-looking spindle cell lesions arising in the breast should be considered, the fascicular variant of pseudoangiomatous stromal hyperplasia, leiomyoma,

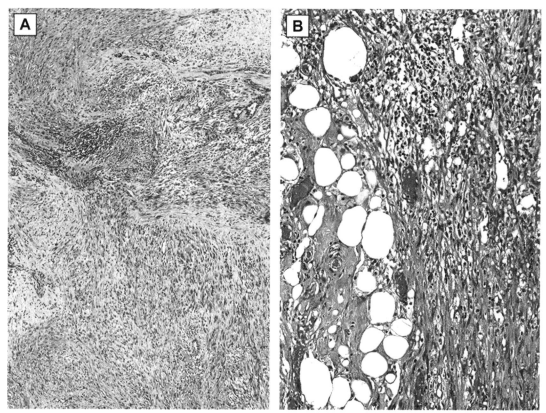

Fig. 2. Reactive spindle cell nodule/exuberant scar. (*A*) Proliferation of spindle cells with the morphologic features of myofibroblasts, arranged in irregular short fascicles and set in loose to fibrous stroma containing lymphocytes (H&E, original magnification × 80). (*B*) The detection of fat necrosis is helpful for a correct interpretation (H&E, original magnification × 150).

inflammatory pseudotumor/inflammatory myofibroblastic tumor, solitary fibrous tumor, and low-grade myofibroblastic sarcoma are most likely to be in the differential diagnosis of myofibroblastoma.[58,60] Most of these lesions can be ruled out by means of immunohistochemistry. Unlike many reactive or neoplastic myofibroblastic lesions that are consistently α-smooth muscle actin–positive, myofibroblastoma usually exhibits the coexpression of desmin and CD34 (see **Fig. 5**), whereas α-smooth muscle actin is variably positive.[58,60] Estrogen/progesterone/androgen receptors, bcl-2, CD99, and CD10 are usually detected but with variable intralesional and/or interlesional expression[58,60] (see **Fig. 5**). Apart from the more eosinophilic cytoplasm of the cells and the more organized fascicular growth pattern, leiomyoma differs by demonstrating diffuse coexpression of desmin, α-smooth muscle actin, and h-caldesmon, whereas CD34 is lacking. Low-grade myofibroblastic sarcoma (also known as low-grade myofibrosarcoma) is a tumor with higher mitotic activity (up

to 35 mitoses per 10 HPFs) that lacks expression of desmin and CD34. Over the past years, several morphologic variants of myofibroblastoma have been recognized[61–69] (**Box 6**). It should be emphasized that some of these represent potential diagnostic pitfalls. In daily practice, the most diagnostically challenging variants are epithelioid/deciduoid-like cell and lipomatous myofibroblastoma. The former are composed of medium-sized to large-sized epithelioid cells with a variable degree of nuclear atypia and a wide variety of growth patterns, such as single cell, single-cell files that may result in a pseudoinfiltrative growth pattern simulating an invasive lobular carcinoma[64,65] (**Fig. 6**). Tumors with larger cells and a deciduoid-like morphology may resemble an invasive apocrine carcinoma or metastatic tumor with epithelioid morphology (carcinoma, melanoma, epithelioid sarcoma, myoepithelioma, rhabdoid tumor, epithelioid malignant peripheral nerve sheath tumor)[66] (**Fig. 7**). The diagnosis of epithelioid/deciduoid-like cell myofibroblastoma is difficult if the epithelioid cell component is the

---

Box 3
Key features of inflammatory pseudotumor/inflammatory myofibroblastic tumor

Definition

- Heterogeneous group of myofibroblastic spindle cell lesions arising spontaneously, with an indolent to intermediate biological potential; similar to its counterpart occurring more frequently in lung and abdominal region

Clinical and radiographic

- Female individuals
- Age (16–86 years)
- Nodule arising spontaneously; rarely after trauma
- Painless nodule (1.0–4.5 cm in greatest diameter)
- Mammography and sonography: nodule with well-defined or ill-defined borders

Gross pathology

- Circumscribed margins
- Firm in consistency
- Gray-tan to whitish or yellow in color

Histopathology

- Circumscribed margins
- Plump spindle cells with the features of myofibroblasts
- None to mild nuclear atypia; only rarely severe nuclear pleomorphism
- Moderate to high cellularity
- Interlacing short bundles; swirling/storiform pattern
- Plasma cells and lymphocytes intermingling with spindle cells
- Low mitotic count (0–3 mitoses per 10 HPF); rarely numerous mitoses
- Loose edematous to fibrous stroma
- Macrophages and a few multinucleated giant cells can be seen

Immunohistochemistry/molecular pathology features

- Positive markers: α-smooth muscle actin, ALK-1 (50% of cases), desmin and cytokeratins can be focally positive
- Negative markers: S-100 protein, CD34, CD21, CD35, estrogen/progesterone receptors, beta-catenin, STAT6
- FISH: ALK gene amplification/rearrangement usually in cases with ALK-1 immunoreactivity

Diagnostic key features

- Fairly circumscribed nodule of α-smooth muscle actin–positive spindle cells with the morphologic features of myofibroblasts, closely intermingling with lymphocytes and plasma cells; ALK-1 expression favors the diagnosis of inflammatory myofibroblastic tumor

Treatment and prognosis

- Complete surgical excision; local recurrence (15%–20% of cases); rarely distant metastases

---

sole cell type present in a small biopsy. The dramatic misdiagnosis of invasive lobular carcinoma in small biopsies is often because the pathologist is not aware of the possibility that myofibroblastoma may be composed predominantly/ exclusively of epithelioid cells (see **Figs. 6** and **7**). In addition, the expression of estrogen/progesterone receptors by the cells of myofibroblastoma is misinterpreted as the luminal-type immunophenotype of an invasive lobular

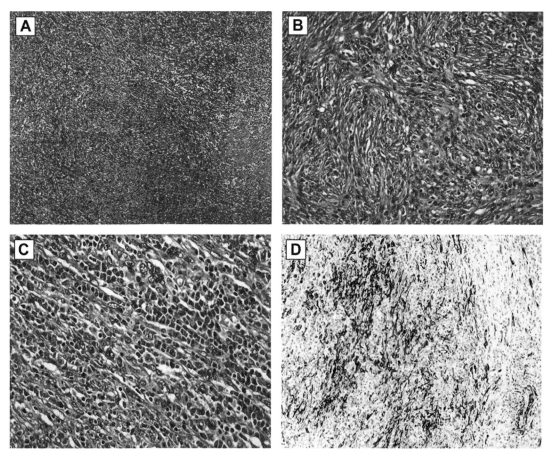

Fig. 3. Inflammatory pseudotumor/inflammatory myofibroblastic tumor. (*A*) Low magnification showing a spindle cell lesion with interspersed inflammatory component (H&E, original magnification ×60). (*B*) Higher-power magnification showing relatively bland-looking spindle cells with swirling pattern (H&E, original magnification ×150). (*C*) Numerous plasma cells are intermixed with spindle cells (hematoxylin and eosin staining; original magnification ×200). (*D*) Most of the spindle cells are stained with α-smooth muscle actin (H&E, original magnification ×100). ALK-1 is negative (not shown).

carcinoma. The correct diagnosis can be confidently rendered if the pathologist correlates the morphologic features with clinical and radiological information.[64,65] There should be a high index of suspicion for myofibroblastoma if the tumor shows pushing and not infiltrative borders, which should prompt the pathologist to perform immunohistochemical analyses, including epithelial and myogenic markers, as well as CD34 (**Box 7**).

Lipomatous myofibroblastoma is a bimorphic tumor with a mature lipomatous component overwhelming the myofibroblastic one.[61,62] Accordingly, this unusual variant of myofibroblastoma is reminiscent of a fibrolipoma or spindle cell lipoma or even desmoid-type fibromatosis at low magnification (**Fig. 8**). Lipomatous myofibroblastoma may represent a diagnostic pitfall in that the spindled cells,

variably admixed with adipocytes, often show a pseudoinfiltrative growth pattern closely reminiscent of desmoid-type fibromatosis or low-grade (fibromatosis-like) spindle cell carcinoma.[61,62] The diagnosis of these 2 tumors should be seriously questioned if the pathologist is dealing with a lesion with well-circumscribed borders. A wide immunohistochemical panel, which includes pancytokeratins, α-smooth muscle actin, desmin, CD34, β-catenin, estrogen/progesterone receptors, and p63, should be performed. Coexpression of desmin, CD34, and estrogen/progesterone receptors, along with the lack of staining with the other aforementioned markers, is consistent with the diagnosis of lipomatous myofibroblastoma.[58, 60–62]

Benign fibroblastic spindle cell tumor is a lesion composed of fibroblast-looking cells, usually haphazardly or focally arranged in short fascicles,

---

Box 4
Key features of pseudoangiomatous stromal hyperplasia (PASH)

Definition

- Hormone-dependent stromal change composed of spindle cells with the morphologic and immuno-histochemical features of fibroblasts/myofibroblasts

Clinical and radiographic

- Often incidental histologic finding associated with benign (hyperplastic epithelial lesions, fibroade-noma, and gynecomastia) or malignant lesions

- Occasionally slowly or rapidly growing mass (nodular PASH)

- Female individuals; more rarely male individuals in association with gynecomastia

- Age (3–70 years); most women are typically premenopausal

- Painless or painful nodule (0.6 to >20 cm in greatest diameter)

- Mammography and sonography: nodule with well-circumscribed borders

Gross pathology (nodular PASH)

- Nodule with circumscribed margins

- Gray-whitish in color

- Occasionally cystic spaces

Histopathology

- Ill-defined margins; well-circumscribed margins (nodular PASH)

- Spindle cells with the features of fibroblasts/myofibroblasts

- Anastomosing, slit-like pseudovascular spaces without red blood cells

- Variable cellularity

- None to mild nuclear atypia

- Focally, more rarely diffuse, fascicular pattern without intervening pseudovascular spaces

- Low mitotic count (1–4 mitoses per 10 HPFs)

- Fibrous to keloid-like stroma

- Extension from perilobular to nonspecialized stroma

Immunohistochemistry

- Positive markers: CD34, bcl-2, and progesterone receptors; variable expression of α-smooth muscle actin, desmin, calponin, and estrogen receptors

- Negative markers: endothelial markers (CD31; ERG), cytokeratins, S-100 protein

Diagnostic key features

- Proliferation of CD34-positive spindle cells forming slit-like pseudovascular spaces; fascicular arrange-ment with myofibroblastoma-like appearance can be seen.

Treatment and prognosis

- Surgical excision; local recurrence (incomplete surgery or multifocal disease in up 20% of cases)

---

and closely admixed with thin or thick collagen fibers[70–75] (**Box 8**; **Fig. 9**). Although similar to myo-fibroblastoma, the cells do not have abundant pale to eosinophilic cytoplasm, lack a diffuse fascicular growth pattern, and are positive only with vimentin and CD34; myogenic markers being absent or only focally expressed.[70–75] Given CD34 expression, some of these tumors in the past have been labeled as "solitary fibrous tumors."[74] Unlike solitary fibrous tumor, benign fibroblastic spindle cell tumor lacks medium-sized blood vessels with hyalinized walls and a branching configuration, as well as STAT-6 immunoreactivity.[76] Occasionally benign fibroblastic spindle cell tumor may

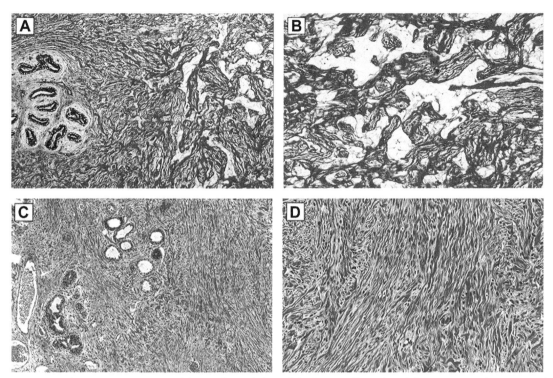

Fig. 4. Pseudoangiomatous stromal hyperplasia. (*A*) Perilobular spindle cell proliferation with formation of pseudovascular spaces (H&E, original magnification ×60). (*B*) In this area, the pseudovascular spaces are large simulating lymphangioma (H&E, original magnification ×100). The cells are negative for CD31 and ERG (not shown). (*C*) Fascicular variant of pseudoangiomatous stromal hyperplasia. The stroma is involved by a proliferation of spindle cells with interspersed thick collagen fibers without evidence of spaces (H&E, original magnification ×60). (*D*) At higher magnification, there is a close resemblance with classic-type myofibroblastoma (H&E, original magnification ×150).

contain a prominent mature fatty component, closely resembling spindle cell lipoma[73] (see **Fig. 9** C, D); however, the former lacks the focal myxoid areas and the ropey collagen fibers characteristically seen in the latter. As benign fibroblastic spindle cell tumor, myofibroblastoma and spindle cell lipoma share partial morphologic and immunohistochemical features, as well as the chromosome 13 rearrangements that lead to loss of the region 13q14 corresponding to the *Rb* gene or *FOXO1* gene, it is likely that they represent variations or transitional phases of the same disease.[77] It has been speculated that these tumors arise from a common precursor cell with the capability of fibroblastic, myofibroblastic and lipomatous differentiation.[7,8,59,60] In addition, the plasticity of this precursor to give rise to spindle, ovoid, or epithelioid/deciduoid cells may explain the heterogeneous morphology of these tumors, especially myofibroblastoma.[7,8,58,60] Although the distinction of myofibroblastoma from benign fibroblastic spindle cell tumors can

be achieved in most cases, there are a few tumors showing hybrid features.[7,8,58,60] In this case, there is no need to go to great lengths to differentiate them, and the generic and descriptive term "*benign spindle cell tumor of the mammary stroma*" is strongly suggested. Although benign spindle cell tumors specific to mammary stroma show morphologic and immunohistochemical overlap with spindle cell tumor–like lesions, there are some diagnostic features helpful in their distinction (**Table 2**). Among the benign spindle cell tumors of the soft tissues, which can occasionally occur in the breast parenchyma, leiomyoma[78–82] (**Fig. 10**), schwannoma/neurofibroma (sporadic or *NF1/NF2*-related),[83–92] spindle cell lipoma,[93–97] solitary fibrous tumor[98–103] (**Fig. 11**), and myxoma[104–108] should be included. These lesions are histologically and immunohistochemically identical to their respective counterpart occurring elsewhere. Their clinicopathologic features are summarized in **Box 9**.

Box 5
Key features of classic-type myofibroblastoma

Definition

• Benign myofibroblastic spindle cell tumor

Clinical and radiographic

• Males and females

• Painless breast nodule (0.5–15 cm in greatest diameter)

• Age (1–87 years); most cases in elderly men and postmenopausal women

• Mammography and sonography: nodule with well-circumscribed borders

Gross pathology

• Firm in consistency

• Whitish in color

• Well-circumscribed, occasionally lobulated, margins

Histopathology

• Well-circumscribed margins; rarely focally infiltrative

• Spindle to epithelioid cells with the features of myofibroblasts

• None to mild nuclear atypia; nuclear pleomorphism in a minority of cases

• Variable cellularity

• Short, straight, haphazardly intersecting fascicles; focal storiform or neural-like pattern

• Low mitotic count (0–2 mitoses per 10 HPFs)

• Thick keloid-like collagen fibers among proliferating cells

• Fibrous stroma; myxoid stromal changes can be prominent in a few cases

• Intratumoral areas of mature adipose tissue can be seen

• Usually no entrapment of ducts/lobules

• Small to medium-sized blood vessels; often hyalinization and foamy macrophages in their walls

• Mast cells variably interspersed among spindle cells

Immunohistochemistry/molecular pathology features

• Positive markers: vimentin, desmin, CD34, estrogen/progesterone/androgen receptors

• Variable expression of α-smooth muscle actin, calponin, CD10, bcl-2, CD99

• Negative markers: cytokeratins, EMA, S-100 protein, ALK-1, β-catenin, STAT6

• FISH: 13q14 deletion (70% of cases)

Diagnostic key features

• Well-circumscribed proliferation of relatively bland-looking spindle to epithelioid myofibroblasts positive to desmin/CD34/estrogen receptor–progesterone receptor (ER-PR), arranged in intersecting short fascicles interrupted by keloid-like collagen fibers

Treatment and prognosis

• Complete surgical excision; clinical indolent course without local recurrence

---

BENIGN SPINDLE CELL LESIONS VERSUS BLAND-LOOKING AGGRESSIVE SPINDLE CELL TUMORS

Although the benign spindle cell lesions represent a relatively uncommon group of diseases, their recognition is crucial to avoid confusion with other bland-looking spindle cell tumors that exhibit potentially aggressive behavior. Among these tumors, the most common are desmoid-type fibromatosis,[109–113] low-grade (fibromatosis-like) spindle cell carcinoma,[114–118] low-grade

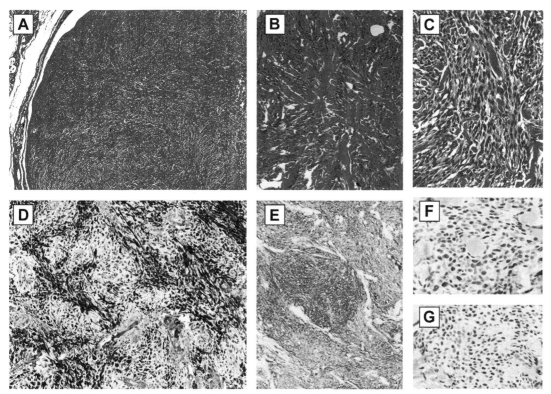

Fig. 5. Myofibroblastoma, classic-type. (*A*) Low magnification showing a well-circumscribed spindle cell tumor with numerous keloid-like collagen fibers (H&E, original magnification ×40). (*B*) The cells are arranged in short fascicles interrupted by keloid-like collagen fibers (H&E, original magnification ×100). (*C*) High magnification: the spindle cells exhibit the morphologic features of myofibroblasts (H&E, original magnification ×200) and are stained with desmin (*D*) (H&E, original magnification ×150), CD34 (*E*) (H&E, original magnification ×150), estrogen (*F*), and progesterone (*G*) receptors (H&E, original magnification [*F*,*G*] ×60).

myofibroblastic sarcoma,[119–122] low-grade fibrosarcoma,[123–127] and dermatofibrosarcoma protuberans.[128–131] The main clinicopathologic features are summarized in **Table 3**.

The differential diagnosis of these tumors includes many benign spindle cell lesions, particularly reactive spindle cell nodule/exuberant scar, nodular fasciitis, inflammatory pseudotumor/inflammatory myofibroblastic tumor, and lipomatous myofibroblastoma. Unlike most of the benign spindle cell lesions, desmoid-type fibromatosis and low-grade (fibromatosis-like) spindle cell carcinoma exhibit, at least focally, infiltrative margins, namely finger-like projections of neoplastic cells into adjacent mammary lobules/ducts and fibroadipose tissue[109–112] (Fig. 12; Fig. 13). The identification of epithelioid-polygonal cells arranged in small cohesive clusters, better highlighted by means of immunohistochemistry (broad-spectrum cytokeratins) is the main diagnostic clue for the diagnosis of low-grade (fibromatosis-like) spindle cell carcinoma[114–118] (Fig. 14). In addition, the demonstration of immunoreactivity for myoepithelial markers, especially p63, in a significant

number of neoplastic cells, irrespective of their morphology, supports the diagnosis of metaplastic carcinoma.[118]

If a lesion has infiltrating margins, along with the absence of any epithelial neoplastic component, ideally confirmed immunohistochemically, desmoid-type fibromatosis should be strongly suspected. Morphologic clues for diagnosis are the proliferation of spindle cells, usually aligned parallel to one another and arranged in long, sweeping fascicles set in a variably fibrous stroma[109–113] (see **Fig. 12**). The nuclei of the neoplastic cells are usually well-spaced, without significant overlapping. Immunohistochemistry, showing immunoreactivity for α-smooth muscle actin, revealing the myofibroblastic nature of the cells, along with nuclear staining for β-catenin (in approximately 80% of cases) is helpful in reaching the correct diagnosis[132] (see **Fig. 12**). Apart from low-grade spindle cell carcinoma, desmoid-type fibromatosis needs to be distinguished from lipomatous myofibroblastoma. This uncommon variant of myofibroblastoma shows areas with pseudoinfiltrative

---

Box 6
Key diagnostic features of morphologic variants of myofibroblastoma

Fibrous/collagenized myofibroblastoma

- Hypocellular tumor with a predominant fibrous stroma

- Keloid-like fibers typical of classic myofibroblastoma are reduced in number

- Irregular slit-like spaces, resembling those seen in pseudoangiomatous stromal hyperplasia

- Focal areas with the features of the classic-type myofibroblastoma

- Differential diagnosis: pseudoangiomatous stromal hyperplasia; inflammatory pseudotumor/inflammatory myofibroblastic tumor with extensive fibrous stroma

Myxoid myofibroblastoma

- Hypocellular tumor with entirely or predominantly myxoid stroma; at low magnification resemblance to myxoma

- Spindle, round, stellate cells

- Mild to moderate nuclear atypia

- Rare mitoses (0–2 mitoses per 10 HPFs)

- Scattered keloid-like collagen fibers within myxoid stroma

- Differential diagnosis: myxoma; nodular mucinosis; nodular fasciitis (myxoid variant); neurofibroma (myxoid variant); mucocele-like tumors; low-grade sarcomas with myxoid stromal changes (myxoid liposarcoma; low-grade myxofibrosarcoma)

Lipomatous myofibroblastoma

- Myofibroblastoma with prominent fatty component

- Well-circumscribed margins

- At low magnification, close resemblance to fibrolipoma, spindle cell lipoma, desmoid-type fibromatosis

- Adipocytes are uniform in size and shape and lack nuclear pleomorphism

- Non-adipocytic component: spindle to epithelioid cells with cytologic features and growth patterns of classic myofibroblastoma

- Adipocytes and spindle cells are variably admixed, often resulting in a finger-like pseudoinfiltrative pattern

- Keloid-like collagen fibers interspersed in the non-adipocytic component

- Mild to moderate nuclear atypia; nuclear pleomorphism rarely seen

- Low mitotic count (0–2 mitoses per 10 HPFs)

- Differential diagnosis: desmoid-type fibromatosis; low-grade (fibromatosis-like) spindle cell carcinoma

Epithelioid/deciduoid myofibroblastoma

- Myofibroblastoma composed exclusively or predominantly (>50% of the entire tumor) of cells with epithelioid or deciduoid-like morphology

- Well-circumscribed margins

- Medium-sized, epithelioid mononucleated or binucleated cells with abundant eosinophilic cytoplasm and round to oval, eccentrically placed nuclei with small evident nucleoli; a minority of spindle cells can be usually identified; occasionally the epithelioid cells are larger and adopt a deciduoid-like or rhabdoid-like appearance

- Mild to moderate degree of nuclear pleomorphism

- Interspersed keloid-like collagen fibers

(Continued)

> **Box 6**
> **Key diagnostic features of morphologic variants of myofibroblastoma (*continued*)**
>
> - Low mitotic count (0–2 mitoses per 10 HPFs)
>
> - Various architectural growth patterns: single cells, single cell files, nests, pseudo-alveolar, solid, trabecular, multinodular
>
> - Variable amount of intratumoral mature fatty component
>
> - Differential diagnosis: invasive lobular carcinoma; epithelioid leiomyoma/leiomyosarcoma; metastatic malignant tumor with epithelioid morphology (melanoma; epithelioid sarcoma; epithelioid variant of malignant peripheral nerve sheath tumor)
>
> Palisaded/Schwannoma-like myofibroblastoma
>
> - Myofibroblastoma with diffuse nuclear palisading and formation of numerous Verocay-like bodies
>
> - At low magnification, a close resemblance to schwannoma
>
> - Minor component of classic-type myofibroblastoma
>
> - Differential diagnosis: schwannoma

fibromatosis-like pattern due to the admixture of the spindle cell component with the lipomatous one that is part of the tumor.[61,62] Unlike desmoid-type fibromatosis, lipomatous myofibroblastoma has pushing borders and the fatty component is not the result of the entrapment of the surrounding adipose tissue.[61,62] Although lipomatous myofibroblastoma and desmoid-type fibromatosis share expression of α-smooth muscle actin, the former is also positive for desmin, CD34, and estrogen/progesterone receptors, which are negative in the latter.[61,62]

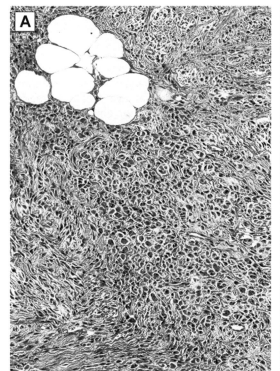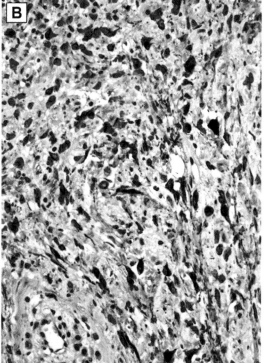

Fig. 6. Epithelioid cell myofibroblastoma. (*A*) Medium-sized epithelioid cells are haphazardly arranged within breast parenchyma. Only a minority of the cells are spindled in shape (*bottom*) (H&E, original magnification ×100). (*B*) Epithelioid cells staining with desmin (H&E, original magnification ×200).

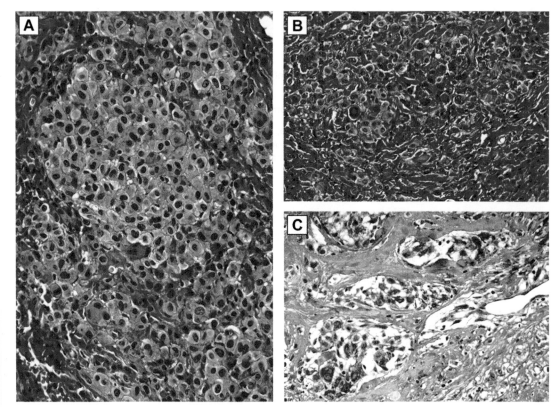

Fig. 7. Deciduoid-like cell myofibroblastoma. (*A*) The tumor is composed of closely packed, large-sized epithelioid cells with large nuclei, very reminiscent of deciduoid cells (H&E, original magnification ×150). (*B*) Some cells are multinucleated and show moderate nuclear pleomorphism. Mitoses are absent (H&E, original magnification ×100). (*C*) Neoplastic cells staining with desmin (H&E, original magnification ×150).

Low-grade myofibroblastic sarcoma can be difficult to distinguish from several other myofibroblastic benign spindle cell lesions in that it usually has relatively circumscribed margins[119–122] and is positive only for α-smooth muscle actin. Morphologic clues to the diagnosis include the presence, at least focally, of moderate nuclear pleomorphism and a high mitotic

---

Box 7
Pitfalls of myofibroblastoma

! All morphologic variants of myofibroblastoma may contain scattered mononucleated or multinucleated atypical cells with moderate to severe nuclear pleomorphism

! Occasionally myofibroblastoma may exhibit focal infiltrative margins

! Epithelioid cell myofibroblastoma may mimic invasive lobular carcinoma

! Deciduoid cell myofibroblastoma may mimic an apocrine invasive carcinoma or a metastatic tumor (melanoma; epithelioid cell sarcoma; rhabdoid tumor)

! Myofibroblastoma with prominent myxoid stroma may mimic other benign or malignant myxoid tumors

! Myofibroblastoma with prominent myxo-edematous stromal changes may mimic pleomorphic hyalinizing angiectatic tumor

! Lipomatous myofibroblastoma may mimic desmoid-type fibromatosis or low-grade (fibromatosis-like) spindle cell carcinoma

! Palisaded myofibroblastoma may mimic schwannoma

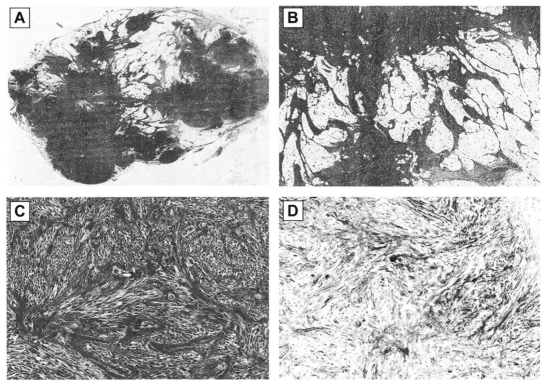

Fig. 8. Lipomatous myofibroblastoma. (*A*) Low magnification showing a fibro-lipomatous tumor with circumscribed borders (H&E, original magnification ×20). (*B*) In some areas the fibrous component shows a fingerlike pseudoinfiltration into the lipomatous component (fibromatosis-like appearance) (H&E, original magnification ×40). (*C*) Higher magnification showing the typical morphologic features of classic-type myofibroblastoma (H&E, original magnification ×80). (*D*) The spindle cells are positive for desmin (H&E, original magnification ×80).

count (from 7 to 35 mitoses per 10 HPFs) (Fig. 15). Low-grade fibrosarcoma of the breast is currently a diagnosis of exclusion. Although the term fibrosarcoma/malignant fibrous histiocytoma has been used in the past, most of these tumors are high-grade spindle cell sarcomas that have not been extensively studied by means of immunohistochemistry and

---

Box 8
Key features of benign fibroblastic spindle cell tumor

Definition

- Benign tumor of spindle cells with the morphologic and immunohistochemical features of fibroblasts

Clinical and radiographic features

- Women; men

- Age (36–83 years)

- Painless breast nodule (2–9 cm in greatest diameter)

- Mammography and sonography: nodule with well-circumscribed borders

Gross pathology

- Firm in consistency

- Whitish in color

- Well-circumscribed margins

(Continued)

Box 8
Key features of benign fibroblastic spindle cell tumor (*continued*)

Histopathology

- Well-circumscribed margins

- Spindle cells with the features of fibroblasts

- None to focally mild nuclear atypia

- Variable cellularity

- Cells haphazardly arranged; focally short, intersecting fascicles

- Low mitotic count (0–2 mitoses per 10 HPFs)

- Thin and thick keloid-like collagen fibers among proliferating cells

- Fibrous stroma

- Intratumoral fatty component; if it is predominant, close resemblance to spindle cell lipoma

- Usually no entrapment of ducts/lobules

- Small-sized blood vessels

Immunohistochemistry

- Positive markers: vimentin, CD34, ER-PRs, focal expression of α-smooth muscle actin can be seen

- Negative markers: desmin, cytokeratins, EMA, S-100 protein, ALK-1, β-catenin, STAT6

Diagnostic key features

- Well-circumscribed proliferation of bland-looking spindle cells with the morphologic and immuno-histochemical features of fibroblasts, arranged in haphazardly intersecting short fascicles with interspersed keloid-like collagen fibers

Treatment and prognosis

- Complete surgical excision; clinical indolent course without local recurrence

---

molecular analyses.[123–125] The term low-grade fibrosarcoma should be restricted to those tumors characterized by bland spindle cell morphology that do not exceed 6 mitoses per 10 HPFs, and the absence of any immunoreactivity, except for vimentin. Based on these strict morphologic and immunohistochemical criteria, the diagnosis of low-grade fibrosarcoma of the breast is rare, with only a few cases reported in the literature.[126,127] Dermatofibrosarcoma protuberans of the breast skin (subcutaneous/dermal location) is a relatively common tumor and its diagnosis is usually straightforward.[128] However, some diagnostic problems may arise when tumor is occasionally located within the breast parenchyma,[129–131] representing an unexpected site for such a tumor. The correct diagnosis is based on the identification of CD34-positive spindle cells diffusely arranged in a storiform growth pattern with infiltration of adjacent breast parenchyma and fibro-fatty tissue[129–131] (**Fig. 16**).

CONCLUDING REMARKS

The diagnosis of a "*benign spindle cell lesion*" of the breast should be made only after ruling out bland-looking, but potentially aggressive spindle cell tumors with which they may be confused. Radiographic features (mammography, ultrasound, and MRI) are nonspecific and they are frequently reported as "suspicious for malignancy," "indeterminate," or "benign." Accordingly, it is not surprising that some benign spindle cells lesions (particularly nodular fasciitis, reactive spindle cell nodule/exuberant scar, inflammatory pseudotumor/inflammatory myofibroblastic tumor, and nodular pseudoangiomatous stromal hyperplasia) are biopsied. An immunohistochemical panel that includes epithelial markers, p63, myogenic markers, CD34, β-catenin, STAT6 and S-100 protein is mandatory. Based on clinical/radiographic, morphologic, and immunohistochemical

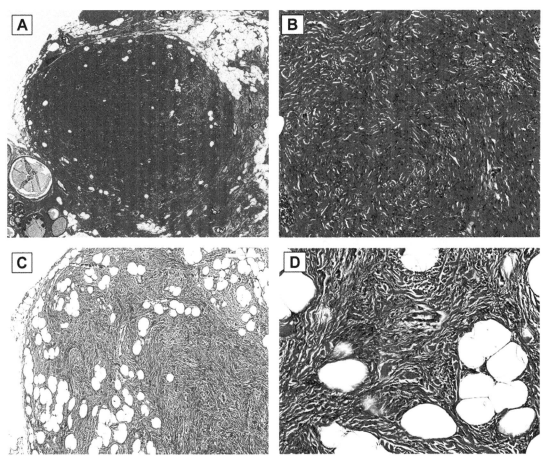

Fig. 9. Benign fibroblastic spindle cell tumor. (*A*) Low magnification showing a fibrous tumor with well-circumscribed borders within the breast parenchyma (H&E, original magnification ×40). (*B*) At higher magnification, the tumor is composed of short fascicles, haphazardly set in fibrous to keloid-like stroma (H&E, original magnification ×80). (*C*) Spindle cell tumor with lipomatous component (H&E, original magnification ×60). (*D*) Spindle cell lipoma-like area is seen (H&E, original magnification ×100).

findings, a correct interpretation of the biopsied lesion can be confidentially achieved in most cases. However, a provisional and descriptive diagnosis of "*bland-looking mesenchymal spindle cell lesion, N.O.S. (not otherwise specified)*" should be made if the immunohistochemical profile is not conclusive, prompting clinicians to excise the entire mass for histologic examination. An awareness of the distinctive morphologic and immunohistochemical features of the different bland-looking spindle cell tumors and tumor-like entities is crucial to ensure that patients receive the correct treatment and prognostic information.

Surgical excision is adequate treatment for benign spindle cell lesions of the breast. However, if the clinicopathologic features are consistent with a diagnosis of nodular fasciitis or pseudoangiomatous stromal hyperplasia, follow-up imaging as an alternative to excisional biopsy has been successfully proposed by some investigators. This is supported by evidence that spontaneous regression has been documented in cases of nodular fasciitis, whereas local recurrence has been reported in some patients who underwent excisional biopsy of pseudoangiomatous stromal hyperplasia. As in other sites, long-term follow-up of patients with inflammatory pseudotumor/inflammatory myofibroblastic tumor and solitary fibrous tumor is advised due to the low risk of local recurrence. Although rare cases of distant metastases from these 2 tumors primarily arising in the breast have been reported in the literature, the illustrations provided by the investigators are not completely convincing.

Table 2
Differential diagnosis of spindle cell tumor–like lesions versus spindle cell tumors specific to mammary stroma

Clinico-pathologic features	NF	RSCN	IP/IMT	PASH	BFSCT	MFB
Clinical/Radiological features	Spontaneous nodule Ill-defined margins	Nodule following biopsy or FNAC Circumscribed margins	Spontaneous nodule Rarely following local trauma	Often microscopic finding Occasionally nodule with circumscribed margins	Spontaneous nodule Well-circumscribed nodule	Spontaneous nodule Well-circumscribed nodule
Histologic Borders	Circumscribed Focally infiltrative	Circumscribed Focally infiltrative	Circumscribed	Ill-defined	Well-circumscribed	Well-circumscribed
Pattern	Short, focally intersecting, fascicles	Intersecting short fascicles; focal storiform pattern	Interlacing short fascicles; swirling storiform pattern	Pseudovascular spaces; short fascicles	Short intersecting fascicles	Short, straight or haphazardly intersecting fascicles
Stroma	Myxoid to fibrous	Delicate collagen fibers	Fibrous to focally edematous	Fibrous	Fibrous Keloid-like collagen fibers	Fibrous to myxoid Keloid-like collagen fibers
Cytology	Spindle cells; foci of extravasated red blood cells and lymphocytes; tissue culture–like appearance	Spindle cells interspersed foamy and hemosiderin-laden macrophages, lymphocytes and plasma cells	Spindle cells admixed with inflammatory cells (lymphocytes, plasma cells)	Spindle cells	Spindle cells	Spindle to ovoid to epithelioid cells
Mitoses	Variable; sometimes numerous	1–4 mitoses per 10 HPFs	0–3 mitoses per 10 HPFs	0–1 mitosis per 10 HPFs	0–2 mitoses per 10 HPFs	2 mitoses per 10 HPFs
Immunophenotype	α-smooth muscle actin+; CD34–; desmin–	α-smooth muscle actin+; CD34–; desmin–	α-smooth muscle actin+; CD34–; desmin–	CD34+; α-smooth muscle actin+; CD31–; ERG–	CD34+; desmin–; α-smooth muscle actin–	Desmin+; CD34+; ER/PR/AR+

Abbreviations: AR, androgen receptors; BFSCT, benign fibroblastic spindle cell tumor; ER, estrogen receptors; FNAC, fine-needle aspiration cytology; HPF, high power field; IP/IMT, inflammatory pseudotumor/inflammatory myofibroblastic tumor; MFB, myofibroblastoma; NF, nodular fasciitis; PASH, pseudoangiomatous stromal hyperplasia; PR, progesterone receptors; RSCN, reactive spindle cell nodule.

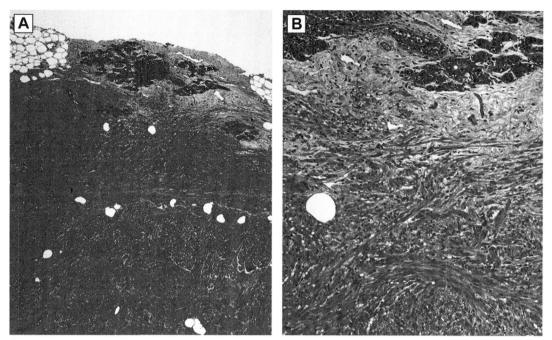

Fig. 10. Leiomyoma. (*A*) Spindle cell tumor with circumscribed borders. A fascicular arrangement of the cells is evident (H&E, original magnification ×60). (*B*) Higher magnification showing cells with the morphologic features of smooth muscle cells, arranged in intersecting fascicles (H&E, original magnification ×100).

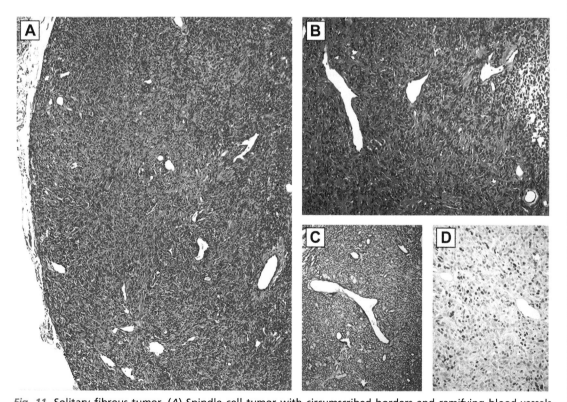

Fig. 11. Solitary fibrous tumor. (*A*) Spindle cell tumor with circumscribed borders and ramifying blood vessels (H&E, original magnification ×60). (*B*) Spindle to ovoid cells embedded into fibrous stroma. Dilated blood vessels with perivascular hyalinization (H&E, original magnification ×80). Neoplastic cells are diffusely stained with CD34 (*C*) (H&E, original magnification ×60) and STAT-6 (*D*) (H&E, original magnification ×80).

Box 9
Key features of benign spindle cell tumors not specific to mammary stroma

Leiomyoma

- Women; rarely in men; age (27–70 years); painless nodule (0.5–13.8 cm in greatest diameter) with well-circumscribed borders at mammography/sonography

- Well-circumscribed nodule, firm in consistency and whitish in color. The cut surface is similar to that seen in uterine leiomyomas

- Interlacing fascicles of deeply eosinophilic spindle-shaped cells with elongated nuclei with blunt ends

- Mitotic activity is absent or low (1–2 mitoses per 10 HPFs)

- Immunohistochemistry: diffuse coexpression of desmin, α-smooth muscle actin and h-caldesmon

Schwannoma/neurofibroma

- Female and male individuals; any age; painless nodule (1–8 cm); encapsulated spindle cell tumors with well-defined margins; occasionally with infiltrative borders

- Schwannoma: alternating Antoni A and B areas; Verocay bodies; hyalinized vessels

- Neurofibroma: sporadic or NF1-related; spindle cells with wavy nuclei set in a myxoid stroma containing isolated keloid-like collagen fibers

- None or rare mitoses (1–2 mitoses per 10 HPF); occasionally moderate nuclear pleomorphism

- Immunohistochemistry: diffuse expression of S100 protein and SOX-10 (schwannoma); variable, often focal, staining with CD34, S100 and SOX-10

Spindle cell lipoma

- Women; age (28–66 years); painless nodule (1.5–3.0 cm); unencapsulated spindle cell tumor admixed with a variable (absent to predominant) mature fatty component and with well-circumscribed margins; focal to diffuse myxoid stromal changes; ropey collagen fibers; floret-like multinucleated cells

- None or rare mitoses (1 mitosis per 10 HPFs)

- Immunohistochemistry: diffuse expression of CD34

Solitary fibrous tumor

- Women; age (41–64 years); painless nodule (1–10 cm)

- Well-circumscribed nodule, firm in consistency and white to grayish in color

- Short fibroblast-like spindle to round/ovoid cells, haphazardly arranged in a fibrous to myxoid stroma

- Mitotic activity: usually 0 to 4 mitoses per 10 HPFs; more than 4 mitoses per 10 HPFs may predict malignant outcome

- Large to small branching vessels, often with perivascular hyalinization

- Immunohistochemistry: diffuse STAT6 and CD34 expression

Myxoma

- Women; more rarely men; age (33–75 years); painless nodule (1.5–5.0 cm)

- Well-circumscribed mass with yellowish, gelatinous appearance

- Spindle to round/stellate-shaped cells set a myxoid stroma containing keloid-like collagen fibers; few small-sized blood vessels

- No mitoses

- Immunohistochemistry: focal staining with α-smooth muscle actin or calponin

Table 3
Differential diagnosis of the most common benign spindle cell tumors

Clinico-pathologic features	Myofibroblastoma	Leiomyoma	Solitary Fibrous Tumor	Spindle Cell Lipoma (Fat-free/poor)	Schwannoma/ Neurofibroma	Myxoma
Clinical/ radiological features	Well-circumscribed nodule	Well-circumscribed nodule	Well-circumscribed nodule	Circumscribed nodule	Well-circumscribed, only focally infiltrative (neurofibroma), margins	Well-circumscribed nodule
Histologic pattern	Myofibroblastic-looking spindle cells arranged in short, straight, or haphazardly intersecting fascicles	Deeply eosinophilic spindle cells with cigar-shaped nuclei, arranged in intersecting fascicles	Short fibroblast-like spindle to round/ ovoid cells, haphazardly arranged; focal storiform pattern	Short fibroblast-looking spindle cells with bipolar cytoplasmic processes, arranged haphazardly or in short bundles	Schwannoma: spindle cells arranged in interlacing fascicles and whorls; palisading nuclei (Verocay bodies); alternating hypercellular (Antoni A areas) and hypocellular (Antoni B) areas Neurofibroma: spindle cells with wavy nuclei, haphazardly arranged in a slightly myxoid stroma containing tick collagen fibers	Fibroblast-like spindle to stellate cells, haphazardly arranged

(continued on next page)

Table 3
(continued)

Clinico-pathologic features	Myofibroblastoma	Leiomyoma	Solitary Fibrous Tumor	Spindle Cell Lipoma (Fat-free/poor)	Schwannoma/ Neurofibroma	Myxoma
Stroma	Fibrous to focally myxoid; keloid-like collagen fibers	Fibrous to focally myxoid	Fibrous to myxoid stroma	Fibrous to predominantly myxoid; ropey collagen fibers	Fibrous to focally myxoid	Myxoid with scattered keloid-like collagen fibers
Mitotic count	0–2 mitosis per 10 HPFs	0–1 mitosis per 50 HPFs	0–4 mitoses per 10 HPFs	0–1 mitosis per 10 HPFs	No mitoses	No mitoses
Vasculature	Small to medium-sized vessels, often with hyalinization of the walls	Small to medium-sized vessels	Large to small branching vessels, often with perivascular hyalinization	Few small or intermediate-sized, thick-walled vessels; more rarely plexiform pattern	Schwannoma: hyalinized vessels	Small-sized vessels
Immunophenotype	Desmin+; CD34+; ER/PR/AR+	α-smooth muscle actin+; desmin+; h-caldesmon+	STAT6+; CD34+	CD34+	S100 protein+; CD34+ (variable)	Focal calponin+

Abbreviations: AR, androgen receptors; ER, estrogen receptors; HPF, high power field; PR, progesterone receptors.

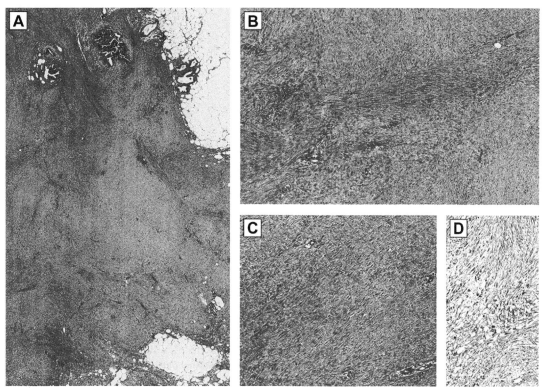

Fig. 12. Desmoid-type fibromatosis. (*A*) Fibrous proliferation infiltrating breast parenchyma (epithelial structures and adipose tissue) (H&E, original magnification ×60). (*B*) Bland-looking spindle cells set in a fibrous stroma, focally arranged in long fascicles (H&E, original magnification ×80). (*C*) The cells, typically aligned parallel, are embedded in abundant fibrous stroma (H&E, original magnification ×100). (*D*) Most of the neoplastic cells show nuclear staining for β-catenin (H&E, original magnification ×100).

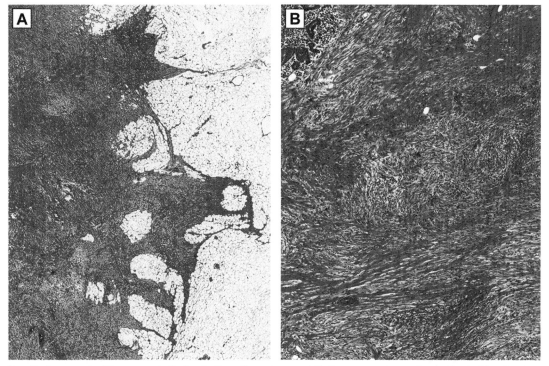

Fig. 13. Low-grade (fibromatosis-like) spindle cell carcinoma. (*A*) The tumor shows finger-like infiltration into adjacent adipose tissue (H&E, original magnification ×60). (*B*) The tumor is composed of bland-looking spindle cells arranged in short fascicles and set in a fibrous stroma (H&E, original magnification ×80).

116

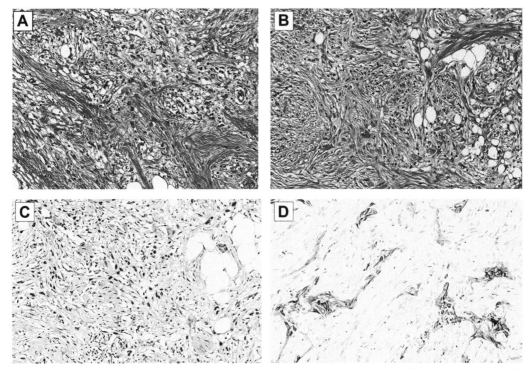

Fig. 14. Low-grade (fibromatosis-like) spindle cell carcinoma. Isolated epithelioid cells (*A*) (H&E, original magnification ×100) or small clusters of cohesive cells are scattered among the spindle cells (*B*) (H&E, original magnification ×150). The spindle cells are positive for p63 (*C*) (H&E, original magnification ×150). Pancytokeratins highlight the small clusters of epithelial cells (*D*) (H&E, original magnification ×150).

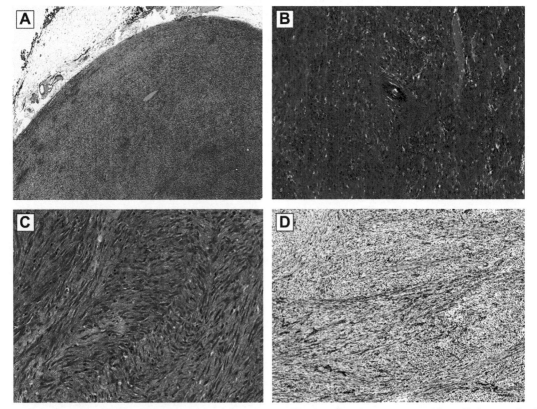

Fig. 15. Low-grade myofibroblastic sarcoma. (*A*) Low magnification showing a tumor with well-circumscribed borders (H&E, original magnification ×40). (*B*) Rare, entrapped epithelial mammary structures are seen (H&E, original magnification ×100). (*C*) The tumor is composed of bland-looking spindle cells with the features of my-ofibroblasts, arranged in fascicles and set in a myxoid stroma (H&E, original magnification ×150). (*D*) The tumor is diffusely positive for α-smooth muscle actin (H&E, original magnification ×80).

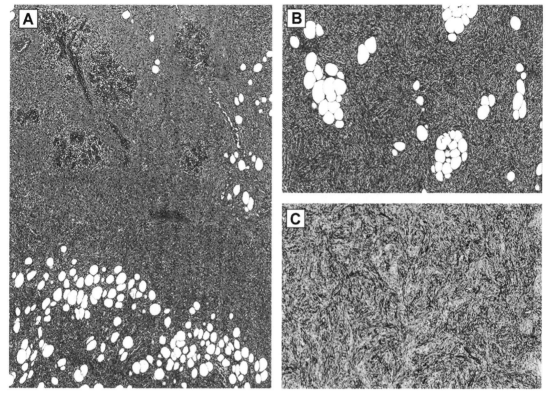

Fig. 16. Dermatofibrosarcoma protuberans. (*A*) Spindle cell tumor infiltrating the breast parenchyma (H&E, original magnification ×80). The neoplastic cells exhibit a diffuse storiform growth pattern (*B*) (H&E, original magnification ×100) and immunostaining for CD34 (*C*) (H&E, original magnification ×150).

REFERENCES

1. Al-Nafussi A. Spindle cell tumours of the breast: practical approach to diagnosis. Histopathology 1999;35:1–13.
2. McMenamin ME, DeSchryver K, Fletcher CD. Fibrous lesions of the breast: a review. Int J Surg Pathol 2000;8:99–108.
3. Brogi E. Benign and malignant spindle cell lesions of the breast. Semin Diagn Pathol 2004;21:57–64.
4. Cheah AL, Billings SD, Rowe JJ. Mesenchymal tumours of the breast and their mimics: a review with approach to diagnosis. Pathology 2016;48:406–24.
5. Rakha EA, Aleskandarany MA, Lee AH, et al. An approach to the diagnosis of spindle cell lesions of the breast. Histopathology 2016;68:33–44.
6. Tay TKY, Tan PH. Spindle cell lesions of the breast—an approach to diagnosis. Semin Diagn Pathol 2017;34(5):400–9.
7. Magro G, Michal M, Bisceglia M. Benign spindle cell tumors of the mammary stroma: diagnostic criteria, classification, and histogenesis. Pathol Res Pract 2001;197:453–66.
8. Magro G, Bisceglia M, Michal M, et al. Spindle cell lipoma-like tumor, solitary fibrous tumor and

myofibroblastoma of the breast: a clinico-pathological analysis of 13 cases in favor of a unifying histogenetic concept. Virchows Arch 2002; 440:249–60.
9. Son YM, Nahm JH, Moon HJ, et al. Imaging findings for malignancy mimicking nodular fasciitis of the breast and a review of previous imaging studies. Acta Radiol Short Rep 2013; 11:2.
10. Yamamoto S, Chishima T, Adachi S. Nodular fasciitis of the breast mimicking breast cancer. Case Rep Surg 2014;2014:747951.
11. Sakuma T, Matsuo K, Koike S, et al. Fine needle aspiration cytology of nodular fasciitis of the breast. Diagn Cytopathol 2015;43:222–9.
12. Rhee SJ, Ryu JK, Kim JH, et al. Nodular fasciitis of the breast: two cases with a review of imaging findings. Clin Imaging 2014;38:730–3.
13. Hayashi S, Yasuda S, Takahashi N, et al. Nodular fasciitis of the breast clinically resembling breast cancer in an elderly woman: a case report. J Med Case Rep 2017;11:57.
14. Paliogiannis P, Cossu A, Palmieri G, et al. Breast nodular fasciitis: a comprehensive review. Breast Care (Basel) 2016;11:270–4.

15. Kang A, Kumar JB, Thomas A, et al. A spontaneously resolving breast lesion: imaging and cytological findings of nodular fasciitis of the breast with FISH showing USP6 gene rearrangement. BMJ Case Rep 2015;2015.

16. Shin C, Low I, Ng D, et al. USP6 gene rearrangement in nodular fasciitis and histological mimics. Histopathology 2016;69:784–91.

17. Pettinato G, Manivel JC, Insabato L, et al. Plasma cell granuloma (inflammatory pseudotumor) of the breast. Am J Clin Pathol 1988;90:627–32.

18. Chetty R, Govender D. Inflammatory pseudotumor of the breast. Pathology 1997;29:270–1.

19. Yip CH, Wong KT, Samuel D. Bilateral plasma cell granuloma (inflammatory pseudotumour) of the breast. Aust N Z J Surg 1997;67:300–2.

20. Sastre-Garau X, Couturier J, Derre J, et al. Inflammatory myofibroblastic tumour (inflammatory pseudotumour) of the breast. Clinicopathological and genetic analysis of a case with evidence for clonality. J Pathol 2002;196:97–102.

21. Zardawi IM, Clark D, Williamsz G. Inflammatory myofibroblastic tumor of the breast. A case report. Acta Cytol 2003;47:1077–81.

22. Ilvan S, Celik V, Paksoy M, et al. Inflammatory myofibroblastic tumor (inflammatory pseudotumor) of the breast. APMIS 2005;113:66–9.

23. Khanafshar E, Phillipson J, Schammel DP, et al. Inflammatory myofibroblastic tumor of the breast. Ann Diagn Pathol 2005;9:123–9.

24. Kim SJ, Moon WK, Kim JH, et al. Inflammatory pseudotumor of the breast: a case report with imaging findings. Korean J Radiol 2009;10: 515–8.

25. Park SB, Kim HH, Shin HJ, et al. Inflammatory pseudotumor (myoblastic tumor) of the breast: a case report and review of the literature. J Clin Ultrasound 2010;38:52–5.

26. Hill PA. Inflammatory pseudotumor of the breast: a mimic of breast carcinoma. Breast J 2010;16:549–50.

27. Vecchio GM, Amico P, Grasso G, et al. Post-traumatic inflammatory pseudotumor of the breast with atypical morphological features: a potential diagnostic pitfall. Report of a case and a critical review of the literature. Pathol Res Pract 2011;207: 322–6.

28. Zhou Y, Zhu J, Zhang Y, et al. An inflammatory myofibroblastic tumour of the breast with ALK overexpression. BMJ Case Rep 2013;2013:4.

29. Zhao HD, Wu T, Wang JQ, et al. Primary inflammatory myofibroblastic tumor of the breast with rapid recurrence and metastasis: a case report. Oncol Lett 2013;5:97–100.

30. Bosse K, Ott C, Biegner T, et al. 23-year-old female with an inflammatory myofibroblastic tumour of the breast: a case report and a review of the literature. Geburtshilfe Frauenheilkd 2014;74:167–70.

31. Markopoulos C, Charalampoudis P, Karagiannis E, et al. Inflammatory myofibroblastic tumor of the breast. Case Rep Surg 2015;2015:705127.

32. Choi EJ, Jin GY, Chung MJ, et al. Primary inflammatory myofibroblastic tumors of the breast with metastasis: radiographic and histopathologic predictive factors. J Breast Cancer 2015;18: 200–5.

33. Talu CK, Çakır Y, Hacıhasanoğlu E, et al. Inflammatory myofibroblastic tumor of the breast coexisting with pseudoangiomatous stromal hyperplasia. J Breast Health 2016;12:171–3.

34. Tabbara SO, Frierson HF Jr, Fechner RE. Diagnostic problems in tissues previously sampled by fine-needle aspiration. Am J Clin Pathol 1991;96: 76–80.

35. Lee KC, Chan JK, Ho LC. Histologic changes in the breast after fine-needle aspiration. Am J Surg Pathol 1994;18:1039–47.

36. Gobbi H, Tse G, Page DL, et al. Reactive spindle cell nodules of the breast after core biopsy or fine-needle aspiration. Am J Clin Pathol 2000;113: 288–94.

37. Garijo MF, Val-Bernal JF, Vega A, et al. Postoperative spindle cell nodule of the breast: pseudosarcomatous myofibroblastic proliferation following endosurgery. Pathol Int 2008;58:787–91.

38. Sciallis AP, Chen B, Folpe AL. Cellular spindled histiocytic pseudotumor complicating mammary fat necrosis. Am J Surg Pathol 2012;36:1571–8.

39. Powell CM, Cranor ML, Rosen PP. Pseudoangiomatous stromal hyperplasia (PASH). A mammary stromal tumor with myofibroblastic differentiation. Am J Surg Pathol 1995;19:270–7.

40. Milanezi MF, Saggioro FP, Zanati SG, et al. Pseudoangiomatous hyperplasia of mammary stroma associated with gynaecomastia. J Clin Pathol 1998;51:204–6.

41. Magro G, Bisceglia M. Myofibroblastoma-like changes in fibro(stromo)-epithelial lesions of the breast: report of two cases. Virch Arch 2005;446:95–6.

42. Virk RK, Khan A. Pseudoangiomatous stromal hyperplasia: an overview. Arch Pathol Lab Med 2010;134:1070–4.

43. Ferreira M, Albarracin CT, Resetkova E. Pseudoangiomatous stromal hyperplasia tumor: a clinical, radiologic and pathologic study of 26 cases. Mod Pathol 2008;21:201–7.

44. Abdull Gaffar B. Pseudoangiomatous stromal hyperplasia of the breast. Arch Pathol Lab Med 2009;133:1335–8.

45. Shehata BM, Fishman I, Collings MH, et al. Pseudoangiomatous stromal hyperplasia of the breast in pediatric patients: an underrecognized entity. Pediatr Dev Pathol 2009;12:450–4.

46. Jones KN, Glazebrook KN, Reynolds C. Pseudoangiomatous stromal hyperplasia: imaging findings

with pathologic and clinical correlation. AJR Am J Radiol 2010;195:1036–42.

47. Gresik CM, Godellas C, Aranha GV, et al. Pseudoangiomatous stromal hyperplasia of the breast: a contemporary approach to its clinical and radiologic features and ideal management. Surgery 2010;148:752–7.

48. Nassar H, Elieff MP, Kronz JD, et al. Pseudoangiomatous stromal hyperplasia (PASH) of the breast with foci of morphologic malignancy: a case of PASH with malignant transformation? Int J Surg Pathol 2010;18:564–9.

49. Almohawes E, Khoumais N, Arafah M. Pseudoangiomatous stromal hyperplasia of the breast: a case report of a 12-year-old girl. Radiol Case Rep 2015;10:1–4.

50. Kelten C, Boyaci C, Leblebici C, et al. Nodule-forming pseudoangiomatous stromal hyperplasia of the breast: report of three cases. J Breast Health 2015; 11:144–7.

51. Krawczyk N, Fehm T, Ruckhäberle E, et al. Diffuse pseudoangiomatous stromal hyperplasia (PASH) causing gigantomastia in a 33-year-old pregnant woman: case report. Breast Care (Basel) 2016;11: 356–8.

52. Lee JW, Jung GS, Kim JB, et al. Pseudoangiomatous stromal hyperplasia presenting as rapidly growing bilateral breast enlargement refractory to surgical excision. Arch Plast Surg 2016;43: 218–21.

53. Protos A, Nguyen KT, Caughran JL, et al. Pseudoangiomatous stromal hyperplasia on core needle biopsy does not require surgical excision. Am Surg 2016;82:117–21.

54. Kelten Talu C, Boyaci C, Leblebici C, et al. Pseudoangiomatous stromal hyperplasia in core needle biopsies of breast specimens. Int J Surg Pathol 2017;25:26–30.

55. Raj SD, Sahani VG, Adrada BE, et al. Pseudoangiomatous stromal hyperplasia of the breast: multimodality review with pathologic correlation. Curr Probl Diagn Radiol 2017;46:130–5.

56. Gleason BC, Hornick JL. Inflammatory myofibroblastic tumours: where are we now? J ClinPathol 2008;61:428–37.

57. Wargotz ES, Weiss SW, Norris HJ. Myofibroblastoma of the breast. Sixteen cases of a distinctive benign mesenchymal tumor. Am J Surg Pathol 1987;11:493–502.

58. Magro G. Mammary myofibroblastoma: a tumor with a wide morphologic spectrum. Arch Pathol Lab Med 2008;132:1813–20.

59. Soyer T, Ayva S, Senyucel MF, et al. Myofibroblastoma of breast in a male infant. Fetal Pediatr Pathol 2012;31:164–8.

60. Magro G. Mammary myofibroblastoma: an update with emphasis on the most diagnostically challenging variants. Histology Histopathology 2016;31:1–23.

61. Magro G, Michal M, Vasquez E, et al. Lipomatous myofibroblastoma: a potential diagnostic pitfall in the spectrum of the spindle cell lesions of the breast. Virchows Arch 2000;437:540–4.

62. Magro G, Longo FR, Salvatorelli L, et al. Lipomatous myofibroblastoma of the breast: case report with diagnostic and histogenetic considerations. Pathologica 2014;106:36–40.

63. Magro G, Amico P, Gurrera A. Myxoid myofibroblastoma of the breast with atypical cells: a potential diagnostic pitfall. Virchows Arch 2007;450:483–5.

64. Magro G. Epithelioid-cell myofibroblastoma of the breast: expanding the morphologic spectrum. Am J Surg Pathol 2009;33:1085–92.

65. Magro G, Vecchio GM, Michal M, et al. Atypical epithelioid cell myofibroblastoma of the breast with multinodular growth pattern: a potential pitfall of malignancy. Pathol Res Pract 2013;209:463–6.

66. Magro G, Gangemi P, Greco P. Deciduoid-like myofibroblastoma of the breast: a potential pitfall of malignancy. Histopathology 2008;52:652–4.

67. Magro G, Foschini MP, Eusebi V. Palisaded myofibroblastoma of the breast: a tumor closely mimicking schwannoma. Report of two cases. Hum Path 2013;44:1941–6.

68. Laforga JB, Escandón J. Schwannoma-like (palisaded) myofibroblastoma: a challenging diagnosis on core biopsy. Breast J 2017;23:354–6.

69. Magro G, Salvatorelli L, Spadola S, et al. Mammary myofibroblastoma with extensive myxoedematous stromal changes: a potential diagnostic pitfall. Pathol Res Pract 2014;210:1106–11.

70. Toker C, Tang CK, Whitely JF, et al. Benign spindle cell breast tumor. Cancer 1981;48:1615–22.

71. Böger A. Benign spindle cell tumor of the male breast. Pathol Res Pract 1984;178:395–9.

72. Chan KW, Ghadially FN, Alagaratnam TT. Benign spindle cell tumour of breast— a variant of spindle cell lipoma or fibroma of breast? Pathology 1984; 16:331–6.

73. Magro G, Bisceglia M, Pasquinelli G. Benign spindle cell tumor of the breast with prominent adipocytic component. Ann Diagn Pathol 1998;2:306–11.

74. Bombonati A, Parra JS, Schwartz GF, et al. Solitary fibrous tumor of the breast. Breast J 2003;9:251.

75. Dragoumis D, Atmatzidis S, Chatzimavroudis G, et al. Benign spindle cell tumor not otherwise specified (NOS) in a male breast. Int J Surg Pathol 2010; 18:575–9.

76. Magro G, Angelico G, Leone G, et al. Solitary fibrous tumor of the breast: report of a case with emphasis on diagnostic role of STAT6 immunostaining. Pathol Res Pract 2016;212:463–7.

77. Magro G, Righi A, Casorzo L, et al. Mammary and vaginal myofibroblastomas are genetically related

lesions: fluorescence in situ hybridization analysis shows deletion of 13q14 region. Hum Pathol 2012;43:1887–93.

78. Jones MW, Norris HJ, Wargotz ES. Smooth muscle and nerve sheath tumors of the breast. A clinico-pathologic study of 45 cases. Int J Surg Pathol 1994;2:85–92.

79. Ende L, Mercado C, Axelrod D, et al. Intraparen-chymal leiomyoma of the breast: a case report and review of the literature. Ann Clin Lab Sci 2007;37:268–73.

80. Minami S, Matsuo S, Azuma T, et al. Parenchymal leiomyoma of the breast: a case report with special reference to magnetic resonance imaging findings and an update review of literature. Breast Cancer 2011;18:231–6.

81. Vecchio GM, Cavaliere A, Cartaginese F, et al. Intraparenchymal leiomyoma of the breast: report of a case with emphasis on needle core biopsy-based diagnosis. Pathologica 2013;105:122–7.

82. Granic M, Stefanovic-Radovic M, Zdravkovic D, et al. Intraparenchimal leiomyoma of the breast. Arch Iran Med 2015;18:608–12.

83. Charu V, Cimino-Mathews A. Peripheral nerve sheath tumors of the breast. Semin Diagn Pathol 2017;34(5):420–6.

84. Bellezza G, Lombardi T, Panzarola P, et al. Schwan-noma of the breast: a case report and review of the literature. Tumori 2007;93:308–11.

85. Gultekin SH, Cody HS, Hoda SA. Schwannoma of the breast. South Med J 1996;89:238–9.

86. Murat A, Kansiz F, Kabakus N, et al. Neurofibroma of the breast in a boy with neurofibromatosis type 1. Clin Imaging 2004;28:415–7.

87. Lee EK, Kook SH, Kwag HJ, et al. Schwannoma of the breast showing massive exophytic growth: a case report. Breast 2006;15:562–6.

88. Dialani V, Hines N, Wang Y, et al. Breast schwan-noma. Case Rep Med 2011;2011:930841.

89. Thejaswini M, Padmaja K, Srinivasamurthy V, et al. Solitary intramammary schwannoma mimicking phylloides tumor: cytological clues in the diag-nosis. J Cytol 2012;29:258–60.

90. Parikh Y, Sharma KJ, Parikh SJ, et al. Intramam-mary schwannoma: a palpable breast mass. Radiol Case Rep 2016;11:129–33.

91. Jeyaretna DS, Oriolowo A, Smith ME, et al. Solitary neurofibroma in the male breast. World J Surg On-col 2007;5:23.

92. Thompson S, Kaplan SS, Poppiti RJ, et al. Solitary neurofibroma of the breast. Radiol Case Rep 2012;7:462.

93. Lew WY. Spindle cell lipoma of the breast: a case report and literature review. Diagn Cytopathol 1993;9:434–7.

94. Smith DN, Denison CM, Lester SC. Spindle cell li-poma of the breast. A case report. Acta Radiol 1996;37:893–5.

95. Mulvany NJ, Silvester AC, Collins JP. Spindle cell li-poma of the breast. Pathology 1999;31:288–91.

96. Abd el-All HS. Breast spindle cell tumours: about eight cases. Diagn Pathol 2006;22(1):13.

97. Jaffar R, Zaheer S, Vasenwala SM, et al. Spindle cell lipoma breast. Indian J Pathol Microbiol 2008;51:234–6.

98. Khalifa MA, Montgomery EA, Azumi N, et al. Soli-tary fibrous tumors: a series of lesions, some in un-usual sites. South Med J 1997;90:793–9.

99. Falconieri G, Lamovec J, Mirra M, et al. Solitary fibrous tumor of the mammary gland: a potential pitfall in breast pathology. Ann Diagn Pathol 2004;8:121–5.

100. Meguerditchian AN, Malik DA, Hicks DG, et al. Sol-itary fibrous tumor of the breast and mammary my-ofibroblastoma: the same lesion? Breast J 2008;14:287–92.

101. Yang LH, Dai SD, Li QC, et al. Malignant solitary fibrous tumor of breast: a rare case report. Int J Clin Exp Pathol 2014;7:4461–6.

102. Salemis NS. Solitary fibrous tumor of the breast: A case report and the review of the literature. Breast J 2017, [Epub ahead of print].

103. Tsai SY, Hsu CY, Chou YH, et al. Solitary fibrous tumor of the breast: a case report and review of the literature. J Clin Ultrasound 2017;45:350–4.

104. Tyler GT. Report of a case of pure myxoma of the breast. Ann Surg 1915;61:121–7.

105. Chan YF, Yeung HY, Ma L. Myxoma of the breast: report of a case and ultrastrucutural study. Pathol-ogy 1986;18:153–7.

106. Balci P, Kabakci N, Isil T, et al. Breast myxoma: radiologic and histopathologic features. Breast J 2007;13:88–90.

107. Magro G, Cavanaugh B, Palazzo J. Clinico-patho-logical features of breast myxoma: report of a case with histogenetic considerations. Virch Arch 2010;456:581–6.

108. Nel J, O'Donnell M, Bradley R. Myxoma of the breast in a male patient. Breast J 2016;22:468–9.

109. Wargotz ES, Norris HJ, Austin RM, et al. Fibroma-tosis of the breast. A clinical and pathological study of 28 cases. Am J Surg Pathol 1987;11:38–45.

110. Rosen PP, Ernsberger D. Mammary fibromatosis. A benign spindle-cell tumor with significant risk for local recurrence. Cancer 1989;63:1363–9.

111. Devouassoux-Shisheboran M, Schammel MD, Man YG, et al. Fibromatosis of the breast: age-correlated morpho-functional features of 33 cases. Arch Pathol Lab Med 2000;124:276–80.

112. Magro G, Gurrera A, Scavo N, et al. Fibromatosis of the breast: a clinical, radiological and pathological study of 6 cases. Pathologica 2002;94:238–46.

113. Wongmaneerung P, Somwangprasert A, Watcharachan K, et al. Bilateral desmoid tumor of the breast: case series and literature review. Int Med Case Rep J 2016;9:247–51.

114. Wargotz ES, Deos PH, Norris HJ. Metaplastic carcinomas of the breast, II: spindle cell carcinoma. Hum Pathol 1989;20:732–40.

115. Gobbi H, Simpson JF, Borowsky A, et al. Metaplastic breast tumors with a dominant fibromatosis-like phenotype have a high risk of local recurrence. Cancer 1999;85:2170–82.

116. Sneige N, Yaziji H, Mandavilli SR, et al. Low-grade (fibromatosis-like) spindle cell carcinoma of the breast. Am J Surg Pathol 2001;25:1009–16.

117. Carter MR, Hornick JL, Lester S, et al. Spindle cell (sarcomatoid) carcinoma of the breast: a clinicopathologic and immunohistochemical analysis of 29 cases. Am J Surg Pathol 2006;30:300–9.

118. Dwyer JB, Clark BZ. Low-grade fibromatosis-like spindle cell carcinoma of the breast. Arch Pathol Lab Med 2015;139:552–7.

119. Taccagni G, Rovere E, Masullo M, et al. Myofibrosarcoma of the breast: review of the literature on myofibroblastic tumors and criteria for defining myofibroblastic differentiation. Am J Surg Pathol 1997;21:489–96.

120. Gocht A, Bösmüller HC, Bässler R, et al. Breast tumors with myofibroblastic differentiation: clinicopathological observations in myofibroblastoma and myofibrosarcoma. Pathol Res Pract 1999;195:1–10.

121. Lucin K, Mustać E, Jonjić N. Breast sarcoma showing myofibroblastic differentiation. Virch Arch 2003;443:222–4.

122. Morgan PB, Chundru S, Hatch SS, et al. Uncommon malignancies: case 1. Low-grade myofibroblastic sarcoma of the breast. J Clin Oncol 2005;23:6249–51.

123. Roberson GV. Fibrosarcoma of the breast. J Ark Med Soc 1973;69:257–65.

124. Pollard SG, Marks PV, Temple LN, et al. Breast sarcoma. A clinicopathologic review of 25 cases. Cancer 1990;66:941–4.

125. Adem C, Reynolds C, Ingle JN, et al. Primary breast sarcoma: clinicopathologic series from the Mayo Clinic and review of the literature. Br J Cancer 2004;91:237–41.

126. Jones MW, Norris HJ, Wargotz ES, et al. Fibrosarcoma-malignant fibrous histiocytoma of the breast. A clinicopathological study of 32 cases. Am J Surg Pathol 1992;16:667–74.

127. Lee JY, Kim DB, Kwak BS, et al. Primary fibrosarcoma of the breast: a case report. J Breast Cancer 2011;14:156–9.

128. Lee SJ, Mahoney MC, Shaughnessy E. Dermatofibrosarcoma protuberans of the breast: imaging features and review of the literature. AJR Am J Roentgenol 2009;193:W64–9.

129. Özcan TB, Hacıhasanoğlu E, Nazlı MA, et al. A rare breast tumor: dermatofibrosarcoma protuberans. J Breast Health 2016;12:44–6.

130. Valli R, Rossi G, Natalini G, et al. Dermatofibrosarcoma protuberans of the breast: a case report. Pathologica 2002;94:310–3.

131. Ramakrishnan V, Shoher A, Ehrlich M, et al. Atypical dermatofibrosarcoma protuberans in the breast. Breast J 2005;11:217–8.

132. Lee AH. Recent developments in the histological diagnosis of spindle cell carcinoma, fibromatosis and phyllodes tumour of the breast. Histopathology 2008;52:45–57.

Lobular Carcinoma In Situ

Hannah Y. Wen, MD, PhD*, Edi Brogi, MD, PhD

KEYWORDS

- Pleomorphic lobular carcinoma in situ • Variant lobular carcinoma in situ • E-cadherin • p120
- *CDH1* • Core biopsy

Key points

- Lobular carcinoma in situ (LCIS) is a risk factor *and* a nonobligate precursor lesion.
- LCIS shows loss of E-cadherin and diffuse cytoplasmic staining for p120 catenin.
- The most frequent chromosome alteration in LCIS is deletion of 16q; the most common somatic mutations in LCIS affect *CDH1* (gene encoding for E-cadherin).
- Surgical excision can be safely spared in patients with classic LCIS diagnosed on needle core biopsy with concordant imaging and pathologic findings.
- Surgical excision is recommended for LCIS with variant or pleomorphic morphology, and for classic LCIS with discordant imaging and/or pathologic findings.

ABSTRACT

Lobular carcinoma in situ (LCIS) is a risk factor and a nonobligate precursor of breast carcinoma. The relative risk of invasive carcinoma after classic LCIS diagnosis is approximately 9 to 10 times that of the general population. Classic LCIS diagnosed on core biopsy with concordant imaging and pathologic findings does not mandate surgical excision, and margin status is not reported. The identification of variant LCIS in a needle core biopsy specimen mandates surgical excision, regardless of radiologic-pathologic concordance. The presence of variant LCIS close to the surgical margin of a resection specimen is reported, and reexcision should be considered.

OVERVIEW

Foote and Stewart[1] first described lobular carcinoma in situ (LCIS) in 1941 as a rare form of mammary cancer originating in lobules and terminal ducts. They reported all the key morphologic features of LCIS that still hold true and accurate today: (1) LCIS is an incidental microscopic finding: "There is no way in which a clinical diagnosis of lobular carcinoma in situ can be made"... "There is no way by which it can be recognized grossly"; (2) LCIS has characteristic morphologic features: "The cells lose polarity, varying in shape while maintaining surprisingly uniform size"; (3) LCIS is multifocal: "it is always a disease of multiple foci." The aforementioned features characterize the so called "classic" form of LCIS. Even though classic LCIS constitutes both a risk factor *and* a nonobligate precursor of invasive breast cancer, it is currently managed as a benign lesion, and does not require complete removal and/or evaluation of margin status. Hormonal chemoprevention is recommended for patients with classic LCIS. In the eighth edition of the TNM staging by the American Joint Committee on Cancer (AJCC),[2] LCIS is no longer staged as Tis.[3]

Disclosure: The authors declare they have no conflict interest to disclose.
Department of Pathology, Memorial Sloan Kettering Cancer Center, 1275 York Avenue, New York, NY 10065, USA
* Corresponding author.
E-mail address: weny@mskcc.org

EPIDEMIOLOGY

Classic LCIS usually is an incidental finding in a breast needle core biopsy or surgical excision specimen targeting another lesion. It is therefore difficult to estimate the actual incidence of LCIS. LCIS is identified in 0.5% to 1.5% of benign breast biopsies[4–6] and in 1.8% to 2.5% of all breast biopsies.[4,7] In a population-based study using data from the Surveillance, Epidemiology, and End Results (SEER) program,[8] the incidence of LCIS in women without prior history of in situ or invasive breast carcinoma increased from 0.90 per 100,000 person-years in 1978 to 1980 to 3.19 per 100,000 person-years in 1996 to 1998.[8,9] The increased incidence of LCIS is likely due to the increased use of mammographic screening and biopsy of mammographically indeterminate or suspicious lesions. Age-specific incidence analysis revealed that the magnitude of the increase was highest among women ages ≥50 years, the age group most likely to participate in routine mammographic screening.[9]

CLINICAL FEATURES

LCIS occurs predominantly in premenopausal women, with mean and median age at diagnosis of 49 and 50 years, respectively (range 20s–80s).[10–13] LCIS is multicentric in 60% to 80% of patients[14] and bilateral in 20% to 60%.[11,15,16] Classic LCIS is clinically and mammographically occult, although recent studies report an association with grouped amorphous or granular mammographic calcifications,[13,17] or heterogeneous non-masslike enhancement with persistent enhancement kinetics on MRI.[17] LCIS variants, such as pleomorphic LCIS and LCIS with central necrosis, are usually detected mammographically due to associated pleomorphic calcifications, or can present as a mass lesion with or without associated calcifications.[13,18–25]

HISTOPATHOLOGY

CLASSIC LOBULAR CARCINOMA IN SITU

LCIS is a proliferation centered in the terminal ductal lobular units (TDLUs), and consists of neoplastic cells that fill and expand most (>50%) of the acini (Fig. 1). Pagetoid extension into the terminal ducts with growth of LCIS cells underneath the ductal epithelium is also common. The cross-section of a duct with pagetoid involvement by LCIS has a characteristic "cloverleaf" pattern (Fig. 2). Classic LCIS is a monomorphic, dyshesive proliferation of nonpolarized cells with round to oval shape, inconspicuous cytoplasm. The nuclei are located in the center of the cells, and are small, round to oval, with smooth nuclear membrane and inconspicuous nucleoli (Fig. 3). Cell borders are indistinct. Intracytoplasmic vacuoles are common, and signet-ring cell formation can occur (Fig. 4). Mitotic activity is absent to exceedingly rare.

The cells of classic LCIS can have scant cytoplasm ("small cells" or "type A" cells)[10] or be a bit larger ("large cell" type or "type B"),[10] with

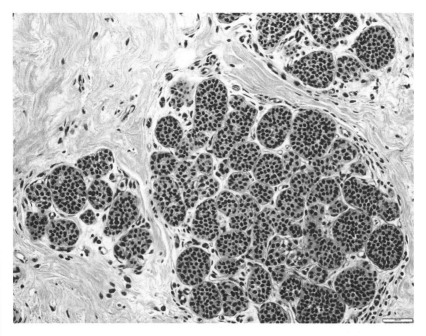

Fig. 1. LCIS, classic type. The acini are expanded by monomorphic, evenly spaced dyshesive cells with low-grade nuclear atypia. Magnification ×200.

Fig. 2. LCIS, classic type, with pagetoid growth in a duct. Magnification ×200.

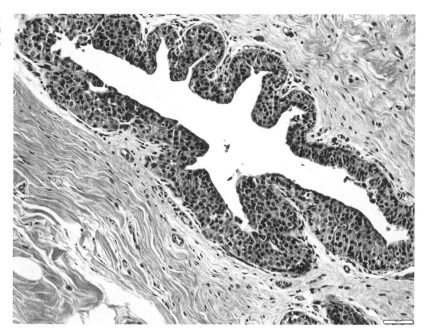

slightly more abundant cytoplasm, slightly larger nuclei and more prominent nucleoli (**Fig. 5**). The 2 cell types can coexist in the same patient, in the same breast, and even in the same lobule. In the absence of necrosis or marked nuclear pleomorphism, LCIS composed predominantly of large cells is best classified as classic LCIS.

The term lobular neoplasia refers to a morphologic spectrum of lesions including atypical lobular hyperplasia (ALH) and classic LCIS. The cells composing ALH are morphologically indistinguishable from those of classic LCIS, but the proliferation is limited to less than 50% of the acini of the terminal duct lobular units and none of the acini is markedly expanded (**Fig. 6**).[6,26] ALH has similar genetic alterations and immunohistochemical profile as classic LCIS, and the 2 lesions often coexist. ALH is associated with a fourfold to fivefold increase in the risk of subsequent breast carcinoma.

Fig. 3. LCIS, classic type with small cells (type A cells). Dyshesive and nonpolarized cells, with scant cytoplasm, monotonous, round to oval nuclei, with regular nuclear membrane, uniform chromatin, and inconspicuous nucleoli. Magnification ×400.

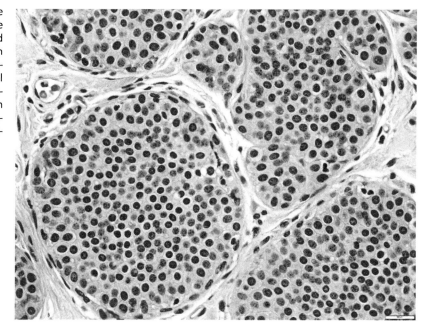

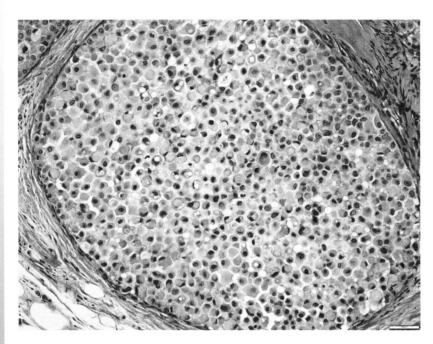

Fig. 4. LCIS with signet-ring cells. Magnification ×400.

LOBULAR CARCINOMA IN SITU VARIANTS

Pleomorphic Lobular Carcinoma In Situ

The term "pleomorphic" was first used to qualify a variant of invasive lobular carcinoma (ILC) showing the infiltrative pattern characteristic of classic ILC (single cell files or targetoid arrangement of dyshesive cells), but having marked nuclear pleomorphism.[27–30] Compared with classic ILC, pleomorphic ILC (P-ILC) consists of larger cells with round to ovoid shape, abundant cytoplasm, and large hyperchromatic nuclei that tend to be located slightly off-center, and have prominent nucleoli (Fig. 7). Binucleation is common. The cytoplasm is often eosinophilic, and slightly granular or foamy. Intracytoplasmic vacuoles similar

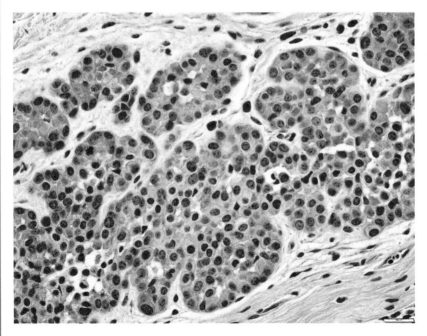

Fig. 5. LCIS, classic type with large cells (type B cells). The cells are slightly larger than type A cells (compare with Fig. 3), have more cytoplasm, slightly larger but uniform nuclei, with scattered nucleoli. Magnification ×400.

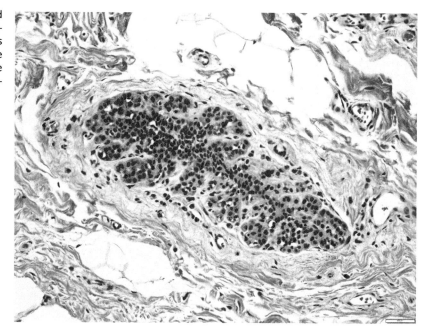

Fig. 6. ALH. Small round dyshesive cells, cytologically similar to the cells of classic LCIS, involve fewer than 50% of the acinar spaces. Magnification ×200.

to those seen in classic ILC are common. Mitotic activity is evident. Some P-ILCs show apocrine differentiation.

Pleomorphic LCIS (P-LCIS) was first described by Frost and colleagues[31] in 1996. The investigators reported a case of P-ILC with extensive in situ component that was morphologically similar to the P-ILC, centered in the lobules or with pagetoid extension into ducts. Middleton and colleagues[32] identified P-LCIS in 17 of 38 cases (45%) of P-ILC. Sneige and colleagues[22] studied 10 cases of P-LCIS without associated invasive carcinoma and 14 cases of P-LCIS with associated P-ILC, and found the histologic features of P-LCIS to be similar in cases with and without invasive carcinoma. Classic LCIS coexisted with P-LCIS in more than 40% of the cases.[22] Central necrosis and calcifications are common in

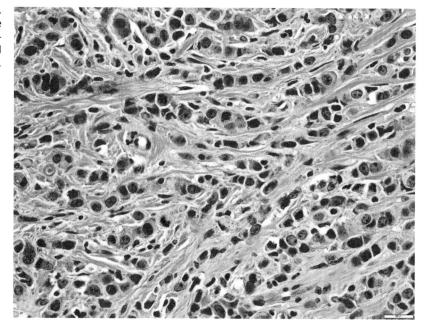

Fig. 7. Pleomorphic ILC. ILC with single-file growth pattern, dyshesive cells, and marked nuclear pleomorphism. Magnification ×400.

P-LCIS (Fig. 8), and mitoses are evident. In contrast to classic LCIS, P-LCIS is often detected mammographically as an area of calcifications, architectural distortion, and less frequently, as a mass lesion with or without associated calcifications.[20,22,23,25,33,34] Patients with P-LCIS tend to be significantly older than patients with classic LCIS,[20,23,34] and most are postmenopausal.[20,23,25] Some investigators further categorize P-LCIS into apocrine and nonapocrine types.[23] The cells of apocrine P-LCIS have abundant eosinophilic cytoplasm, and are frequently binucleated. Apocrine P-LCIS seems to be more common in postmenopausal women.[23]

Due to its solid growth pattern, marked nuclear pleomorphism, and presence of necrosis and calcifications, P-LCIS closely mimics ductal carcinoma in situ (DCIS) (Fig. 9). However, the cells of P-LCIS are dyshesive, lack true cell polarity, and do not form secondary lumina. Immunohistochemical stains for E-cadherin and p120 can help resolve the differential diagnosis of P-LCIS versus DCIS in ambiguous cases (see the "Immunohistochemistry" section).

Lobular Carcinoma In Situ with Necrosis (Also Known as "Florid" Lobular Carcinoma In Situ)

LCIS with necrosis refers to a proliferative lesion that exhibits the cytologic features of classic LCIS, including cell dyshesion and type A or type B morphology, but is characterized by massive expansion of the acini (at least 50 cells across the diameter of an acinus) and central necrosis (Fig. 10), which are incompatible with the diagnosis of classic LCIS. The necrotic foci often harbor calcifications. This lesion is also referred as "florid" LCIS.[24,35] LCIS with necrosis also tends to occur at an older age than classic LCIS, and is commonly associated with invasive carcinoma.[19] Fadare and colleagues[19] reported 18 cases of LCIS with comedo-type necrosis, 12 (67%) of which had associated invasive carcinoma, most commonly ILC with classic morphology. Like P-LCIS, LCIS with necrosis closely mimics solid DCIS. Among the 18 cases of LCIS with comedo-type necrosis reported by Fadare and colleagues,[19] 2 had initial diagnosis of DCIS on core biopsy. Immunohistochemical stains for E-cadherin and p120 can be useful to confirm the diagnosis in cases with ambiguous morphology (see the "Immunohistochemistry" section).

IMMUNOHISTOCHEMISTRY

E-CADHERIN

Rasbridge and colleagues[36] first reported the loss of E-cadherin expression in ILC in 1993. In the same year, several other investigators reported similar findings, as well as complete or partial loss of E-cadherin in LCIS and ALH.[37,38] E-cadherin, a member of the cadherin family, is a calcium-dependent cell-cell adhesion glycoprotein in epithelial cells.[39,40] E-cadherin is encoded by the CDH1 gene, located on chromosome 16q22.1.[41] Using polymerase chain reaction (PCR)/single-strand conformation polymorphism

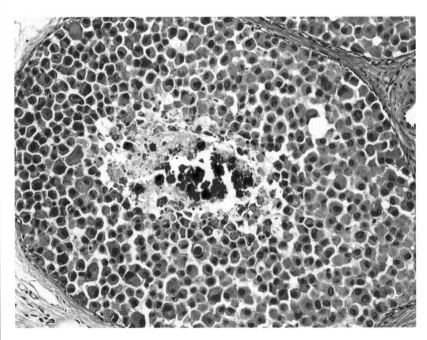

Fig. 8. LCIS, pleomorphic type. Dyshesive proliferation of round to oval cells with abundant cytoplasm, large eccentric nuclei with irregular nuclear membrane, coarse chromatin, and prominent nucleoli. Foci of necrosis with calcifications are common. Magnification ×200.

Fig. 9. DCIS, with solid growth pattern, high nuclear grade and necrosis. Magnification ×200.

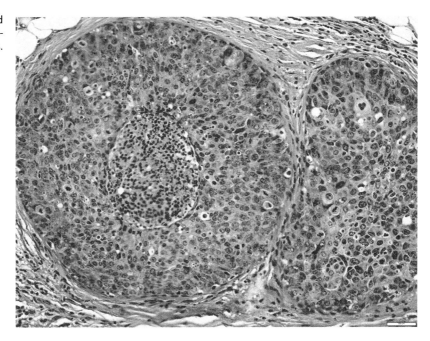

assay, Berx and colleagues[41,42] detected truncation mutations in the extracellular domain of E-cadherin, in combination with loss of heterozygosity (LOH) of chromosome 16q22.1 containing the *CDH1* gene in more than 50% of the ILCs examined. The same truncating mutations and LOH of the wild-type allele was also identified in LCIS.[43]

By immunohistochemistry, normal mammary glands, DCIS, and most invasive ductal carcinomas (IDCs) show strong and continuous membranous staining for E-cadherin (**Fig. 11**). In contrast, ILC and LCIS, including all LCIS variants, are characterized by loss or aberrant expression of the E-cadherin protein (**Fig. 12**). Immunohistochemical stain for E-cadherin is routinely used to distinguish lobular from ductal lesions, and is especially useful in separating LCIS variants from DCIS in cases with ambiguous morphology

Fig. 10. LCIS with central necrosis. This proliferation of cells morphologically indistinguishable from those of classic LCIS, is associated with massive acinar expansion (50 or more cells across the diameter of an expanded acinus) and central necrosis. Magnification ×200.

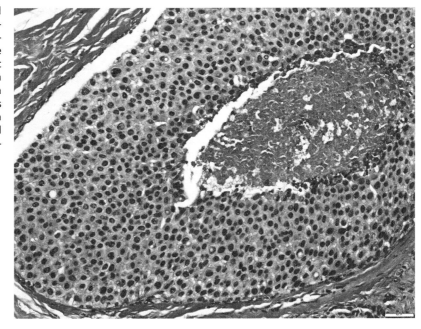

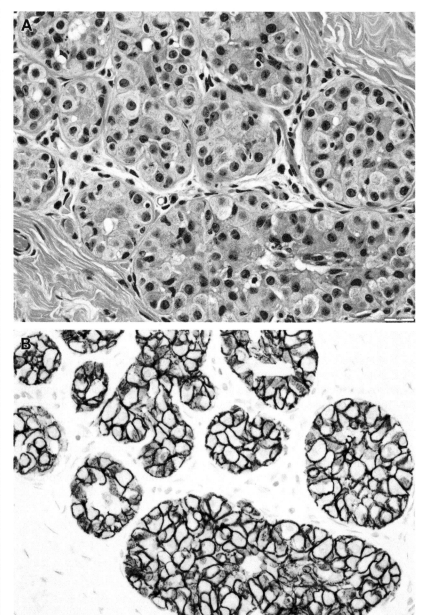

Fig. 11. DCIS, extending to lobules. (*A*) Hematoxylin-eosin (H&E) stain. (*B*) Immunohistochemical stain for E-cadherin. The cells show strong membranous staining for E-cadherin, consistent with ductal phenotype. Magnification ×200.

(**Figs. 13** and **14**). Most cases of LCIS demonstrate complete loss of E-cadherin staining (see **Fig. 14**B), but in some cases of LCIS, attenuated E-cadherin expression is observed, with scattered cells showing dotlike discontinuous and weak membranous staining or patchy cytoplasmic staining (see **Fig. 13**B).

The results of immunohistochemical staining should always be interpreted in the context of morphologic findings. Aberrant E-cadherin staining patterns have been documented in invasive mammary carcinoma and LCIS.[44–48] In particular, the finding of membranous E-cadherin with attenuated intensity does not preclude the diagnosis of LCIS in cases with conventional lobular morphology, and is attributed to presence of dysfunctional E-cadherin protein.[45,47]

Fig. 12. LCIS, pleomorphic type, with central necrosis. (*A*) H&E stain. (*B*) Immunohistochemical stain for E-cadherin. The LCIS cells are negative for E-cadherin. Magnification ×200.

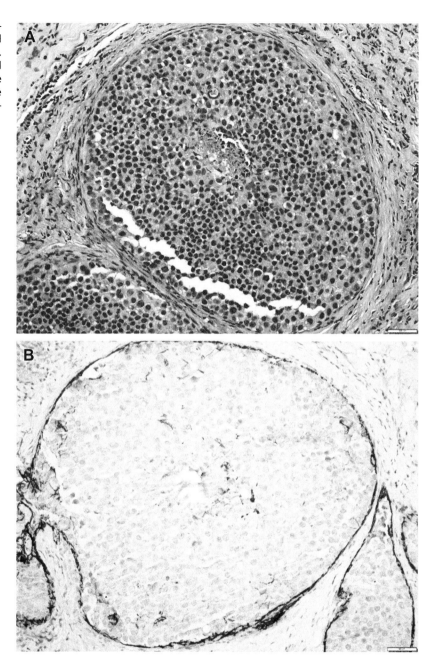

P120-CATENIN

p120, a tyrosine kinase substrate, interacts with E-cadherin and catenins and is required for cadherin-mediated cell-cell adhesion.[49–52] Cadherins are both necessary and sufficient to recruit p120 to the cell membrane.[52] In cells lacking functional cadherins, p120 is located in the cytoplasm (**Fig. 15**).[52] Sarrio and colleagues[53] reported cytoplasmic localization of p120 in all stages of lobular neoplasia, including ALH, LCIS, ILC, and metastatic lobular carcinoma. The investigators analyzed 326 breast biopsies using tissue microarrays, including 219 IDC, 69 ILC, 29 ALH, and 9 LCIS.[53] Immunohistochemical stain for p120 showed diffuse cytoplasmic staining in 90% (26/29) of ALH and 100% (9/9) of LCIS.[53] In contrast, ductal carcinoma showed reduced membranous staining for p120 but no cytoplasmic distribution.[53]

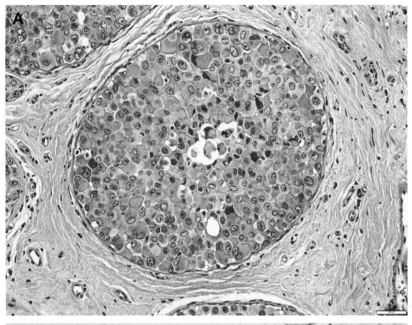

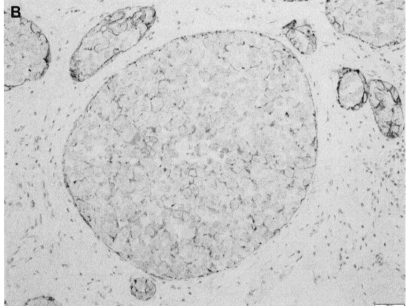

Fig. 13. P-LCIS, apocrine type. (*A*) H&E stain. (*B*) Immunohistochemical stain for E-cadherin. The cells are dyshesive, with abundant eosinophilic granular cytoplasm, large nuclei, and prominent nucleoli. Instead of complete loss of E-cadherin expression, the cells composing P-LCIS in this case show focal incomplete, attenuated, and granular membranous staining for E-cadherin. Magnification ×200.

Cytoplasmic location of p120 was significantly associated with the absence of E-cadherin expression. Using an MDA-231 breast cancer cell line that is negative for E-cadherin due to promoter hypermethylation, the investigators demonstrated that restored expression of E-cadherin induced a shift of p120 protein from the cytoplasm to the membrane, where p120 colocalized with reexpressed E-cadherin.[53] Dabbs and colleagues[54] evaluated the diagnostic utility of p120 in 64 ILC (49 classic and 15 pleomorphic) and 62 IDC. They documented loss of E-cadherin and intense cytoplasmic staining of p120 in all ILC cases. The immunostaining pattern for E-cadherin and p120 correlated with histology in 100% of the cases.[54] Based on these findings, the investigators

Fig. 14. LCIS with massive acinar expansion and central necrosis. (*A*) H&E stain. (*B*) Immunohistochemical stain for E-cadherin. This variant form of lobular carcinoma in situ closely mimics solid DCIS. The LCIS cells are completely negative for E-cadherin. Magnification ×200.

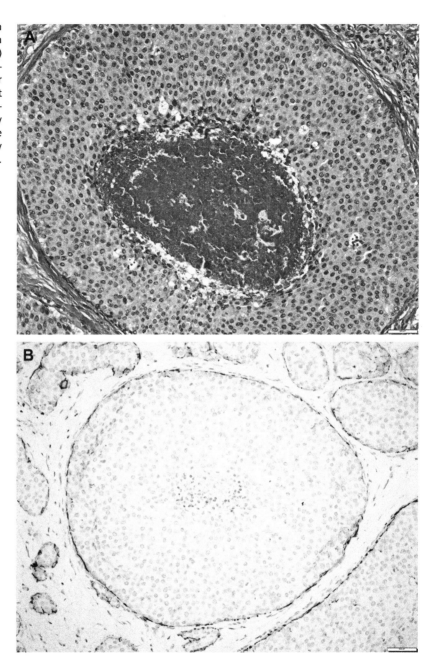

concluded cytoplasmic staining of p120 is a useful, positive marker for lobular neoplasia.[54] Diffuse cytoplasmic staining pattern for p120 is also observed in P-LCIS.[55]

ESTROGEN RECEPTOR, PROGESTERONE RECEPTOR, AND HUMAN EPIDERMAL GROWTH FACTOR RECEPTOR 2

Classic LCIS is usually positive for estrogen receptor (ER) and/or progesterone receptor (PR) and negative for human epidermal growth factor receptor 2 (HER2).[56] Immunohistochemical stains were performed in a subset of LCIS samples from patients enrolled in National Surgical Adjuvant Breast and Bowel Project (NSABP) Protocol B-17,[56] and all cases tested were positive for ER and PR, and negative for HER2.[56] In P-LCIS, ER is positive in 72% to 100% of the cases, PR in 50% to 100% of cases, and HER2 is overexpressed in 1% to 41% of the cases.[20,22,23,32,33] In a study of

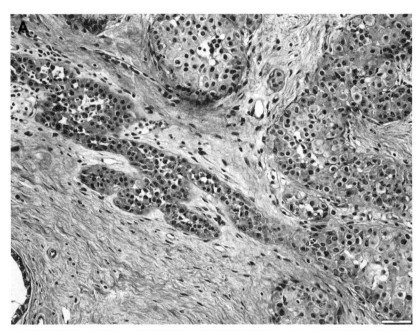

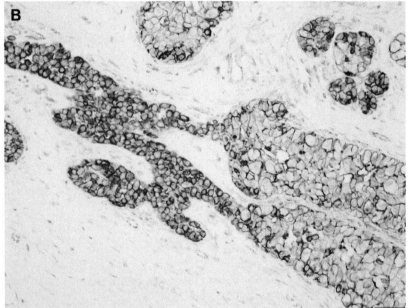

Fig. 15. A case with both LCIS (*left*) and DCIS (*right*). (*A*) H&E stain. (*B*) Immunohistochemical stain for p120. It demonstrates cytoplasmic expression of p120 in the LCIS and membranous staining in DCIS. Magnification ×200.

31 cases of P-LCIS, including 13 P-LCIS with apocrine morphology,[23] ER and PR expression was detected in all nonapocrine P-LCIS, but only in 20% of apocrine P-LCIS.[23] HER2 overexpression was identified in 13% of all P-LCIS, and was restricted to the apocrine P-LCIS.[23] At present, there is no recommendation to test and report ER, PR, and HER2 status in LCIS.

DIFFERENTIAL DIAGNOSIS AND DIAGNOSTIC PITFALLS

LOBULAR CARCINOMA IN SITU VARIANTS MIMIC SOLID DUCTAL CARCINOMA IN SITU

P-LCIS and LCIS with necrosis exhibit histologic features usually seen in DCIS, which may lead to possible misdiagnosis as DCIS with solid morphology. Sullivan and colleagues[57] retrospectively performed E-cadherin staining in a series of core biopsies with original diagnoses of solid DCIS. Ten (13.3%) of 75 cases were reclassified as LCIS, including 9 LCIS variants (5 P-LCIS and 4 LCIS with necrosis) and 1 classic LCIS.[57] LCIS variants display some morphologic features characteristic of LCIS, such as dyshesive growth, lack of microacinar formation, intracytoplasmic lumina and signet-ring cell morphology. The identification of any of these morphologic features in an intraductal solid proliferation should raise the differential diagnosis of LCIS variant. The latter diagnosis can be confirmed using immunohistochemical stains for E-cadherin and p120. LCIS shows loss of membranous staining for E-cadherin and diffuse cytoplasmic accumulation of p120. The management of patients with variant LCIS and no invasive carcinoma remains highly controversial, especially with respect to radiation therapy. Information regarding the clinical follow-up of patients with diagnosis of P-LCIS remains extremely limited, but a few small series suggest that P-LCIS tends to recur locally with or without associated invasion. Some series found lower recurrence rates in patients treated with radiation therapy.[20,25,34]

CLASSIC LOBULAR CARCINOMA IN SITU INVOLVING COLLAGENOUS SPHERULOSIS MIMICS LOW-GRADE CRIBRIFORM DUCTAL CARCINOMA IN SITU

Collagenous spherulosis, first described by Clement and colleagues[58] in 1987, is a benign lesion consisting of globoid deposits of variably collagenized matrix surrounded by basement membrane and myoepithelium. This alteration is often associated with myoepithelial hyperplasia. Collagenous spherulosis is usually an incidental microscopic finding, but in some cases can be detected mammographically due to associated calcifications.[59] LCIS often involves foci of collagenous spherulosis, in a pattern that can mimic low-grade cribriform DCIS (Fig. 16).[59–62] The key morphologic features distinguishing LCIS in collagenous spherulosis from low-grade cribriform DCIS, first reported by Sgroi and Koerner,[60] include the myoepithelial nature of the cells surrounding the spaces, the presence of basement membranelike material within the pseudoglandular spaces, and the dyshesive growth of the neoplastic cells that show cytomorphology of classic LCIS. Resetkova and colleagues[59] reviewed 59 cases of collagenous spherulosis, and found LCIS involving collagenous spherulosis in 15 of 59 cases, including 4 cases initially misinterpreted as DCIS by the submitting pathologist.[59]

LOBULAR CARCINOMA IN SITU INVOLVING SCLEROSING ADENOSIS MIMICS INVASIVE LOBULAR CARCINOMA

Sclerosing adenosis is a benign sclerosing alteration of the TDLU, characterized by distortion of acini and glands due to abundant deposition of periglandular basement membrane and stromal sclerosis (Fig. 17). Myoepithelial hyperplasia and epithelial calcifications are common. Sclerosing adenosis can be a focal finding, or it may diffusely involve the breast. Sclerosing adenosis is often detected mammographically due to associated calcifications or a mass lesion. Classic LCIS often involves foci of sclerosing adenosis, in an arrangement that can closely simulate invasive carcinoma (Fig. 18). The absence of stromal desmoplasia, the presence of a thick basement membrane, and retained myoepithelial cells around the sclerosed glands and tubules are useful diagnostic clues. Immunohistochemical stains for myoepithelial markers can be used in difficult cases (see Fig. 18B).

GENETICS

Lakhani and colleagues[63] first reported LOH on chromosomes 16q, 17q, 17p, and 13q in LCIS, using microdissection, polymorphic DNA markers and PCR assay. Comparative genomic hybridization (CGH) analysis of LCIS revealed a low average rate of copy number changes and no evidence of amplifications. The most frequent chromosome alteration in LCIS is the loss of 16q, followed by gain of 1q.[64–68] Other recurrent genetic alterations include loss of 16p, 17p, and 22q.[64] LCIS and ALH have similar patterns of genomic alterations.[64] LCIS/ALH and ILC share some common chromosome alterations; however, the average number of copy number changes in LCIS/ALH is significantly lower than in ILC and invasive carcinoma in general.[64] Loss of 16q is also the most common genetic alteration in low-grade DCIS,[69–71] tubular carcinoma, well-differentiated invasive carcinoma,[72] and premalignant lesions, such as atypical ductal hyperplasia (ADH)[73,74] and columnar cell changes with atypia.[75] In contrast, high-grade DCIS and poorly differentiated invasive carcinoma, show high frequency of amplifications (17q12, 11q13) and a higher average rate of genetic imbalances, suggesting distinct evolutional pathways between low-grade and high-grade tumors.[70] Comparing copy number alterations of LCIS, DCIS, and associated invasive carcinoma,

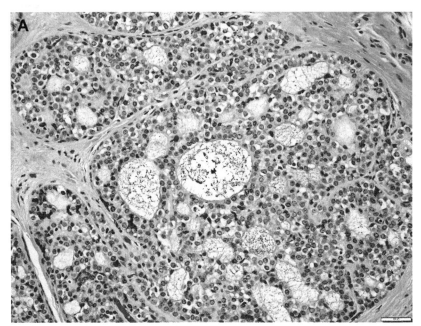

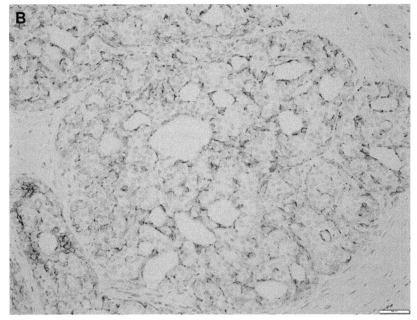

Fig. 16. LCIS involving collagenous spherulosis mimicking cribriform DCIS. (*A*) H&E stain. (*B*) Immunohistochemical stain for E-cadherin. Note the basement membrane-like material in the lumen and the dyshesive growth pattern of the neoplastic cells. The absent of immunoreactivity for E-cadherin in the neoplastic cells confirms the lobular phenotype. Magnification ×200.

Buerger and colleagues[65] proposed that LCIS and low-grade DCIS are closely related neoplastic lesions evolving from a single cell clone. Columnar cell changes, LCIS/ALH, low-grade DCIS, tubular carcinoma, ILC and well-differentiated IDC not only frequently coexist,[76,77] but also exhibit similar immunophenotypes[78] and clonal relationships,[79,80] supporting the hypothesis that these lesions are members of a family of low-grade lesions of the breast, including precursor lesions, in situ

and invasive carcinoma with low-grade morphology (see the article by Laura C. Collins's article, "Precursor Lesions of the Low Grade Breast Neoplasia Pathway," elsewhere in this issue).[76,78]

P-LCIS shares similar genomic alterations as classic LCIS, including 16q loss and 1q gain,[23,81] but shows higher numbers of genetic alterations. In particular, apocrine P-LCIS displays additional recurrent changes, such as amplification of the

Fig. 17. Sclerosing adenosis. Magnification ×200.

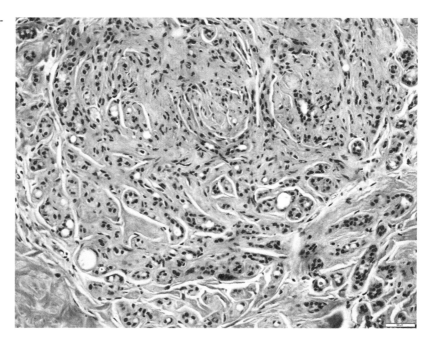

HER2 gene at 17q11.2 to 17q12, gain of 16p, loss of 8p and amplification of *cyclin D1* gene at 11q13.3.[23]

Genomic analyses reveal a clonal relationship and similar mutation profile between LCIS and synchronous or metachronous invasive carcinoma, supporting the role of LCIS as a precursor to invasive carcinoma.[67,82–86] Hwang and colleagues[67] analyzed 24 samples containing synchronous ipsilateral LCIS and ILC by microdissection and array CGH, and found 16q loss and 1q gain to be the most common alterations in LCIS and ILC, occurring in 100% and 90% of paired samples respectively.[67] In 14 of 24 cases, synchronous LCIS and ILC were found to be more similar to each other than to any of the other lesion pairings, calculated by weighted similarity scores.[67] Aulmann and colleagues[82] analyzed 9 paired cases of LCIS and subsequent ipsilateral invasive breast carcinoma (5 ILCs and 4 IDCs) by microdissection and mitochondrial D-loop sequencing. Clonal relationships were observed in 3 of the 5 LCIS/ILC pairs, whereas all 4 IDCs appeared to be clonally unrelated to the LCIS.[82] Andrade and colleagues[83] assessed clonal relationships by single nucleotide polymorphism array in 17 cases of LCIS and synchronous carcinoma, including 9 ILCs, 4 DCIS, and 4 IDCs. Seven (41%) pairs across all matched lesion types were found to be clonal. These studies demonstrated that at least a subset of LCIS represents a precursor of invasive carcinoma.

Targeted capture massively parallel sequencing and whole exome sequencing analyses identified a similar repertoire of somatic mutations in synchronous LCIS and ILC.[84–86] The most frequent somatic mutations in LCIS and ILC are *CDH1* (56% and 66%, respectively), *PIK3CA* (41% and 52%, respectively), and *CBFB* (12% and 19%, respectively).[84] The mutation of *CDH1* gene is in keeping with the loss of E-cadherin expression, a hallmark of lobular carcinoma. In addition to allele loss at *CDH1* locus (16q22.1) and somatic mutations of *CDH1* gene, epigenetic alterations such as promoter hypermethylation can also lead to downregulation or silencing of E-cadherin.[87–90]

Germline mutation of *CDH1* is associated with familial early-onset, poorly differentiated, diffuse gastric cancer,[91] and increased risk of lobular breast cancer.[92–95] In women with *CDH1* germline mutation, the estimated cumulative risk by age 80 years is more than 80% for gastric cancer, and 39% to 60% for breast cancer.[94–97] Annual breast MRI starting at age of 30 years is recommended for breast cancer surveillance in this group of women.[98]

NATURAL HISTORY AND PROGNOSIS

LCIS is a risk factor *and* a nonobligate morphologic precursor of invasive breast carcinoma. McDivitt and colleagues[99] reported a follow-up study of 50 patients with LCIS treated with local

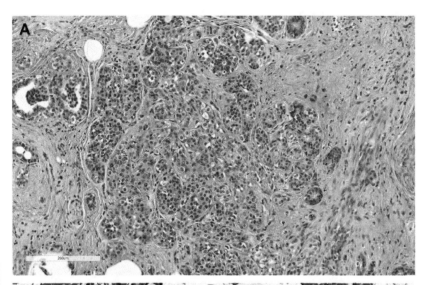

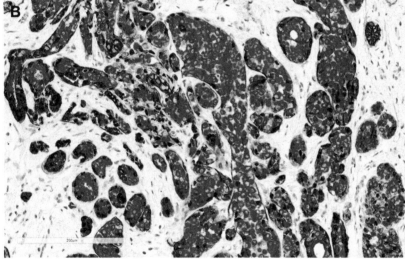

Fig. *18.* LCIS involving sclerosing adenosis. (*A*). H&E stain. (*B*). Immuno-histochemical stain for ADH5. ADH5 stain demonstrates the presence of myoepithelial cells surrounding adenosis and LCIS.

excision. The cumulative risk of subsequent invasive breast carcinoma was 8% after 5 years, 15% after 10 years, 27% after 15 years, 35% after 20 years, and more than 50% after 23 years.[99] The cumulative risk of contralateral breast cancer was 10% after 10 years, 15% after 15 years, and 25% after 20 years.[99] Several other long-term follow-up studies also indicated an increased incidence of breast cancer in both the ipsilateral and contralateral breasts in patients with LCIS.[4–6,10,100,101] In a recent long-term follow-up study of 1060 women with LCIS and median follow-up of 81 months (range, 6–368 months), 150 patients developed 168 breast cancers (63% ipsilateral, 25% contralateral, 12% bilateral). The annual incidence of breast carcinoma in women with LCIS was 2%.[12]

The subsequent breast carcinoma included DCIS (35%), IDC (29%), ILC (27%), and other types of invasive carcinoma (9%). The relative risk of subsequent breast carcinoma in patients with LCIS is 9 to 10 times greater than that in the general population.[5,6,101] The relative risk of invasive breast carcinoma after diagnosis of ALH is 3 to 5 times that of general population,[6,26,102,103] approximately one-half that of LCIS.[6] Analysis of SEER data revealed the minimum cumulative risk of developing invasive breast carcinoma after LCIS was 7.1% at 10 years, with equal predisposition in both breasts.[104] In a long-term follow-up study of 161 women with index diagnosis of ALH, 25 (16%) developed invasive breast cancer that arose in the ipsilateral breast in 17 cases

(68%) and in the contralateral breast in 5 cases (20%) with known laterality.[103] The relative risk of breast cancer in women with ALH and no other atypical lesion was 2.6 (95% confidence interval [CI] 1.7–3.9, *P*<.0001).[103] Most invasive carcinomas that developed in women with ALH had low Nottingham grade and excellent survival.[105] The distinction between ALH and LCIS remains valuable for the purpose of patient counseling.

MANAGEMENT

Historically, mastectomy was recommended for women with LCIS, based on the observation that there is an increased risk of subsequent invasive breast cancer.[1,7,16,100] Haagensen and colleagues[10] pioneered the concept that "when it (LCIS) occurs alone without accompanying infiltrating carcinoma, it is a distinctive benign disease which predisposes to subsequent carcinoma" and advocated a more conservative approach of close follow-up as an alternative to mastectomy. Currently, there is a general agreement that LCIS represents both a risk factor *and* a nonobligate precursor of breast cancer. Observation alone is the preferred management option. Counseling for chemoprevention with tamoxifen or aromatase inhibitors is recommended.

The National Comprehensive Cancer Network (NCCN) guidelines recommend follow-up of patients with physical examinations every 6 to 12 months and annual diagnostic mammograms.[106] In the eighth edition of the AJCC staging system, LCIS has been removed from the staging classification system and is no longer included in the pathologic tumor in situ (pTis) category.[3]

Results of randomized controlled clinical trials support the use of tamoxifen or aromatase inhibitors for risk reduction among women at increased risk of breast cancer. The National Surgical Adjuvant Breast and Bowel Project (NSABP) Breast Cancer Prevention Trial (P-1) demonstrated that subsequent risk of invasive breast cancer can be significantly reduced by tamoxifen.[107] In the NSABP P-1 trial, women (n = 13,388) at increased risk for breast cancer were randomly assigned to receive placebo (n = 6707) or 20 mg/d tamoxifen (n = 6681) for 5 years. Patients with increased breast cancer risk were defined as 60 years of age or older, or 35 to 59 years of age with a 5-year predicted risk for breast cancer of at least 1.66%, or those with a history of LCIS.[107] Tamoxifen reduced the risk of invasive breast cancer by 49%.[107] The National Cancer Institute of Canada Clinical Trials Group Mammary Prevention.3 Trial (NCIC CTG MAP.3) is a randomized, placebo-controlled, double-blind trial of exemestane for breast cancer prevention in postmenopausal women.[108] Postmenopausal women were eligible if they had at least one of the following risk factors: age 60 years or older, Gail risk score greater than 1.66%, prior ADH or ALH or LCIS on breast biopsy, or prior DCIS treated with mastectomy. A total of 4560 women were randomized to either exemestane (2285 patients) or placebo (2275 patients).[108] At a median follow-up of 35 months, exemestane reduced the relative incidence of invasive breast cancers by 65%, from 0.55% to 0.19%.[108] King and colleagues[12] reported a 29-year longitudinal single institution experience with LCIS. Among 1060 patients with LCIS without concurrent breast cancer diagnosed between 1980 and 2009, 1004 chose surveillance with (n = 173) or without (n = 831) chemoprevention.[12] The overall cumulative cancer incidence at 15 years was 26%, with a 2% annual incidence of breast cancer. The 10-year cumulative cancer risks in women with or without chemoprevention were 7% and 21%, respectively. In multivariate analysis, chemoprevention was the only clinical factor associated with breast cancer risk reduction.[12] The American Society of Clinical Oncology Clinical Practice guidelines recommend that the use of chemoprevention should be discussed as an option to reduce the risk of breast cancer in high-risk patients.[109]

The natural history of P-LCIS remains poorly characterized. Due to the rarity of P-LCIS without concurrent invasive carcinoma, reports of the natural history of P-LCIS are anecdotal. No randomized prospective clinical trial data are available. Currently there is no consensus regarding the treatment recommendations for P-LCIS. A survey sent to self-identified breast surgeons revealed that in cases of P-LCIS present at the surgical margins, 53% of the surgeons would not reexcise, 23% sometimes would reexcise, and 24% would always reexcise.[110] All published series on outcomes of P-LCIS are retrospective and adjuvant therapy was not uniform (**Table 1**).[20,25,34,111] According to the 2012 WHO consensus classification, "in the absence of better information on the natural history of pleomorphic LCIS, caution should be exercised in recommending more aggressive management strategies, such as excision to negative margins or mastectomy as a routine practice after a diagnostic surgical biopsy reveals pleomorphic LCIS."[111] According to the NCCN guidelines,[106] "Some variants of LCIS (pleomorphic LCIS) may have a similar biological behavior to that of DCIS. Clinicians may consider complete excision with negative margins for pleomorphic LCIS, but this may lead to high mastectomy rate without proven clinical benefit. There are no data to support using radiotherapy in this setting".[106]

Table 1
Characteristics and outcomes of patients with pure P-LCIS in the published series

Authors, Year	No. of Patients	Surgery	Margin Clearance				Additional Therapy			Median Follow-up, Month	Recurrence Rate
			At Margin	<1 mm	1.1–2 mm	>2 mm	CP	XRT	CP + XRT		
Downs-Kelly et al,[111] 2011	26	BCS	6 (23%)	7 (27%)	4 (15%)	9 (35%)	6 (23%)	4 (15%)	6 (23%)	46	1 (3.8%) (had positive margin)
Khoury et al,[20] 2014	31	BCS 29 (94%) TM 2 (6%)	9 (29%)	No data	No data	No data	11 (35%)	3 (10%)	No data	55.6	6 (19.4%) (4 had positive margin)
Flanagan et al,[25] 2015	12	BCS	No data	4 (30%)	No data	No data	3 (25%)	1 (8%)	No data	49	None
De Brot et al,[34] 2017	7	BCS	2 (29%)	3 (43%)	No data	No data	1 (14%)	0	0	67	4 (57%)

Abbreviations: BCS, breast conserving surgery; CP, chemoprevention; TM, total mastectomy; XRT, radiation therapy.

The management of patients with classic LCIS or ALH diagnosed at needle core biopsy with radiologic-pathologic concordant findings is also debated and is the subject of an article by Benjamin C. Calhoun's article, "Core Needle Biopsy of the Breast: An Evaluation of Contemporary Data," elsewhere in this issue. In brief, the past decade has seen the publication of studies with careful radiologic-pathologic correlation and acceptably low upgrade rates (1%–4.4%) at surgical excision of classic LCIS or ALH diagnosed at needle core biopsy with radiologic-pathologic concordant findings.[112–119] A recent prospective multi-institutional trial (TBCRC 020) revealed a 1% (1/74; 95% CI 0.01–7) upgrade rate for cases with central pathology review.[120] These results have demonstrated that routine excision is not indicated for patients with classic LCIS or ALH on core biopsy and concordant imaging findings. As specified in the 2016 consensus guidelines by the American Society of Breast Surgeons, "we no longer advocate *routine* excision of ALH or LCIS when the radiological and pathologic diagnoses are concordant, and no other lesions requiring excision are present."[121]

LCIS variants (pleomorphic LCIS or LCIS with necrosis) diagnosed on core biopsy require surgical excision. The reported upgrade rates were 25% to 30%.[25,33,57,122] The NCCN guidelines recommend surgical excision for pleomorphic LCIS and classic LCIS with discordant imaging findings.[106]

SUMMARY

The relative risk of invasive carcinoma after a diagnosis of classic LCIS is approximately 9 to 10 times that of general population. LCIS and ILC share common copy number alterations and somatic mutations. A subset of LCIS is clonally related to synchronous or subsequent invasive breast carcinoma. Classic LCIS diagnosed at needle core biopsy with concordant imaging and pathologic findings does not mandate surgical excision. Active surveillance and chemoprevention are management options for classic LCIS. The finding of variant LCIS at needle core biopsy warrants surgical excision. The management of patients with variant LCIS and no invasive carcinoma on excision is the subject of debate.

REFERENCES

1. Foote FW, Stewart FW. Lobular carcinoma in situ: a rare form of mammary cancer. Am J Pathol 1941; 17:491–6, 3.

2. Amin MB, Edge SB. AJCC Cancer Staging Manual. 8th Edition. Springer; 2017.

3. Giuliano AE, Connolly JL, Edge SB, et al. Breast cancer—major changes in the American Joint Committee on Cancer eighth edition cancer staging manual. CA Cancer J Clin 2017;67(4):290–303.

4. Wheeler JE, Enterline HT, Roseman JM, et al. Lobular carcinoma in situ of the breast. Long-term followup. Cancer 1974;34:554–63.

5. Andersen JA. Lobular carcinoma in situ of the breast. An approach to rational treatment. Cancer 1977;39:2597–602.

6. Page DL, Kidd TE Jr, Dupont WD, et al. Lobular neoplasia of the breast: higher risk for subsequent invasive cancer predicted by more extensive disease. Hum Pathol 1991;22:1232–9.

7. Giordano JM, Klopp CT. Lobular carcinoma in situ: incidence and treatment. Cancer 1973;31:105–9.

8. Li CI, Anderson BO, Daling JR, et al. Changing incidence of lobular carcinoma in situ of the breast. Breast Cancer Res Treat 2002;75:259–68.

9. Li CI, Daling JR, Malone KE. Age-specific incidence rates of in situ breast carcinomas by histologic type, 1980 to 2001. Cancer Epidemiol Biomarkers Prev 2005;14:1008–11.

10. Haagensen CD, Lane N, Lattes R, et al. Lobular neoplasia (so-called lobular carcinoma in situ) of the breast. Cancer 1978;42:737–69.

11. Beute BJ, Kalisher L, Hutter RV. Lobular carcinoma in situ of the breast: clinical, pathologic, and mammographic features. AJR Am J Roentgenol 1991;157:257–65.

12. King TA, Pilewskie M, Muhsen S, et al. Lobular carcinoma in situ: a 29-year longitudinal experience evaluating clinicopathologic features and breast cancer risk. J Clin Oncol 2015;33:3945–52.

13. Maxwell AJ, Clements K, Dodwell DJ, et al. The radiological features, diagnosis and management of screen-detected lobular neoplasia of the breast: findings from the Sloane Project. Breast 2016;27:109–15.

14. Powers RW, O'Brien PH, Kreutner A Jr. Lobular carcinoma in situ. J Surg Oncol 1980;13:269–73.

15. Hutter RV, Snyder RE, Lucas JC, et al. Clinical and pathologic correlation with mammographic findings in lobular carcinoma in situ. Cancer 1969;23:826–39.

16. Hutter RV. The management of patients with lobular carcinoma in situ of the breast. Cancer 1984;53:798–802.

17. Scoggins M, Krishnamurthy S, Santiago L, et al. Lobular carcinoma in situ of the breast: clinical, radiological, and pathological correlation. Acad Radiol 2013;20:463–70.

18. Georgian-Smith D, Lawton TJ. Calcifications of lobular carcinoma in situ of the breast: radiologic-pathologic correlation. AJR Am J Roentgenol 2001;176:1255–9.

19. Fadare O, Dadmanesh F, Alvarado-Cabrero I, et al. Lobular intraepithelial neoplasia [lobular carcinoma in situ] with comedo-type necrosis: A clinicopathologic study of 18 cases. Am J Surg Pathol 2006;30: 1445–53.

20. Khoury T, Karabakhtsian RG, Mattson D, et al. Pleomorphic lobular carcinoma in situ of the breast: clinicopathological review of 47 cases. Histopathology 2014;64:981–93.

21. Sapino A, Frigerio A, Peterse JL, et al. Mammographically detected in situ lobular carcinomas of the breast. Virchows Arch 2000;436:421–30.

22. Sneige N, Wang J, Baker BA, et al. Clinical, histopathologic, and biologic features of pleomorphic lobular (ductal-lobular) carcinoma in situ of the breast: a report of 24 cases. Mod Pathol 2002;15: 1044–50.

23. Chen YY, Hwang ES, Roy R, et al. Genetic and phenotypic characteristics of pleomorphic lobular carcinoma in situ of the breast. Am J Surg Pathol 2009;33:1683–94.

24. Shin SJ, Lal A, De Vries S, et al. Florid lobular carcinoma in situ: molecular profiling and comparison to classic lobular carcinoma in situ and pleomorphic lobular carcinoma in situ. Hum Pathol 2013; 44:1998–2009.

25. Flanagan MR, Rendi MH, Calhoun KE, et al. Pleomorphic lobular carcinoma in situ: radiologic-pathologic features and clinical management. Ann Surg Oncol 2015;22:4263–9.

26. Page DL, Dupont WD, Rogers LW, et al. Atypical hyperplastic lesions of the female breast. A long-term follow-up study. Cancer 1985;55: 2698–708.

27. Dixon JM, Anderson TJ, Page DL, et al. Infiltrating lobular carcinoma of the breast. Histopathology 1982;6:149–61.

28. Page DL, Anderson TJ. Diagnostic histopathology of the breast. Philadelphia: WB Saunders; 1987.

29. Eusebi V, Magalhaes F, Azzopardi JG. Pleomorphic lobular carcinoma of the breast: an aggressive tumor showing apocrine differentiation. Hum Pathol 1992;23:655–62.

30. Weidner N, Semple JP. Pleomorphic variant of invasive lobular carcinoma of the breast. Hum Pathol 1992;23:1167–71.

31. Frost AR, Tsangaris TN, Silverberg SG. Pleomorphic lobular carcinoma in situ. AJSP: Reviews & Reports 1996;1:27–31.

32. Middleton LP, Palacios DM, Bryant BR, et al. Pleomorphic lobular carcinoma: morphology, immunohistochemistry, and molecular analysis. Am J Surg Pathol 2000;24:1650–6.

33. Chivukula M, Haynik DM, Brufsky A, et al. Pleomorphic lobular carcinoma in situ (PLCIS) on breast core needle biopsies: clinical significance and immunoprofile. Am J Surg Pathol 2008;32:1721–6.

34. De Brot M, Koslow Mautner S, Muhsen S, et al. Pleomorphic lobular carcinoma in situ of the breast: a single institution experience with clinical follow-up and centralized pathology review. Breast Cancer Res Treat 2017;165(2):411–20.

35. Hoda SA, Brogi E, Koerner FC, et al. Rosen's breast pathology. 4th edition. Wolters Kluwer; 2014.

36. Rasbridge SA, Gillett CE, Sampson SA, et al. Epithelial (E-) and placental (P-) cadherin cell adhesion molecule expression in breast carcinoma. J Pathol 1993;169:245–50.

37. Gamallo C, Palacios J, Suarez A, et al. Correlation of E-cadherin expression with differentiation grade and histological type in breast carcinoma. Am J Pathol 1993;142:987–93.

38. Moll R, Mitze M, Frixen UH, et al. Differential loss of E-cadherin expression in infiltrating ductal and lobular breast carcinomas. Am J Pathol 1993;143:1731–42.

39. Yoshida-Noro C, Suzuki N, Takeichi M. Molecular nature of the calcium-dependent cell-cell adhesion system in mouse teratocarcinoma and embryonic cells studied with a monoclonal antibody. Dev Biol 1984;101:19–27.

40. Nagafuchi A, Shirayoshi Y, Okazaki K, et al. Transformation of cell adhesion properties by exogenously introduced E-cadherin cDNA. Nature 1987;329:341–3.

41. Berx G, Staes K, van Hengel J, et al. Cloning and characterization of the human invasion suppressor gene E-cadherin (CDH1). Genomics 1995;26:281–9.

42. Berx G, Cleton-Jansen AM, Strumane K, et al. E-cadherin is inactivated in a majority of invasive human lobular breast cancers by truncation mutations throughout its extracellular domain. Oncogene 1996;13:1919–25.

43. Vos CB, Cleton-Jansen AM, Berx G, et al. E-cadherin inactivation in lobular carcinoma in situ of the breast: an early event in tumorigenesis. Br J Cancer 1997;76:1131–3.

44. Harigopal M, Shin SJ, Murray MP, et al. Aberrant E-cadherin staining patterns in invasive mammary carcinoma. World J Surg Oncol 2005;3:73.

45. Da Silva L, Parry S, Reid L, et al. Aberrant expression of E-cadherin in lobular carcinomas of the breast. Am J Surg Pathol 2008;32:773–83.

46. Choi YJ, Pinto MM, Hao L, et al. Interobserver variability and aberrant E-cadherin immunostaining of lobular neoplasia and infiltrating lobular carcinoma. Mod Pathol 2008;21:1224–37.

47. Dabbs DJ, Schnitt SJ, Geyer FC, et al. Lobular neoplasia of the breast revisited with emphasis on the role of E-cadherin immunohistochemistry. Am J Surg Pathol 2013;37:e1–11.

48. Canas-Marques R, Schnitt SJ. E-cadherin immunohistochemistry in breast pathology: uses and pitfalls. Histopathology 2016;68:57–69.

49. Reynolds AB, Daniel J, McCrea PD, et al. Identification of a new catenin: the tyrosine kinase

substrate p120cas associates with E-cadherin complexes. Mol Cell Biol 1994;14:8333–42.

50. Shibamoto S, Hayakawa M, Takeuchi K, et al. Association of p120, a tyrosine kinase substrate, with E-cadherin/catenin complexes. J Cell Biol 1995;128:949–57.

51. Daniel JM, Reynolds AB. The tyrosine kinase substrate p120cas binds directly to E-cadherin but not to the adenomatous polyposis coli protein or alpha-catenin. Mol Cell Biol 1995;15:4819–24.

52. Thoreson MA, Anastasiadis PZ, Daniel JM, et al. Selective uncoupling of p120(ctn) from E-cadherin disrupts strong adhesion. J Cell Biol 2000;148:189–202.

53. Sarrio D, Perez-Mies B, Hardisson D, et al. Cytoplasmic localization of p120ctn and E-cadherin loss characterize lobular breast carcinoma from preinvasive to metastatic lesions. Oncogene 2004;23:3272–83.

54. Dabbs DJ, Bhargava R, Chivukula M. Lobular versus ductal breast neoplasms: the diagnostic utility of p120 catenin. Am J Surg Pathol 2007;31:427–37.

55. Dabbs DJ, Kaplai M, Chivukula M, et al. The spectrum of morphomolecular abnormalities of the E-cadherin/catenin complex in pleomorphic lobular carcinoma of the breast. Appl Immunohistochem Mol Morphol 2007;15:260–6.

56. Fisher ER, Costantino J, Fisher B, et al. Pathologic findings from the National Surgical Adjuvant Breast Project (NSABP) Protocol B-17. Five-year observations concerning lobular carcinoma in situ. Cancer 1996;78:1403–16.

57. Sullivan ME, Khan SA, Sullu Y, et al. Lobular carcinoma in situ variants in breast cores: potential for misdiagnosis, upgrade rates at surgical excision, and practical implications. Arch Pathol Lab Med 2010;134:1024–8.

58. Clement PB, Young RH, Azzopardi JG. Collagenous spherulosis of the breast. Am J Surg Pathol 1987;11:411–7.

59. Resetkova E, Albarracin C, Sneige N. Collagenous spherulosis of breast: morphologic study of 59 cases and review of the literature. Am J Surg Pathol 2006;30:20–7.

60. Sgroi D, Koerner FC. Involvement of collagenous spherulosis by lobular carcinoma in situ. Potential confusion with cribriform ductal carcinoma in situ. Am J Surg Pathol 1995;19:1366–70.

61. Hill P, Cawson J. Collagenous spherulosis with lobular carcinoma in situ: a potential diagnostic pitfall. Pathology 2007;39:361–3.

62. Eisenberg RE, Hoda SA. Lobular carcinoma in situ with collagenous spherulosis: clinicopathologic characteristics of 38 cases. Breast J 2014;20:440–1.

63. Lakhani SR, Collins N, Sloane JP, et al. Loss of heterozygosity in lobular carcinoma in situ of the breast. Clin Mol Pathol 1995;48:M74–8.

64. Lu YJ, Osin P, Lakhani SR, et al. Comparative genomic hybridization analysis of lobular carcinoma in situ and atypical lobular hyperplasia and potential roles for gains and losses of genetic material in breast neoplasia. Cancer Res 1998;58:4721–7.

65. Buerger H, Simon R, Schafer KL, et al. Genetic relation of lobular carcinoma in situ, ductal carcinoma in situ, and associated invasive carcinoma of the breast. Mol Pathol 2000;53:118–21.

66. Etzell JE, Devries S, Chew K, et al. Loss of chromosome 16q in lobular carcinoma in situ. Hum Pathol 2001;32:292–6.

67. Hwang ES, Nyante SJ, Yi Chen Y, et al. Clonality of lobular carcinoma in situ and synchronous invasive lobular carcinoma. Cancer 2004;100:2562–72.

68. Mastracci TL, Shadeo A, Colby SM, et al. Genomic alterations in lobular neoplasia: a microarray comparative genomic hybridization signature for early neoplastic proliferation in the breast. Genes Chromosomes Cancer 2006;45:1007–17.

69. Tsuda H, Fukutomi T, Hirohashi S. Pattern of gene alterations in intraductal breast neoplasms associated with histological type and grade. Clin Cancer Res 1995;1:261–7.

70. Buerger H, Otterbach F, Simon R, et al. Comparative genomic hybridization of ductal carcinoma in situ of the breast-evidence of multiple genetic pathways. J Pathol 1999;187:396–402.

71. Fujii H, Szumel R, Marsh C, et al. Genetic progression, histological grade, and allelic loss in ductal carcinoma in situ of the breast. Cancer Res 1996;56:5260–5.

72. Buerger H, Otterbach F, Simon R, et al. Different genetic pathways in the evolution of invasive breast cancer are associated with distinct morphological subtypes. J Pathol 1999;189:521–6.

73. Lakhani SR, Collins N, Stratton MR, et al. Atypical ductal hyperplasia of the breast: clonal proliferation with loss of heterozygosity on chromosomes 16q and 17p. J Clin Pathol 1995;48:611–5.

74. Tsuda H, Takarabe T, Akashi-Tanaka S, et al. Pattern of chromosome 16q loss differs between an atypical proliferative lesion and an intraductal or invasive ductal carcinoma occurring subsequently in the same area of the breast. Mod Pathol 2001;14:382–8.

75. Simpson PT, Gale T, Reis-Filho JS, et al. Columnar cell lesions of the breast: the missing link in breast cancer progression? A morphological and molecular analysis. Am J Surg Pathol 2005;29:734–46.

76. Abdel-Fatah TM, Powe DG, Hodi Z, et al. High frequency of coexistence of columnar cell lesions, lobular neoplasia, and low grade ductal carcinoma in situ with invasive tubular carcinoma and invasive lobular carcinoma. Am J Surg Pathol 2007;31:417–26.

77. Brandt SM, Young GQ, Hoda SA. The "Rosen Triad": tubular carcinoma, lobular carcinoma in situ, and columnar cell lesions. Adv Anat Pathol 2008;15:140–6.

78. Abdel-Fatah TM, Powe DG, Hodi Z, et al. Morphologic and molecular evolutionary pathways of low nuclear grade invasive breast cancers and their putative precursor lesions: further evidence to support the concept of low nuclear grade breast neoplasia family. Am J Surg Pathol 2008;32:513–23.

79. Aulmann S, Elsawaf Z, Penzel R, et al. Invasive tubular carcinoma of the breast frequently is clonally related to flat epithelial atypia and low-grade ductal carcinoma in situ. Am J Surg Pathol 2009; 33:1646–53.

80. Wagner PL, Kitabayashi N, Chen YT, et al. Clonal relationship between closely approximated low-grade ductal and lobular lesions in the breast: a molecular study of 10 cases. Am J Clin Pathol 2009;132:871–6.

81. Reis-Filho JS, Simpson PT, Jones C, et al. Pleomorphic lobular carcinoma of the breast: role of comprehensive molecular pathology in characterization of an entity. J Pathol 2005;207:1–13.

82. Aulmann S, Penzel R, Longerich T, et al. Clonality of lobular carcinoma in situ (LCIS) and metachronous invasive breast cancer. Breast Cancer Res Treat 2008;107:331–5.

83. Andrade VP, Ostrovnaya I, Seshan VE, et al. Clonal relatedness between lobular carcinoma in situ and synchronous malignant lesions. Breast Cancer Res 2012;14:R103.

84. Sakr RA, Schizas M, Carniello JV, et al. Targeted capture massively parallel sequencing analysis of LCIS and invasive lobular cancer: repertoire of somatic genetic alterations and clonal relationships. Mol Oncol 2016;10:360–70.

85. Begg CB, Ostrovnaya I, Carniello JV, et al. Clonal relationships between lobular carcinoma in situ and other breast malignancies. Breast Cancer Res 2016;18:66.

86. Shah V, Nowinski S, Levi D, et al. PIK3CA mutations are common in lobular carcinoma in situ, but are not a biomarker of progression. Breast Cancer Res 2017;19:7.

87. Yoshiura K, Kanai Y, Ochiai A, et al. Silencing of the E-cadherin invasion-suppressor gene by CpG methylation in human carcinomas. Proc Natl Acad Sci U S A 1995;92:7416–9.

88. Graff JR, Herman JG, Lapidus RG, et al. E-cadherin expression is silenced by DNA hypermethylation in human breast and prostate carcinomas. Cancer Res 1995;55:5195–9.

89. Droufakou S, Deshmane V, Roylance R, et al. Multiple ways of silencing E-cadherin gene expression in lobular carcinoma of the breast. Int J Cancer 2001;92:404–8.

90. Sarrio D, Moreno-Bueno G, Hardisson D, et al. Epigenetic and genetic alterations of APC and CDH1 genes in lobular breast cancer: relationships with abnormal E-cadherin and catenin expression

and microsatellite instability. Int J Cancer 2003; 106:208–15.

91. Guilford P, Hopkins J, Harraway J, et al. E-cadherin germline mutations in familial gastric cancer. Nature 1998;392:402–5.

92. Keller G, Vogelsang H, Becker I, et al. Diffuse type gastric and lobular breast carcinoma in a familial gastric cancer patient with an E-cadherin germline mutation. Am J Pathol 1999;155:337–42.

93. Guilford PJ, Hopkins JB, Grady WM, et al. E-cadherin germline mutations define an inherited cancer syndrome dominated by diffuse gastric cancer. Hum Mutat 1999;14:249–55.

94. Pharoah PD, Guilford P, Caldas C, International Gastric Cancer Linkage Consortium. Incidence of gastric cancer and breast cancer in CDH1 (E-cadherin) mutation carriers from hereditary diffuse gastric cancer families. Gastroenterology 2001;121:1348–53.

95. Kaurah P, MacMillan A, Boyd N, et al. Founder and recurrent CDH1 mutations in families with hereditary diffuse gastric cancer. JAMA 2007;297:2360–72.

96. Fitzgerald RC, Hardwick R, Huntsman D, et al. Hereditary diffuse gastric cancer: updated consensus guidelines for clinical management and directions for future research. J Med Genet 2010;47:436–44.

97. Hansford S, Kaurah P, Li-Chang H, et al. Hereditary diffuse gastric cancer syndrome: CDH1 mutations and beyond. JAMA Oncol 2015;1:23–32.

98. van der Post RS, Vogelaar IP, Carneiro F, et al. Hereditary diffuse gastric cancer: updated clinical guidelines with an emphasis on germline CDH1 mutation carriers. J Med Genet 2015;52:361–74.

99. McDivitt RW, Hutter RV, Foote FW Jr, et al. In situ lobular carcinoma. A prospective follow-up study indicating cumulative patient risks. JAMA 1967; 201:82–6.

100. Hutter RV, Foote FW Jr. Lobular carcinoma in situ. Long term follow-up. Cancer 1969;24:1081–5.

101. Rosen PP, Kosloff C, Lieberman PH, et al. Lobular carcinoma in situ of the breast. Detailed analysis of 99 patients with average follow-up of 24 years. Am J Surg Pathol 1978;2:225–51.

102. Dupont WD, Page DL. Risk factors for breast cancer in women with proliferative breast disease. N Engl J Med 1985;312:146–51.

103. Page DL, Schuyler PA, Dupont WD, et al. Atypical lobular hyperplasia as a unilateral predictor of breast cancer risk: a retrospective cohort study. Lancet 2003;361:125–9.

104. Chuba PJ, Hamre MR, Yap J, et al. Bilateral risk for subsequent breast cancer after lobular carcinoma-in-situ: analysis of surveillance, epidemiology, and end results data. J Clin Oncol 2005;23:5534–41.

105. McLaren BK, Schuyler PA, Sanders ME, et al. Excellent survival, cancer type, and Nottingham grade after atypical lobular hyperplasia on initial breast biopsy. Cancer 2006;107:1227–33.

106. National Comprehensive Cancer Network Version 2. 2017. Available at: https://www.nccn.org. Accessed April 6, 2017.

107. Fisher B, Costantino JP, Wickerham DL, et al. Tamoxifen for prevention of breast cancer: report of the National Surgical Adjuvant Breast and Bowel Project P-1 Study. J Natl Cancer Inst 1998;90:1371–88.

108. Goss PE, Ingle JN, Ales-Martinez JE, et al. Exemestane for breast-cancer prevention in postmenopausal women. N Engl J Med 2011;364:2381–91.

109. Visvanathan K, Hurley P, Bantug E, et al. Use of pharmacologic interventions for breast cancer risk reduction: American Society of Clinical Oncology clinical practice guideline. J Clin Oncol 2013;31:2942–62.

110. Blair SL, Emerson DK, Kulkarni S, et al. Breast surgeon's survey: no consensus for surgical treatment of pleomorphic lobular carcinoma in situ. Breast J 2013;19:116–8.

111. Downs-Kelly E, Bell D, Perkins GH, et al. Clinical implications of margin involvement by pleomorphic lobular carcinoma in situ. Arch Pathol Lab Med 2011;135:737–43.

112. Nagi CS, O'Donnell JE, Tismenetsky M, et al. Lobular neoplasia on core needle biopsy does not require excision. Cancer 2008;112:2152–8.

113. Hwang H, Barke LD, Mendelson EB, et al. Atypical lobular hyperplasia and classic lobular carcinoma in situ in core biopsy specimens: routine excision is not necessary. Mod Pathol 2008;21:1208–16.

114. Rendi MH, Dintzis SM, Lehman CD, et al. Lobular in-situ neoplasia on breast core needle biopsy: imaging indication and pathologic extent can identify which patients require excisional biopsy. Ann Surg Oncol 2012;19:914–21.

115. Murray MP, Luedtke C, Liberman L, et al. Classic lobular carcinoma in situ and atypical lobular hyperplasia at percutaneous breast core biopsy: outcomes of prospective excision. Cancer 2013;119: 1073–9.

116. Chaudhary S, Lawrence L, McGinty G, et al. Classic lobular neoplasia on core biopsy: a clinical and radio-pathologic correlation study with follow-up excision biopsy. Mod Pathol 2013;26:762–71.

117. D'Alfonso TM, Wang K, Chiu YL, et al. Pathologic upgrade rates on subsequent excision when lobular carcinoma in situ is the primary diagnosis in the needle core biopsy with special attention to the radiographic target. Arch Pathol Lab Med 2013;137:927–35.

118. Susnik B, Day D, Abeln E, et al. Surgical outcomes of lobular neoplasia diagnosed in core biopsy: prospective study of 316 cases. Clin Breast Cancer 2016;16:507–13.

119. Menon S, Porter GJ, Evans AJ, et al. The significance of lobular neoplasia on needle core biopsy of the breast. Virchows Arch 2008;452:473–9.

120. Nakhlis F, Gilmore L, Gelman R, et al. Incidence of adjacent synchronous invasive carcinoma and/or ductal carcinoma in-situ in patients with lobular neoplasia on core biopsy: results from a prospective multi-institutional registry (TBCRC 020). Ann Surg Oncol 2016;23:722–8.

121. The American Society of Breast Surgeons Consensus Statements. Available at: https://www.breastsurgeons.org/new_layout/about/statements/index.php#consensus_statements. Accessed November 2, 2016.

122. Carder PJ, Shaaban A, Alizadeh Y, et al. Screen-detected pleomorphic lobular carcinoma in situ (PLCIS): risk of concurrent invasive malignancy following a core biopsy diagnosis. Histopathology 2010;57:472–8.

Ancillary Prognostic and Predictive Testing in Breast Cancer
Focus on Discordant, Unusual, and Borderline Results

Kimberly H. Allison, MD

KEYWORDS

- ER testing • HER2 testing • Fluorescence in situ hybridization (FISH) • Molecular testing
- Breast cancer • OncotypeDX • Predictive testing

ABSTRACT

Ancillary testing in breast cancer has become standard of care to determine what therapies may be most effective for individual patients with breast cancer. Single-marker tests are required on all newly diagnosed and newly metastatic breast cancers. Markers of proliferation are also used, and include both single-marker tests like Ki67 as well as panel-based gene expression tests, which have made more recent contributions to prognostic and predictive testing in breast cancers. This review focuses on pathologist interpretation of these ancillary test results, with a focus on expected versus unexpected results and troubleshooting borderline, unusual, or discordant results.

ROLE OF ANCILLARY TESTS IN BREAST CANCER TREATMENT

OVERVIEW

To serve as a valued member of a breast cancer treatment team, today's practicing surgical pathologist needs to learn to think like a "diagnostic oncologist" with an in-depth understanding of the treatment implications of the details of the their cancer diagnoses.[1–6] This is especially critical when performing or interpreting additional prognostic and predictive markers because these have become the primary branch-point in clinical decision-making algorithms for breast cancer treatment. The pathologist's role in the breast cancer treatment team has changed from just rendering a diagnosis of breast cancer, to providing translation and integration of all the available biologic information on an individual patient's cancer, such that the treatment team and patient can make individualized treatment decisions for each unique case (**Fig. 1**).

Key Points
ROLE OF ANCILLARY TESTING IN BREAST CANCER

- Breast cancer treatment guidelines organize patients into different treatment groups on the basis of hormone receptor and HER2 test results
- The 8th edition of the American Joint Committee on Cancer staging manual adds a clinical Prognostic Staging system that includes traditional TNM plus results of ancillary tests

Disclosure Statement: No disclosures.
Department of Pathology, Stanford University School of Medicine, 300 Pasteur Drive, Lane 235, Stanford, CA 94305, USA
E-mail address: allisonk@stanford.edu

Surgical Pathology 11 (2018) 147–176
https://doi.org/10.1016/j.path.2017.09.006

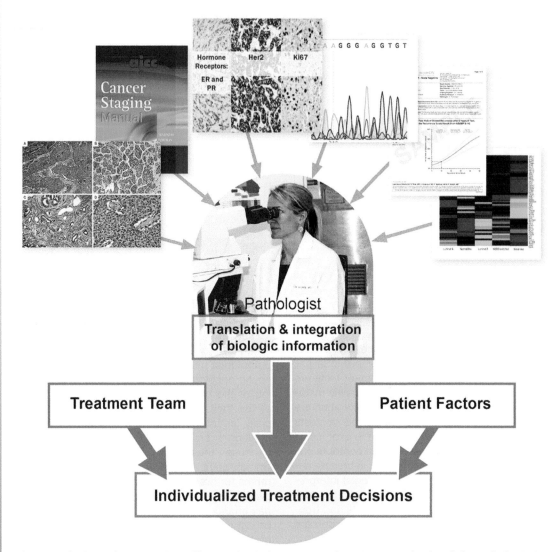

Fig. 1. Predictive and prognostic ancillary testing in breast cancer have increasingly placed the pathologist in a new role as a "diagnostic oncologist" who performs, interprets, and integrates pathology data on each patient's tissue such that individualized treatment decisions can be made.

Most breast cancer treatment guidelines, such as the National Comprehensive Cancer Network (NCCN) guidelines and St Gallen recommendations, are organized by hormone receptor and human epidermal growth factor receptor 2 (HER2) status.[7–9] It is critical that these test results are correct because treatment algorithms are different for breast cancers grouped into the following categories: (1) estrogen receptor (ER)-positive, HER2-negative, (2) ER-positive, HER2-positive, (3) ER-negative, HER2-positive, and (4) negative for ER and HER2.[10] Molecular data on gene expression also support segregation of breast cancers into similar groups with hormone receptor expression associated with the luminal molecular subtypes, HER2 overexpression associated with the HER2-enriched subtype and the

"triple-negative" breast cancers associated with the basal-like molecular subtype.[11–18] However, the overlap of these groups as defined by gene expression versus traditional immunohistochemistry (IHC)/in situ hybridization (ISH) is imperfect.[19] In addition, gene expression profiling results are subject to variability by testing platform and are currently not as accessible as traditional testing methods.[20–22] As such, most treatment guidelines use the well-validated, traditional hormone receptor and HER2 biomarkers (as assessed by IHC or ISH) as the basis for treatment recommendations. A rough overview of how these ancillary markers are associated with clinical and pathologic characteristics, as well as the gene expression/molecular subtypes, is shown in **Fig. 2**.

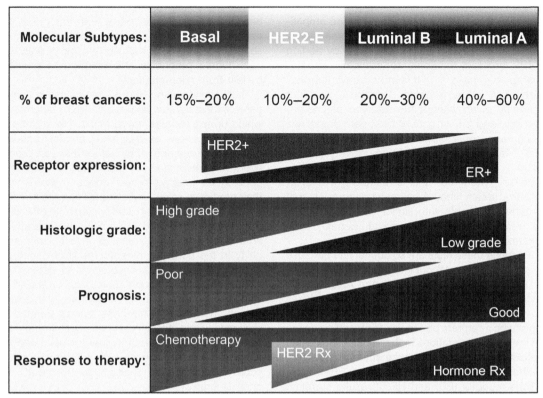

Molecular Subtypes:	Basal	HER2-E	Luminal B	Luminal A
% of breast cancers:	15%–20%	10%–20%	20%–30%	40%–60%
Receptor expression:	HER2+			ER+
Histologic grade:	High grade			Low grade
Prognosis:	Poor			Good
Response to therapy:	Chemotherapy	HER2 Rx		Hormone Rx

Fig. 2. Breast cancers can be segregated into groups with common clinical and pathologic features on the basis of their hormone receptor and HER2 expression. These generally align with the 4 main gene expression–based molecular subtypes of breast cancer.

Hormone receptor and HER2 results are well recognized as powerful prognostic tools that add prognostic value beyond the traditional TNM stage. In fact, the eighth edition of the American Joint Committee on Cancer (AJCC) staging system has completely revised breast cancer clinical staging into "prognostic staging" groups on the basis of traditional TNM combined with hormone receptor, HER2, grade, and OncoytpeDX testing (if available/applicable).[23–25] By incorporating these markers of the biology of the breast cancer, the hope is that these stage groupings will more accurately reflect overall prognosis. Using this new system, breast cancers with the same TNM pathologic stage will be further stratified into clinical prognostic stages. For example, a triple-negative breast cancer would have a higher prognostic stage than an ER-positive, HER2-negative breast cancer with the same TNM characteristics. This new prognostic staging system is complex, is considered a working document, and will likely undergo additional revisions because improved treatment strategies in each of these groupings can alter prognosis.

In addition to providing overall treatment and prognostic groupings, hormone receptor and HER2 testing makes a patient with breast cancer a candidate for specific therapies. It has been well

established that patients with breast cancers with hormone receptor expression are more likely to benefit from treatment with hormone-targeting therapies like tamoxifen, aromatase inhibitors, or ovarian suppression/ablation than those without hormone receptor expression.[26–28] Although the decision to treat or not is binary, the amount of hormone receptor expression as well as the degree of response to treatment is not necessarily binary and can be more of a spectrum.[29] This has particular relevance when setting the standards for a positive versus a negative result and reporting standards, because setting a threshold for positive necessarily creates borderline/gray zone results when close to a threshold. For example, although 1% of cells with weak (1+) staining is the standard threshold for ER staining (per College of American Pathologists [CAP]/American Society of Clinical Oncology [ASCO] guidelines) as determined by the lower limit of patients who receive some benefit from hormonal therapies, this low a threshold may not be the ideal definition for an ER-positive versus ER-negative breast cancer for overall treatment guidelines.[30–34]

It has also been well established that patients with breast cancers that overexpress the growth factor receptor HER2, primarily by gene amplification, can have significant survival benefit in this aggressive form of breast cancer by adding HER2-targeted therapies to standard chemotherapy regimens.[35–40] It is important to emphasize that HER2-targeted therapies are not currently given without the addition of chemotherapy, and breast cancer treatment guidelines encourage consideration of chemotherapy plus HER2-targeted regimens even in very limited extent, lymph node–negative, HER2-positive disease. Therefore, the threshold for HER2-positive ideally should be maintained such that groups of patients with similar results are likely to receive significant survival benefit from treatment.

Because these tests are so critical and because of earlier concerns about interlaboratory variability in ER and HER2 results, CAP and ASCO jointly established both HER2 and ER testing guidelines to help ensure standardization.[41–44] Every pathologist who interprets breast tissue should be aware of the recommendations in these guidelines when validating or interpreting these stains. In addition, pathologists should be aware of how ER/progesterone receptor (PR) and HER2 results correlate with the histologic findings and be able to recognize and troubleshoot discordant, borderline, or unusual results.

Although hormone receptor and HER2 testing can help define which cancers may respond to targeted therapies, predicting which will respond to chemotherapy is more challenging, but is often aided by ancillary tests measuring proliferation rates. Hormone receptor–negative cancers (both HER2-positive and HER2-negative) are generally high grade and have high proliferative rates. Patients with hormone receptor–negative cancers derive significant benefit from chemotherapy and high rates of response to neoadjuvant chemotherapy are seen.[45] In these ER-negative cancers, response to neoadjuvant chemotherapy is also highly predictive of long-term outcomes, with patients who achieve complete pathologic response having very high long-term cure rates.[46–50] However, in ER-positive breast cancers the benefit of chemotherapy is not always as clear. In addition, neoadjuvant chemotherapy response is less predictive of long-term outcomes in ER-positive cancers. For example, ER-positive/HER2-positive breast cancers often receive chemotherapy plus HER2-targeted therapies, but are less likely to have a complete pathologic response to neoadjuvant treatment than ER-negative/HER2-positive breast cancers. In the large group of ER-positive/HER2-negative breast cancers, the question of chemotherapy benefit is most challenging. It is in this group of patients that proliferation rate testing can aid in separating out which patients are more likely to have worse prognosis and therefore a greater benefit from chemotherapy.

There are a variety of prognostic assays using gene expression signatures to help determine which breast cancers are at higher risk of recurrence. However, assays that predict patient benefit from chemotherapy (rather than just prognosis) have become the most widely adopted by oncologists treating breast cancer because of their predictive value. OncotypeDX and MammaPrint are the assays most widely used, both of which can now be performed on formalin-fixed paraffin-embedded tissue. These assays have their primary utility in the hormone receptor–positive cancers, and are often used by oncologists to determine which ER-positive, lymph node–negative patients with breast cancer may *not* benefit from the addition chemotherapy to hormone therapy treatment regimens. Thus, these tests are most frequently used when chemotherapy is being considered in ER-positive breast cancer, with a low recurrence score supporting a decision to "opt-out" of chemotherapy.

Although both OncotypeDX and MammaPrint assays have many genes in their panels (21 for OncotypeDX and 70 for MammaPrint), their recurrence risk scores are heavily weighted by the proliferation-related genes in their panels. This makes sense because traditional chemotherapy targets more rapidly dividing cells. Multigene prognostic assays are now endorsed by the ASCO, St Gallen, and NCCN guidelines as tests providing information that could assist therapeutic decision-making in ER-positive cancers. This review focuses primarily on OncotypeDX testing because it is currently the most common panel-based test used in breast cancer decision-making in the United States.

OVERVIEW OF EVALUATION OF DISCORDANT RESULTS

Discordant ER and HER2 results can fall into several categories, as summarized in Table 1. In each of these categories, examples of types of discordance are listed and a few examples of possible causes (not comprehensive). In general, discordant results will be more common in cases with borderline results near a positive threshold (such as weakly positive ER expression), cases with heterogeneous findings, and cases with unusual result categories (particularly in HER2 fluorescence in situ hybridization [FISH] testing). These can be valid discordances that are

Table 1
Evaluation of discordant ER or HER2 results

Type of Discordance	Examples for ER	Examples for HER2
Discordance of ER or HER2 status with histology/clinico-pathologic findings	Result: ER-negative results (0% staining by IHC) for grade 1 invasive cancers (ductal or lobular), pure tubular or pure mucinous cancers. Possible causes: Incorrect initial histologic classification, false-negative IHC result, specimen mix-up	Result: HER2-positive results (3+ by IHC) for grade 1 invasive cancers (ductal or lobular), pure tubular or pure mucinous cancers Possible causes: Incorrect initial histologic classification, false-positive IHC result, specimen mix-up
Discordance between testing methods (same sample)	Result: ER-positive result by IHC but negative by RT-PCR quantitative result using 21-gene recurrence assay (OncoytpeDX) Possible causes: Borderline positive result, low cancer cellularity causing false-negative RT-PCR result, false-positive IHC result due to overstaining	Result: HER2-negative by IHC (1+) but positive by FISH. Possible causes: False-negative IHC due to tissue handling factors, unusual FISH-positive category (such as ratio >2.0 but mean HER2 signals per cell <4.0), mutations in HER2 protein causing IHC antibody to not recognize it
Discordance with prior results (same patient, different samples)	Result: ER-positive primary and ER-negative metastatic disease Possible causes: True result caused by heterogeneity of ER expression or loss of ER expression with disease progression, false-negative result in metastatic sample due to tissue handling issues, or metastatic cancer is non-breast	Result: HER2-negative on core biopsy and HER2-positive on excision. Possible causes: True result caused by heterogeneity for HER2, unusual or borderline/equivocal results, false-negative initial result, different testing methods
Discordance between laboratories	Result: Weak ER expression results (1%–10%, 1+) by Lab 1 and negative (<1%) by Lab 2 Possible causes: Borderline result, different scoring methodology (such as digital image analysis), different test methodology	Result: HER2-negative in Lab 1 and positive in Lab 2 Possible causes: Differences in tests used (eg, IHC, CISH, FISH), unusual or borderline/equivocal results, different scoring methods

Abbreviations: CISH, chromogenic in situ hybridization; ER, estrogen receptor; FISH, fluorescence in situ hybridization; HER2, human epidermal growth factor receptor 2; IHC, immunohistochemistry; RT-PCR, reverse-transcriptase polymerase chain reaction.

explained by those factors creating unusual testing scenarios. These discordances can be challenging to explain to clinicians expecting straightforward results, but pathology expertise can be especially helpful in guiding treatment decisions in these situations.

Review of the original hematoxylin-eosin (H&E) findings for confirmation of histologic discordances can uncover disagreements with the original reporting of histologic characteristics as well as specimen mix-ups. Repeat testing on the same or additional samples can also be helpful in resolving some challenging cases.

In addition to these considerations, when a false-positive or false-negative test result is suspected, possible preanalytic, analytical, and postanalytic causes of test failure should be explored. Common preanalytic explanations include prolonged ischemic times (CAP recommends <1 hour), decalcification processes and inadequate fixation (CAP recommends 6–72 hours with appropriate sectioning to ensure penetration) causing false-negative results. Analytical factors include test methodology differences and standards. Postanalytic factors include test interpretation criteria and methods (such as digital image analysis, or variability in how FISH cells are selected for counting) and variability due to the interpreter (such as overinterpretation of IHC stain intensity for HER2).

HORMONE RECEPTOR STAINS

Key Points
HORMONE RECEPTOR TESTING IN
BREAST CANCER

- Positivity for ER/PR makes a patient a candidate for hormonal therapies.

- Clinical treatment algorithms for ER-positive versus ER-negative disease are very different.

- CAP/ASCO guidelines exist for performance and interpretation of ER testing in breast cancer.

- The threshold for ER and PR positivity is very low (1% of cells with 1 + weak staining) and requires careful examination at lower power to detect.

- Pathologists should report the percent and intensity of the ER and PR stains.

- Very weakly positive high-grade breast cancers may behave more similarly to hormone receptor–negative cancers (but they are still reported as positive).

- Grade 1 ductal or lobular carcinomas, pure mucinous, and tubular carcinomas should be ER-positive. If not, the result is discordant and the case should be further evaluated to explain the discordance.

- Some low-grade breast cancers/lesions are expected to be hormone receptor–negative such as the following:
  - Adenoid cystic carcinoma
  - Low- grade metaplastic carcinomas (eg, adenosquamous carcinomas, fibromatosislike)
  - Secretory carcinoma
  - Well-differentiated apocrine carcinomas
  - Microglandular adenosis
  - Metastatic malignancies

FUNCTION OF HORMONE RECEPTORS

ER and PR are nuclear receptors that, when combined with their hormonal ligands, can bind to DNA targets to cause hormone-related transcription. These play a role in normal breast development,

differentiation and lactation. There are 2 forms of ER: ER-alpha (encoded by the *ESR1* gene on chromosome 6) and ER-beta (encoded by the *ESR2* gene on chromosome 14). ER-alpha is the most critical receptor in breast cancer and mutations in this protein can cause resistance to endocrine therapy. It is activated when bound to 17-beta-estradiol (estrogen) and causes transcription of many genes typically expressed by luminal breast cancers. Immunohistochemistry antibodies used in clinical laboratories recognize the ER-alpha receptor, since ER-beta is not currently indicated as a prognostic or predictive marker in breast cancer.

PR expression is activated by binding to progesterone, which causes transcription of PR-related genes. PR expression appears to be regulated by ER-alpha and when activated these hormone receptors interact to direct chromatin remodeling that may have antiproliferative effects. Because is it extremely rare for an invasive breast cancer to have PR expression in the absence of ER expression, PR has predominantly prognostic/predictive implications in the setting of ER-positive disease. ER-positive invasive cancers with low to absent PR expression are typically higher grade and more proliferative, sometimes also HER2-positive ("luminal B" characteristics), features associated with a worse prognosis and worse response to hormone therapy. There are multiple proposed mechanisms of PR loss in ER-positive disease that may account for these findings, including abnormal ER-alpha signaling pathways, loss of the *PR* gene, and downregulation by HER2.[51]

INTERPRETATION OF HORMONE RECEPTOR STAINS

ER and PR expression in both normal breast and ER-positive breast cancers should be nuclear. Normal breast epithelium can serve as an internal positive control, with ER and PR expression variably present in luminal but not myoepithelial cells. Columnar cell change and low-grade in situ proliferations are more uniformly ER-positive than background breast tissue and apocrine metaplasia is typically ER-negative. ER can also be present in some stromal cells, smooth muscle cells of the areola and in lymphocytes. In some cases an internal positive control may not be present. An external control should always be evaluated and include appropriately positive and negative tissues.

An invasive breast cancer should be evaluated for both the intensity and percentage of cells with nuclear ER and PR expression. There can be regional variability in hormone receptor expression and the percentage reported should reflect the percentage of positive cells in the entire sample of the invasive cancer tested (not the just area of highest expression). When the intensity is variable it can be reported as a range or an average intensity, with many systems using a 0, 1+, 2+, and 3+ range. Different scoring systems can be used to combine the intensity and percentage information for an overall score (such as an H or Allred score); however, these are not required but both percentage and intensity should be clearly reported in all cases. In addition to reporting percent and intensity results, an interpretation as ER-positive or PR-positive or PR-negative should also be included in the report.

According to the 2010 CAP/ASCO ER and PR Testing in Breast Cancer Guidelines, breast cancers with as few as 1% of cells with weak intensity for ER or PR staining should be considered ER-positive because of evidence of potential benefit from endocrine therapy.[26,27,31] To identify focal or weak levels of hormone receptor expression, low-power scanning of results is often insufficient for detection. Therefore, in cases that appear negative on low-power, a higher-power scan of the slide is also appropriate to rule out a weakly hormone receptor–positive case. It can be clinically useful to report low ER or PR expressing cancers (1%–10% positive) as "weakly positive" or "focally positive" to differentiate these cases as borderline with a negative result (see later in this article for more discussion on borderline ER results).

PR expression tends to vary more than ER expression, and this helps account for the effectiveness of PR to further stratify ER-positive cases into different prognostic categories (although specific PR thresholds for this purpose are not well-validated).[52] The specific antibody used also has been reported to have an effect on the range of hormone receptor positivity.[53] With the use of rabbit monoclonal antibodies, ER expression is more bimodal, with reports of fewer cases in the intermediate percentage range using SP1.[54] Some studies even report these antibodies have better correlation with clinical response to hormone therapy. However, there is also the concern that some antibodies may be too sensitive, with classification of too many cases as positive that otherwise have characteristics more in keeping with a triple-negative cancer. The UK Neqas program highlighted issues with the PgR rabbit monoclonal antibody SP2 causing false-positive tests because of oversensitivity.[55]

Digital image analysis interpretation of hormone receptor stains has become more frequent and can provide an objective measure of the required quantitative and semiquantitative reporting measures. However, the quantitative imaging analysis system used must be appropriately calibrated for high concordance with the gold standard validated manual methodologies and is subject to additional pitfalls, such as counting staining in nonepithelial cells or in situ components, detection threshold variability, and variability in the regions of interest analyzed. As such, pathologist oversight and final interpretation of the digital result on every case is essential before reporting results on a clinical breast cancer case. There are currently no published guidelines for digital image analysis in ER, but if used, it is also subject to CAP/ASCO ER guidelines standards, such as validation procedures and proficiency testing standards.

EXPECTED VERSUS UNEXPECTED HORMONE RECEPTOR RESULTS

It is essential to have a strong understanding of which types of breast cancers are expected to be hormone receptor–positive or hormone receptor–negative so that discordant results can be further investigated and potential errors detected. Although PR can be variable and results may not be easily predicted, ER tends to produce more predictable results, thereby facilitating recognition of discordant results when encountered. Invasive cancers considered extremely likely to be ER-positive include classic low-grade (Nottingham grade 1) invasive ductal and lobular carcinomas (Fig. 3A, B). In addition, special histologic subtypes, such as pure tubular carcinoma, pure mucinous carcinoma, and pure cribriform carcinomas should be uniformly ER-positive (PR can be variable to negative). These cancers are treated as good prognosis subtypes with minimal therapeutic interventions. If these subtypes are ER-negative (or HER2-positive), potential causes of a false-negative ER result or re-review for misclassification of a pure histologic type or an error in grading, should be considered. In addition, low-grade ductal carcinoma in situ, encapsulated papillary carcinomas, and solid papillary carcinomas are all expected to be uniformly ER-positive. In the rare situation that a cancer in one of these categories is ER-negative with no other explanation after further workup, the report should include a statement about the unusual nature of the result, that additional testing be considered (on additional tissue samples if available) and that the cancer may not behave as expected for a cancer with the histologic characteristics by which it was characterized.

ER-negative cancers tend to be higher grade; however, ER expression in a high-grade in situ or invasive cancer is not necessarily considered a discordant result. Higher-grade cancers do more often have heterogeneity or weak ER expression and can have variable results with different assays if close to the threshold for positive. For example, in our laboratory we have seen low ER-positive breast cancers (1%–30% weak ER expression) that have negative quantitative ER results by

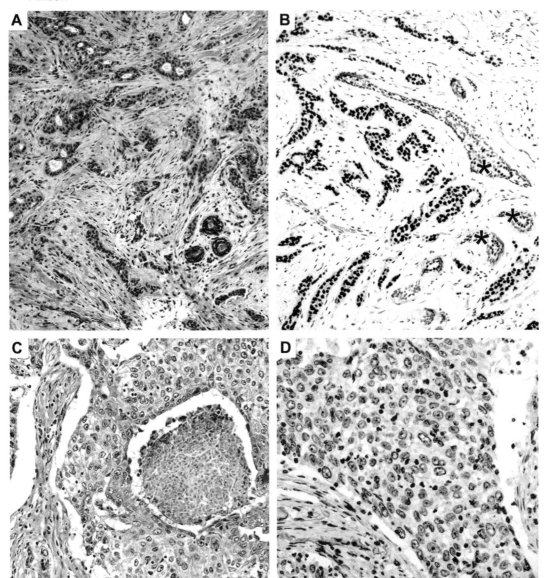

Fig. 3. Examples of ER expression patterns in breast cancer. A and B show a low-grade invasive ductal carcinoma (*A*, H&E stain, original magnification ×200) with strong, uniform ER expression by IHC as expected (*B*, ER stain, original magnification ×200). The asterisks annotate some of the normal ducts serving as a positive internal control (should have variable but strong staining). If a grade 1 ductal or lobular cancer or a pure tubular, mucinous, or cribriform carcinoma is ER-negative, this is considered a discordant result and the case should be worked up further. C and D show a high-grade breast carcinoma with histologic features on (H&E, original magnification ×400) (*C*) associated with the basal-like molecular subtype of breast cancer (high-grade cells with sheetlike growth and areas of necrosis) but with weak ER expression by IHC (*D*, original magnification ×400). With a threshold for positive of only 1% of cells with weak staining, weak ER-positive/HER2-negative high-grade cancers will be classified as ER-positive breast cancers but it may be more appropriate in some cases to treat similar to a triple-negative breast cancer.

reverse-transcriptase polymerase chain reaction (RT-PCR)–based OncoytpeDX testing or a negative result by quantitative image analysis. This discordance can be explained by the differences in testing methodology and an initial borderline positive result. Although manually interpreted IHC is still the gold standard, the clinical relevance of very weak ER expression is not entirely clear. Borderline or weakly positive ER cancers can be problematic for treating

clinicians because any level of ER expression ≥1% may exclude a patient from treatments or clinical trials intended for triple-negative cancers only. Recent evidence has shown that most weak ER-positive cancers have histopathologic features (high-grade, sheetlike growth, areas of necrosis) and molecular profiles more similar to the basal-like intrinsic subtype of breast cancer than luminal subtypes (**Fig. 3**C, D).[30,32–34] A recent meta-analysis of retrospective clinical outcomes data on cancers with 1% to 9% ER expression found that borderline/weak ER-expressing cancers gained no significant survival benefit from endocrine therapy, but did have a slightly better overall prognosis than ER-negative (<1%) cancers.[32] Although prospective data are still lacking, using other clinical-pathologic factors to make clinical decisions may be useful in this borderline ER+ group. Grade, patient age, PR status, and molecular subtype assays (such as PAM-50 or BluePrint) may be useful to consider in this setting on a case by case basis. The 2010 CAP/ASCO ER testing guidelines will likely be updated in the near future and there are proposals for the guidelines panel to address the topic of treatment decisions in weak ER-positive breast cancers.

Although low-grade ductal and lobular cancers should be hormone receptor–positive, there are some lower-grade breast cancers that are commonly negative for ER and PR (and HER2). These include adenoid cystic carcinoma, secretory carcinoma, low-grade adenosquamous carcinomas, well-differentiated squamous carcinomas, low-grade apocrine carcinomas and low-grade fibromatosislike metaplastic carcinoma. It can be useful to comment that this is an expected result that is considered concordant with these special histologic subtypes, some of which have a good prognosis despite their ER negativity. In addition, microglandular adenosis is another low-grade, infiltrative-appearing hormone receptor–negative process that is triple-negative. Because microglandular adenosis (which is negative for myoepithelial stains) can mimic invasive low-grade ductal or tubular carcinomas, it should be a consideration in an ER-negative tubule-forming infiltrative process. Last, metastatic malignancies should be considered in lesions that have unusual histologic patterns for breast cancer (such as invasive papillary, large gland forming, or low-grade neuroendocrine) and are ER-negative.[56] Primary breast lymphomas and sarcomas are also triple-negative and should be considered in the appropriate clinical/histologic context.

Consideration for Additional Testing

Core needle biopsies are the preferred sample on which to perform ER, PR, and HER2 testing because these samples are more likely to have minimal ischemic times and well-controlled fixation. In addition, decisions on neoadjuvant treatment can be made before surgery when indicated. However, in the setting of a negative initial core biopsy result, consideration for additional testing on the surgical sample should be made in certain settings, which are summarized in **Box 1**.

Box 1
When to consider additional hormone receptor or human epidermal growth factor receptor 2 (HER2) testing on a subsequent sample after initial core biopsy results

Initial core biopsy result is borderline, insufficient, equivocal, unusual, or discordant with histologic or clinical findings

Cancer is high grade (grade 3) and was negative for HER2 on initial core

Heterogeneity of grade or morphology noted on the surgical sample

Limited initial sample on core biopsy

Doubt about specimen handling of initial core biopsy sample (long ischemic time, short time in fixative, alterative fixative used)

Pathologist suspects testing error on initial core biopsy

Validation

CAP requires proof of initial validation of any new ER/PR antibody with a previously clinically validated test. There should be at least 90% concordance with previously validated ER-positive results and at least 95% concordance with previously validated ER-negative results. In addition, proficiency testing should be ongoing (at least twice/year) with at least 90% performance on graded challenges.

INTERPRETATION OF HUMAN EPITHELIAL GROWTH FACTOR RECEPTOR 2 RESULTS

Key Points
HUMAN EPITHELIAL GROWTH FACTOR RECEPTOR 2 TESTING IN BREAST CANCER

- HER2-positive breast cancers have a more aggressive clinical behavior.

- A positive HER2 test makes a patient a candidate for HER2-targeted therapies, which are typically only offered in conjunction with chemotherapy.

- HER2 status can either be determined by protein expression (IHC) or gene amplification (ISH).

- CAP/ASCO guidelines exist for performance and interpretation of HER2 testing in breast cancer; it is anticipated these will be updated in 2017.

- HER2 IHC test interpretation requires analysis of the completeness and intensity of cell membrane staining with results expressed as 0 to 1+ (negative), 2+ (equivocal), and 3+ (positive), but pathologists should also be aware of unusual staining patterns.

- HER2 ISH test results typically are either straightforward/"classic" negative (ratio <2.0 and average HER2 signals per cell <6.0) or positive (ratio ≥2.0 and average HER2 signals per cell ≥6.0) but unusual result categories with less clear clinical implications also exist of which the pathologist should be aware.

- Grade 1 ductal or lobular carcinomas, pure mucinous and tubular carcinomas should be HER2-negative. If not, the result is discordant and the case should be further evaluated to explain the discordance.

FUNCTION

HER2 is a member of a family of growth factor receptors (including HER1/EGFR, HER3, and HER4) that regulate normal cell proliferation, development, and survival. It is located on the cell surface in normal breast epithelium. When activated by ligand binding, a conformational change occurs in the HER2 protein that promotes receptor dimerization, which in turn activates an intracellular tyrosine kinase portion of the protein. This activation then regulates intracellular signaling through MAP-kinase and PI3-kinase pathways. In breast cancers, amplification of the *HER2* gene (*ERBB2)* is the primary mechanism by which the HER2 protein will be overexpressed at the cell surface. This protein overexpression then can result in promotion of more aggressive cancer biology due to increases in cancer proliferation, cell motility, and angiogenesis. HER2 also serves as an ideal target for antibody-based therapies because it is located on the cancer cell surface and is present in much higher levels than in normal cells. There are a number of HER2-targeted therapies available today, some of which are used in combination with the first (and still standard) anti-HER2 biologic therapy, trastuzumab (Herceptin).[37,57] One of these agents, pertuzumab, is currently approved by the Food and Drug Administration (FDS) to be used only in combination with trastuzumab + chemotherapy in the neoadjuvant setting.[38] As mentioned previously, use of neoadjuvant therapy is an indication for determination of biomarker status on core needle biopsy. However, additional testing on a surgical specimen can be useful as well and is discussed as follows.

TESTING METHODOLOGIES

HER2 can be assessed using IHC to test for protein overexpression or by in situ hybridization (ISH) to test for gene amplification. Because IHC is readily available and lower cost/overhead, many laboratories use IHC as the first test performed and if there is an equivocal result reflex the case to ISH testing (either in-house or at a reference laboratory). It is also acceptable to do ISH testing as a first line or to use both tests on all cases (dual testing). In the proposed 2017 update of the CAP/ASCO HER2 testing guidelines (which had an open comment period in June of 2017), a greater emphasis on using IHC to guide interpretation and testing of unusual ISH categories was proposed. When used appropriately and according to guidelines, these 2 testing methodologies can inform each other and be a useful way to detect unusual cases (such as HER2 heterogeneity) and potential errors in this important test.

INTERPRETATION OF HUMAN EPIDERMAL GROWTH FACTOR RECEPTOR 2 IMMUNOHISTOCHEMISTRY

A work-aid to HER2 IHC interpretation criteria is presented in **Fig. 4**, with an emphasis on the main aspects of evaluating the stain: (1) if the staining is membranous and complete versus incomplete/partial, (2) the intensity of the stain, and (3) the percentage of the cells with these features. There are 4 main IHC result categories (0, 1+, 2+, and 3+), in addition to the possibility of an indeterminate result, with 0 to 1+ results interpreted as negative for overexpression, 2+ results interpreted as equivocal and 3+ results reported as positive for overexpression. Minor wording changes were made to interpretation of the 2+ category after the 2013 guidelines were published and are to be included in the 2017 update.[58–60] These included elimination of the contradictory terms "circumferential" and "incomplete" and the switch to the FDA-approved terminology "weak and moderate complete membrane staining observed in greater than 10% of tumor cells" as the standard definition of a 2+ result.

Critical to the appropriate determination of HER2 IHC status is the evaluation of the stain intensity, with overinterpretation of stain intensity as one of the most common causes of a HER2 IHC-positive, ISH-negative discordance.[61] Comparison of stain intensity with negative (0–1+) and positive (3+) controls should serve as a reference for intensity measures. In addition, a practical approach is to use the magnification rule, which takes into account the magnification of the lens required to identify the staining as follows: using

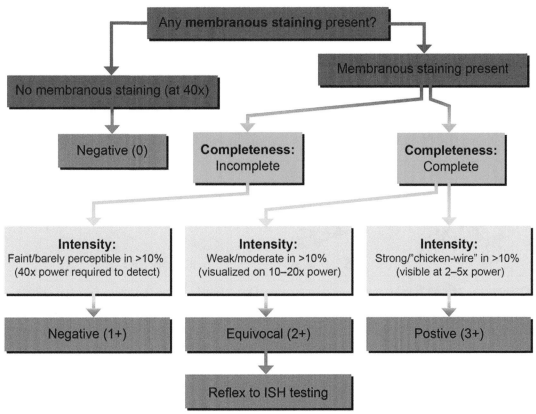

Fig. 4. Work-aid flow diagram for interpreting HER2 IHC. HER2 expression on the cell membrane is evaluated including both the completeness of the membrane staining and the intensity of the staining. Intensity of the stain can be very subjective so standardizing evaluation by magnification the staining is visible by can be useful in addition to comparison to a range of 0, 1+, 2+, and 3+ controls.

a ×10 ocular, if staining is noted with a ×2 to ×5 objective it can be considered strong intensity, staining detected using a ×10 to ×20 objective considered weak-moderate and staining detected only on ×40 faint/barely perceptible.[62,63]

UNUSUAL STAINING PATTERNS

Unusual HER2 IHC staining patterns can present an interpretative challenge. Cases with granular, cytoplasmic staining (**Fig. 5**A) can make it difficult to interpret the degree of membranous staining present and should be considered IHC equivocal so that ISH testing can be performed for more definitive characterization. Cases with significant crush artifact (as in **Fig. 5**B) can produce a similar problem, with disruption of the membranous stain that can be overinterpreted as positive; these cases should be interpreted as IHC *indeterminate* if the crush artifact interferes with the ability to evaluate membranous staining in a significant portion of the invasive cancer. IHC indeterminate cases due to crush artifact can often yield a determinant result when reflexed to ISH. Another unusual pattern of IHC

staining is moderate-strong but incomplete staining, sometimes in a baso-lateral pattern. Although this staining pattern is considered HER2-positive in the gastrointestinal tract, incomplete membrane staining in a breast cancer might place this result in the 1+, negative category. However, this is another unusual staining pattern that should be considered equivocal and reflexed to ISH testing because some breast cancers with this pattern can have HER2 gene amplification. **Fig. 5**C shows an example of a micropapillary breast cancer that has this staining pattern and was HER2 amplified by FISH. The IHC for this case was interpreted as IHC equivocal, with an unusual staining pattern. **Fig. 5**D shows a tubule-forming breast cancer that has a strong basal-pattern of staining that could also be categorized as IHC equivocal (with an unusual staining pattern) but was negative for HER2 gene amplification by FISH.

Although most cases have uniform HER2 IHC expression, a small percentage (<1%–2%) of cases will have heterogeneity for HER2 overexpression.[64–66] If there are clustered areas of 3+ IHC staining cells that represent more than

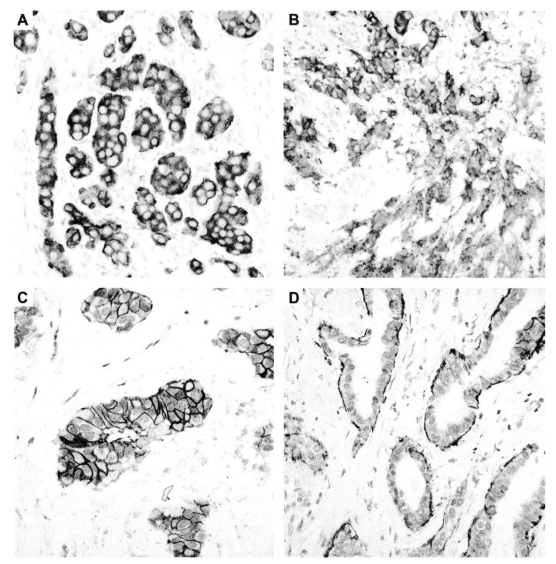

Fig. 5. Unusual HER2 IHC staining patterns. (*A*) shows a breast cancer with granular cytoplasmic staining for HER2. This can obscure membranous staining and should be interpreted as 2+, equivocal, by IHC with further testing by ISH methods indicated. (*B*) shows a HER2 IHC stain result in an area in which crush artifact precludes accurate interpretation. Cases with abundant artifact should be interpreted as indeterminate and additional testing by ISH pursued. (*C*) shows an example of a micropapillary breast carcinoma with predominantly incomplete membranous staining but with strong intensity. Because these cases can have HER2 gene amplification (as this case did by FISH testing), this unusual pattern can be classified as 2+, equivocal by IHC. (*D*) shows a well-differentiated, grade 1, invasive ductal carcinoma with strongly but incomplete HER2 IHC staining with only basal staining present. This case was interpreted as 2+, equivocal, with an unusual staining pattern, but was HER2-negative by FISH testing (as expected for a grade 1 ductal carcinoma) [H&E, original magnification [*A–D*], ×400].

10% of the cancer tested, then the case can be reported as HER2-positive; if less than 10% of the total area of the invasive cancer tested, the case is technically considered IHC equivocal. When a heterogeneous case is reflexed to ISH testing, care should be taken to indicate to the individual counting the ISH test those areas that had 3+ expression levels; these areas should be counted and reported separately if the ISH test also supports a HER2 heterogeneous cancer. The report for a HER2 heterogeneous case should include the percentage of the overall sample that is HER2-positive, which can vary from block to block, occasionally accounting for discordant results between tissue samples.[67] Fig. 6A, B shows a case with HER2 IHC heterogeneity that had 3+ staining by IHC in less than 10% of the initial tissue sample from the primary breast cancer (an

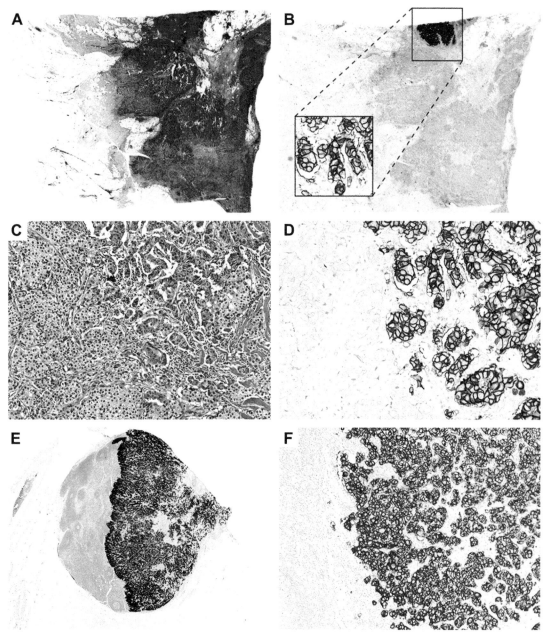

Fig. 6. An example of a case with clustered heterogeneity for HER2 overexpression by IHC. (*A*) (H&E, original magnification ×1) and (*B*, original magnification ×1) (HER2 IHC) show low-power images of an invasive ductal carcinoma with less than 10% of cells with circumferential, intense membrane staining for HER2 (3+). This sample was called HER2 equivocal because the 3+ population represented less than 10% of the total sample tested; however, the pathologist sent additional tissue blocks of the primary breast cancer (*C, D*, H&E, original magnification *C* ×100, *D* ×200) and metastatic cancer to the lymph node (*E, F*) for HER2 testing. The second block of the primary (*C*, H&E) had 3+ HER2 staining in approximately 50% of the sample, which can be reported as HER2-positive by IHC. Interestingly, the carcinoma metastatic to the lymph node (*E*, H&E, original magnification ×2) was uniformly (100%) HER2 3+ positive by IHC (*F*, H&E, original magnification ×100).

equivocal result). Subsequent testing of a second tissue block showed 50% 3+ IHC HER2 staining (a positive result) (**Fig. 6**C, D) and a positive lymph node showed 100% 3+ IHC HER2 staining (**Fig. 6**E, F). Although the clinical significance of heterogeneity for HER2 is currently unclear, these

patients are considered eligible for HER2-targeted therapies.

Per the CAP/ASCO guidelines, HER2 IHC should not be performed on unstained slides that have been cut more than 6 weeks before testing. **Fig. 7**A, B shows an example of a case that had

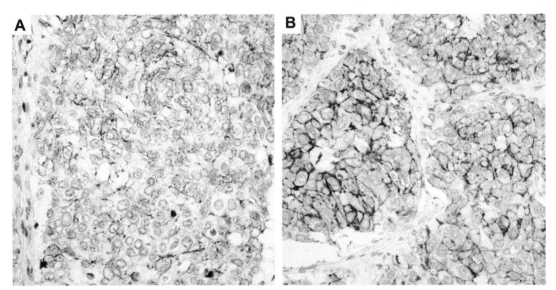

Fig. 7. An example of the effect of time since unstained sections were cut from the tissue block on HER2 expression. Sections from the same tissue block were stained for HER2. Only 1+ staining was noted after more than 6 weeks elapsed since cutting the unstained sections from the tissue block (as shown in *A*). However, 2+ staining is present when the test is run on freshly cut unstained sections (*B*) [H&E, original magnification *A, B* ×400].

only 1+ staining on slides cut more than 6 weeks before testing (panel A) with subsequent freshly cut slides resulting in 2+ staining (panel B). This case had low-level HER2 gene amplification by FISH.

Guidelines for using quantitative image analysis (QIA) for HER2 IHC test interpretation in breast cancer are under way (or published already at the time of release of this article). These guidelines should serve as a useful guide for those using QIA to help control for variability in pathologist interpretation of HER2 IHC results, but the standards in the original HER2 testing guidelines still apply in the QIA setting and pathologist oversight of the final reported result will be required.

An important component of interpretation of HER2 (similar to ER and PR) is correlation of the results with the other histopathologic findings in an individual case. See later in this article on expected versus unexpected results (and **Table 1**) for further discussion on this important component of interpretation.

INTERPRETATION OF HUMAN EPIDERMAL GROWTH FACTOR RECEPTOR 2 IN SITU HYBRIDIZATION TESTING

ISH assays can be either single or dual probe (although single-probe assays are becoming much less common), and can use a variety of probe-detection methods, including FISH, chromogenic methods (CISH), or silver-enhanced (SISH) methods. Guideline recommendations apply to all methods.

In the dual-probe ISH methodology, 1 probe will mark the HER2 gene (located on chromosome 17) and 1 probe will mark the centromere of the same chromosome. The criteria for dual-probe ISH interpretation are based on the ratio of HER2 to centromeric signals as well as the average HER2 signals per cell. Dual-probe ISH results will fall into 1 of 5 result groups, with the vast majority of cases likely to be in group 5 (negative) or group 1 (positive) (**Fig. 8**) (see later in this article for discussion of other result groups).

For single-probe assays, only the average HER2 signals per cell is used. Cases with ≥ 6 average HER2 signals per cell are considered HER2-positive and cases with fewer than 4 average HER2 signals per cell are considered HER2-negative. Cases with ≥ 4 or less than 6 average HER2 signals per cell are considered ISH equivocal and the test is reflexed to other methods of HER2 testing, such as dual-probe ISH. Although considered a valid testing methodology, single-probe ISH assays have largely been replaced by dual-probe assays, so this review focuses on dual-probe ISH.

USUAL OR BORDERLINE RESULTS

Although classic "group 1" HER2 amplification (ratio ≥ 2.0 and ≥ 6 mean HER2 signals per cell) and classic "group 5" nonamplified cases (ratio <2.0 and <4 HER2 signals per cell) are typically straightforward, cases with less common results require

Result Group	Category	Ratio	Mean HER2 signals/cell	Example	CAP/ASCO FISH Interpretation
Group 1	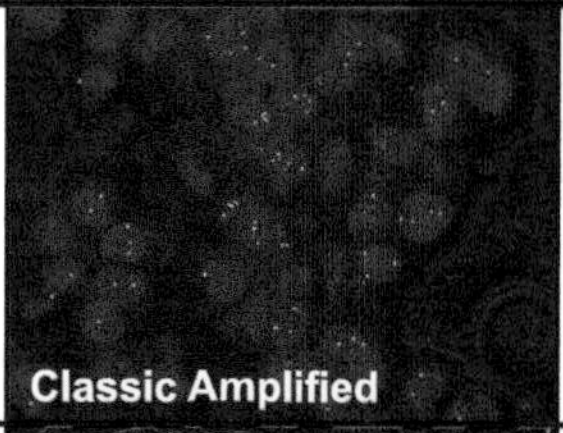 Classic Amplified	≥2.0	≥6.0	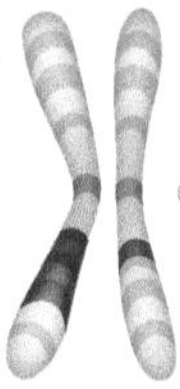 CEP17 HER2	2013: Positive 2017 proposal:Positive
Group 2	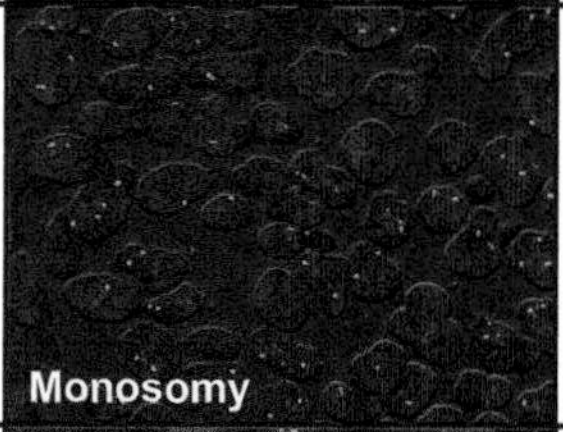 Monosomy	≥2.0	<4.0	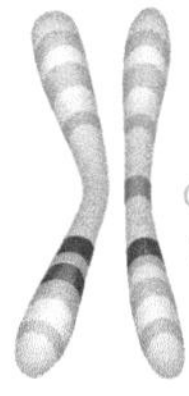 CEP17 HER2	2013: Positive 2017 proposal: Additional work-up required[a] → Negative unless concurrent IHC 3+
Group 3	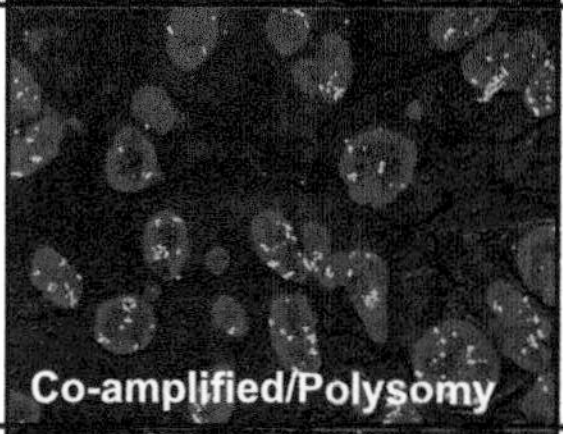 Co-amplified/Polysomy	<2.0	≥6.0	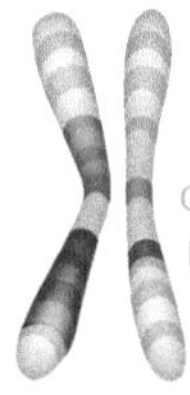 CEP17 HER2	2013: Positive 2017 proposal: Additional work-up required[a] Positive if concurrent IHC 2+ or 3+ (otherwise negative)
Group 4	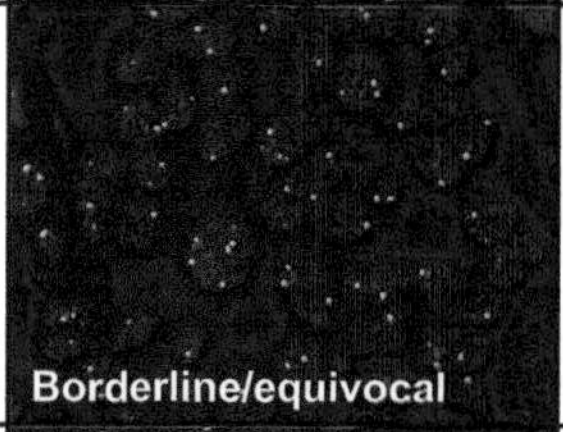 Borderline/equivocal	<2.0	4.0 – 6.0	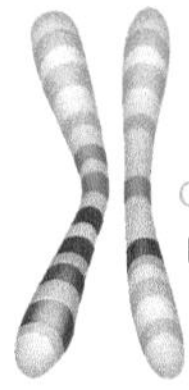 CEP17 HER2	2013: Equivocal 2017 proposal: Additional work-up required[a] → Negative unless concurrent IHC 3+
Group 5	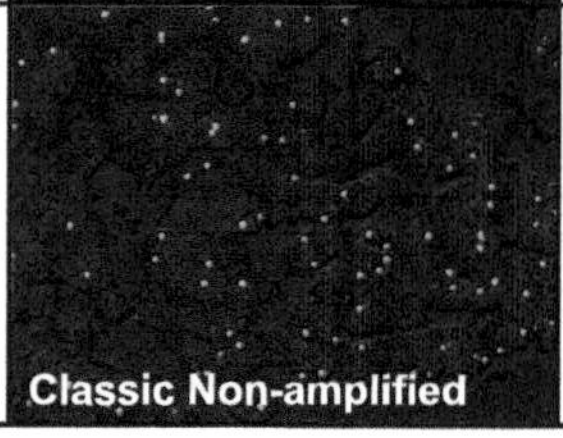 Classic Non-amplified	<2.0	≥6.0	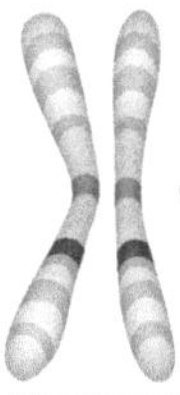 CEP17 HER2	2013: Negative 2017 proposal: Negative

Fig. 8. Dual HER2 ISH results fall into 1 of 5 result groups with different interpretations. Group 1 (classic HER2 amplified) and group 5 (classic HER2 not amplified) categories are most common. Groups 2, 3, and 4 are uncommon but present challenges in interpretation and treatment recommendations because of more limited evidence about their behavior. Both the 2013 HER2 guideline ISH interpretations for groups 2 to 4 as well as the proposed modifications to the 2017 HER2 guidelines update are shown.[a] See text for proposed additional workup.

more consideration and correlation with other factors. In the anticipated 2017 guidelines update, it is proposed that cases with initial ISH results in groups 2 to 4 require additional workup, beginning with correlation with IHC results on the same sample per tissue block. The IHC results are then used to aid in interpretation of the case as HER2-positive or HER2-negative (see the following for specific interpretations for each group). If the IHC is 2+ (equivocal), the ISH test should be evaluated by a second observer, blinded to the previous ISH results, and at least 20 additional cells should be counted. The areas with the strongest IHC staining should be included in this count. If including this new count in the overall ISH results changes the result to another group (such as groups 1 or 5), this new category is used for the final result. However, if the result remains in the same ISH group, the interpretation should be as follows based on the specific ISH result categories:

Group 2 (Ratio ≥2.0 and <4.0 Human Epidermal Growth Factor Receptor 2 Signals per Cell)

Considered NEGATIVE unless the concurrent IHC is 3+ (then considered *positive*). These cases, which often have reduced CEP17 signals or "monosomy" for CEP17, have low HER2 signals per cell but because of the reduced CEP17 signals have a ratio greater than 2.0. Although they were eligible for the initial HER2 clinical trials, such as the HERA trial, they represented a very small percentage of the overall cases (0.8%) so outcome data for this group are limited.[64,68–71] Recent retrospective evaluation of BCIRG trial data indicates that this group does not benefit from trastuzumab and that their outcomes are not worse than standard HER2-negative cancers (group 5) treated with chemotherapy without trastuzumab.[69] In a multi-institution review of unusual HER2 FISH categories, group 2 cases represented 1.4% of cases, and they were frequently ER-positive (79%) and had a spectrum of histologic grades from 13% grade 1% to 44% grade 2% and 43% grade 3.[64] This group also frequently had negative (30%) or equivocal (58%) HER2 IHC results.

Group 3 (Ratio <2.0 and ≥6.0 Human Epidermal Growth Factor Receptor 2 Signals per Cell)

Considered POSITIVE unless concurrent IHC is 0 to 1+ (then considered *negative*). This group has increases in both HER2 and centromere signals, resulting in a ratio less than 2.0 despite elevated average HER2 copy numbers (above 6.0). These results are also uncommon, representing only 0.4% to 3.0% of cases sent for FISH testing in most studies.[64,68–71] These cases were largely excluded from initial clinical trials because they were considered ratio negative and likely to have polysomy for chromosome 17 rather than HER2 gene amplification. The few cases enrolled into the BCIRG-006 adjuvant trastuzumab-trial were insufficient to determine if there was benefit from HER2-targeted therapy. Therefore, clinical outcome data for this group are currently largely limited to trials without HER2-targeted therapy, such as the BCIRG-005 data, which indicated a worse overall and disease-free survival for this group compared with standard (group 5) HER2-negative cases.[69] However, subsequent data supporting that most cases in this group have co-amplification of both the HER2 gene and centromeric regions led the 2013 guidelines to consider these cases ISH-positive.[72–78] More recent evidence supports that this group may be heterogeneous, with some cases having highly amplified results that correlate well with IHC 2 to 3+ protein expression and some that are negative by IHC.[64,71]

Group 4 (Ratio <2.0 and 4.0–6.0 Human Epidermal Growth Factor Receptor 2 Signals per Cell)

Considered NEGATIVE unless concurrent IHC is 3+ (then considered *positive*). Cases in this group were considered HER2 ISH equivocal in the 2013 guidelines, with recommendations for additional testing. The frequency of this result group varies based on the patient population referred for ISH testing, but ranges from 1% to 16% with higher frequencies reported by reference laboratories that receive predominantly IHC 2+ cases than laboratories that perform dual IHC and FISH testing, which report frequencies of 4% to 7%.[64,68–71] Between 2013 and 2017, cases in this result group were often sent for additional testing using alternative probes; however, because of the highly variable results depending on which probes were used and because none of these are clinically validated to identify cases likely to respond to HER2-targeted therapies, the use of alternative probes should not be standard practice.[79,80] Recent data from multiple institutions indicate group 4 cases are typically ER-positive and HER2 IHC-negative (0–1+) or 2+ equivocal, and only rarely 3+ positive.[64,71] Therefore, concurrent IHC results may be best suited to inform interpretation of final FISH results.

Because the clinical outcomes data on response to treatment are still limited for these 3 groups, the guidelines update proposal also recommends including a comment in the report when a group 2 to 4 final result is negative based on IHC results to reflect the limited data available and how IHC was used in the final FISH interpretation. If the case is particularly challenging, consultation with a breast pathology specialist or reference laboratory with expertise in challenging HER2 ISH testing may be helpful. Although the use of alternative probes may be a part of a consultative workup, they are not recommended as a required component of standard practice in the workup of these ISH cases.

EXPECTED VERSUS UNEXPECTED RESULTS

The 2013 update to the CAP/ASCO HER2 Testing Guidelines emphasized the critical role of the pathologist in correlating morphologic and clinical findings with HER2 test results. The guidelines continue to emphasize that the pathologist should recognize HER2 testing results that would be considered discordant that might require additional testing or explanation.[41,59,60] Good prognosis histologic subtypes, such as pure mucinous, pure tubular, pure cribriform or adenoid cystic carcinomas should all be HER2-negative. In addition, grade 1 invasive ductal or lobular carcinomas should also be HER2-negative. A HER2-positive result in any of these settings should prompt further workup including troubleshooting the HER2 test as well as review of the histology. An example of a case that was initially classified as a mucinous carcinoma on core needle biopsy that tested HER2-positive (by both IHC and FISH) is shown in **Fig. 9.** On review, this discordance was explained by misclassification of the histologic subtype. This carcinoma did have areas with mucin production but it also had solid, nonmucinous areas, was Nottingham grade 3 overall, and had a Ki67 proliferative rate of 25%. High-grade carcinomas can produce mucin and if diagnosed as a "mucinous carcinoma," treating clinicians may use treatment recommendations for the good prognosis subtypes (see NCCN guidelines). "High-grade carcinoma with mucin production" was the revised diagnosis for this HER2-positive cancer.

Some histologic discordances may be explained by an unusual HER2 FISH category, such as FISH

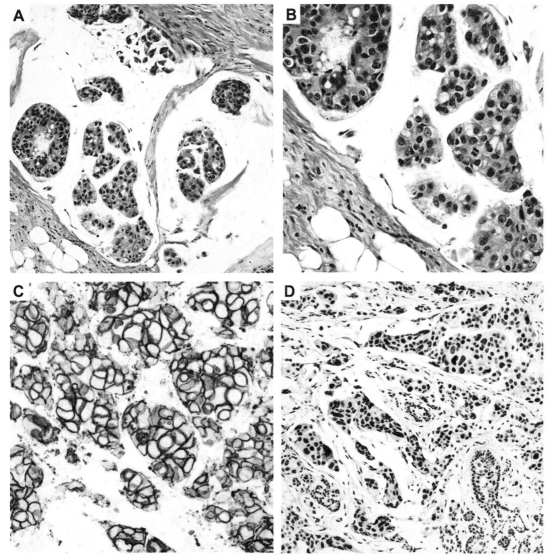

Fig. 9. An example of a case that was initially classified as a mucinous carcinoma on core needle biopsy (*A*, *B* [H&E, original magnification *A*, ×200 *B*, ×400]) that subsequently tested HER2-positive by IHC (*C*, H&E, original magnification ×400) and FISH testing. On review, this discordance was explained by misclassification of the histologic subtype. This carcinoma did have areas with mucin production but it also had solid, nonmucinous areas, was Nottingham grade 3 overall, and had a Ki67 proliferative rate of 25% (*D* [H&E, original magnification ×200]). High-grade carcinomas can produce mucin and if diagnosed as a "mucinous carcinoma," treating clinicians may use treatment recommendations for the good prognosis histologic subtypes. "High-grade carcinoma with mucin production" was the revised diagnosis for this HER2-positive cancer.

group 2, 3, or 4 cases or heterogeneous cases. Very rarely, an IHC-positive, FISH-negative discordance might be explained by other mechanisms of protein overexpression than gene amplification.[81] Also very rarely, an IHC-negative, FISH-positive discordance can be explained by mutations in the portion of the HER2 gene encoding the region of the protein recognized by the IHC antibody, causing a "false-negative" IHC result. If no apparent reason for a discordance is identified, the report should include comments about how unusual the combination of results are and that correlation with results on any additional samples may be indicated.

The typical HER2-positive cancer is intermediate to high grade, often with abundant eosinophilic cytoplasm or apocrine cytology and a high proliferative rate (generally 20% or higher). HER2-positive cancers commonly present in younger patients and often with associated high-grade ductal carcinoma in situ (DCIS). However, these features are not considered specific for HER2 positivity, and as such, a HER2-negative case with these characteristics is not necessarily an unexpected or discordant result. Generally, HER2 amplification and protein overexpression is believed to be stable with disease progression or recurrence, so a case that previously tested positive by one testing methodology is generally expected to be positive by other methods and in subsequent samples. The most obvious exception to this is in HER2 heterogeneous cases, for which HER2 test status can change from tissue sample to tissue sample, as mentioned previously.[67]

Consideration for Additional Testing

Because HER2 status is most often determined on an initial core biopsy sample, there are some scenarios in which additional HER2 testing of the surgical excision might be considered (see **Box 1**). If there are concerns about the initial core biopsy sample not being representative of the final overall tumor, or if the initial core biopsy result was indeterminate, borderline, discordant, or unusual, then the pathologist should consider retesting of the surgical sample. In the initial version of the 2013 HER2 guidelines, it stated that HER2 testing *must* be repeated on the surgical specimen after a negative result on core biopsy if the cancer was grade 3. However, this statement was subsequently revised to state that it *may* be repeated (based on pathologist judgment) but that repeat testing in this setting is not mandatory.[58,59] This revision was based on data showing high HER2-negative concordance rates between core and excision results and the inability of studies to identify a subset of cancers that would benefit from mandatory retesting.[82]

Validation

CAP requires proof of initial validation of any new HER2 test with a previously clinically validated test. Ideally, concordance between IHC and ISH assays should be greater than 90%. Ongoing concordance monitoring should be part of quality assurance. In addition, performing periodic trend analysis can be helpful to ensure the percentage of HER2-positive cases are within range of what is expected for the population being tested. Regional differences in the percentage of HER2-positive cancers have been reported, and it can be helpful to compare laboratories with similar population characteristics with one another.[83,84] In addition, proficiency testing should be ongoing (at least twice/year) with at least 90% performance on graded challenges.

PROLIFERATION MARKERS: KI67 AND PANEL-BASED ASSAYS

Key Points
PROLIFERATION MARKERS IN BREAST CANCER

- Measures of proliferation in breast cancer are used for a variety of purposes including determination of likelihood of response to chemotherapy.

- Ki67 is a relatively inexpensive, in situ IHC test that can estimate the cell proliferation index of a breast cancer; however, there are issues with standardization of scoring methodologies and reproducibility.

- Panel-based gene expression assays developed to predict outcomes in breast cancer are largely driven by proliferation-related genes.

- NCCN guidelines recommend "considering" OncotypeDX testing in ER+, lymph node–negative cancers greater than 0.5 cm to determine which patients may not benefit from the addition of chemotherapy to endocrine therapy. MammaPrint testing is also being used in a similar manner.

- Pathologic factors such as grade, PR levels, and proliferative rate typically correlate with OncotypeDX recurrence scores (RS) at the ends of the pathologic spectrum (cases that are grade 1, PR high, and Ki67 <10% correlate with low RS, whereas cases that are grade 3, PR low, with Ki67 >10% correlate with high RS). However, OncotypeDX RS results are not as easily correlated with pathology factors in cases with intermediate-risk factors (for example: grade 2, low PR, 10%–20% Ki67).

- Further workup should be considered if a *major discordance* is observed between standard pathology results and RS, such as the following:

  o Genomic Health quantitative ER result is negative or much lower than expected based on IHC result AND RS is higher than expected based on grade or proliferation rate.

  o Biopsy site changes or intermixed inflammation may be an explanation.

- Be able to recognize major discordances of ancillary test results with other histopathologic features of a case

- Serve as a consultant on treatment recommendation in cases with borderline or unusual results

Ki67

Different IHC scoring modalities to estimate the percentage of Ki67-positive carcinoma cells have been used, including manual counting of positive and negative cells, "eyeballed" estimates, and digital QIA. Studies have documented significant variability in scores between observers and methodologies.[89,90] In an attempt to further standardize Ki67 interpretation, the International Ki67 in Breast Cancer Working Group (IKBCWG) published recommendations for scoring and has continued to test methods to increase concordance.[91] These initial recommendations included manual counting of a minimum of 500 cells, and ideally at least 1000 cells. However, routinely counting 1000 cells is time-consuming and may be impractical for general practice in every case. Another source of variability is selection of areas to count and whether overall counts should be only hotspots or a more global average. Although correlation between observers is slightly better for global methods, hot spots or "bimodality" of Ki67 expression has been identified as an independent prognostic factor and may be clinically more relevant.[92]

Although digital scoring methods offer some obvious advantages because of the ability to supply a quantitative result, it is still subject to variability based on the detection thresholds set and the regions of interest selected for analysis.[93–95] Digital scoring can also have confounders such as intermixed inflammatory cells, carcinoma in situ, or other proliferating cells, so still requires significant pathologist oversight.

The IKBCWG work also showed that agreement on very high (>20%) or very low (<10%) Ki67 scores is excellent to perfect but that cases with scores between 10% and 20% have the greatest interobserver variability.[96] Given these findings, "eyeballed estimates" may be clinically sufficient for the ends of the spectrum but manual or quantitative digital counting may be especially important in the intermediate Ki67 range, especially for ER-positive cancers. **Fig. 10** (high cellularity) and **Fig. 11** (low cellularity) show examples of regions of cancers with Ki67 results in the 0% to 30% range that have been counted manually to determine the percent positive cells. These figures show how cellularity of the region may influence

Function

Ki67 by IHC is a relatively inexpensive, in situ test that provides an estimate of the number of active cells in the cell cycle. It has been suggested that luminal A and luminal B carcinomas can be stratified by a Ki67 of 13.25%.[85] From a therapeutic standpoint, the proliferative index can provide prognostic information, and help stratify which breast cancers might benefit from chemotherapy, especially in ER-positive cancers.[86] Changes in Ki67 have also been used as a marker of response to neoadjuvant treatments.[87,88] In addition, when the Ki67 score is discordant with other pathologic features such as the Nottingham grade, hormone receptor, or HER2 status of a breast cancer, it can serve as a red flag for additional pathology review. Although pathology practices for scoring Ki67 immunohistochemical stains are currently not standardized, this marker can serve as an inexpensive "first-round" proliferation marker in a breast cancer workup.

Cellular proliferation is also a key driver in the common commercial panel-based gene expression assays such as OncotypeDX and MammaPrint, which include proliferation genes, such as cyclin D1, MIB-1 and others. A summary of the most commonly used panel-based assays is shown in **Table 2**.

Interpretation

Key Points
PATHOLOGIST'S ROLE IN INTERPRETING ANCILLARY TESTS

- Be familiar with testing guidelines or recommendations

- Know interpretation criteria and thresholds for results

- Be familiar with the clinical impact(s) of the test result

Table 2
Common panel-based molecular tests used to predict outcomes in breast cancer

Test (Company)	Centralized Testing?	Number of Genes Tested	Patient Population Validated for	Results Reported	Clinical Utility
OncotypeDX (Genomic Health, Redwood City, CA)	Yes	Expression of 16 cancer-related genes (5 reference genes)	ER+; 0–3 positive lymph nodes	1. Recurrence Score (RS) and low, intermediate or high-risk category 2. Quantitative ER, PR, and HER2 levels (*but not validated for clinical decision-making*)	Estimation of recurrence risk (3 categories) and benefit of chemotherapy (in addition to hormonal therapy)
MammaPrint BluePrint (Agendia, Amsterdam, Netherlands)	Yes	Expression of 70 genes	ER+ or ER−; Stage 1–2, 0–3 positive lymph nodes	1. Low or high recurrence risk categories 2. Molecular subtype 3. Quantitative ER, PR, and HER2 levels (*but not validated for clinical decision-making*)	Estimation of recurrence risk (high vs low): most useful in ER+ patients; and subtype used as outcome indicator
PAM50/Prosigna (NanoString Technologies, Seattle, WA)	No (laboratories can purchase testing system)	Expression of 50 cancer-related genes	ER+, Stage 1–2, lymph node–negative or 1–3 positive lymph nodes	1. Molecular subtype (*only reported in non-US countries*) 2. Risk of Recurrence Score (ROR)	Estimation of recurrence risk (3 categories) and subtype used as outcome indicator

Abbreviations: ER, estrogen receptor; HER2, human epidermal growth factor receptor 2; PR, progesterone receptor.

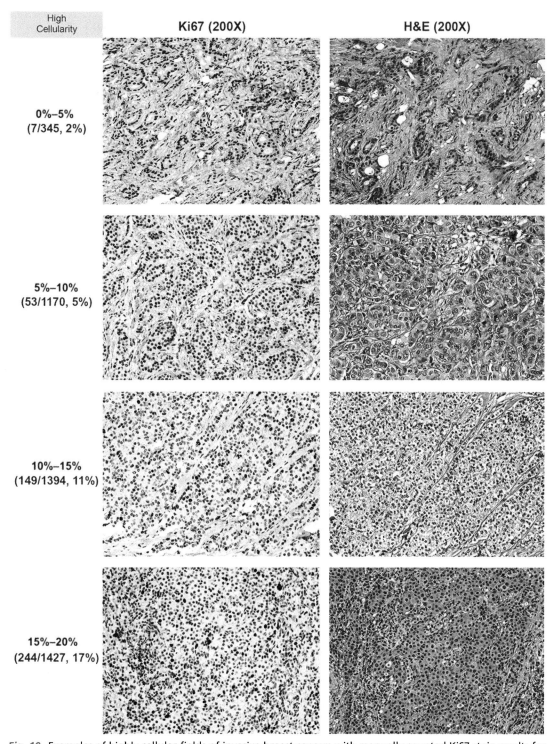

High Cellularity	Ki67 (200X)	H&E (200X)
0%–5% (7/345, 2%)		
5%–10% (53/1170, 5%)		
10%–15% (149/1394, 11%)		
15%–20% (244/1427, 17%)		

Fig. 10. Examples of highly cellular fields of invasive breast cancers with manually counted Ki67 stain results for the field. Examples of well-counted Ki67 fields may help pathologists calibrate their Ki67 estimates.

"eyeballed" estimates and may serve as useful standards when making these estimates. However, some experts have emphasized that treatment decisions for individual patients should not be made based solely on small differences in Ki67 around a specific threshold, and therefore reporting results as ranges may be most appropriate.[97]

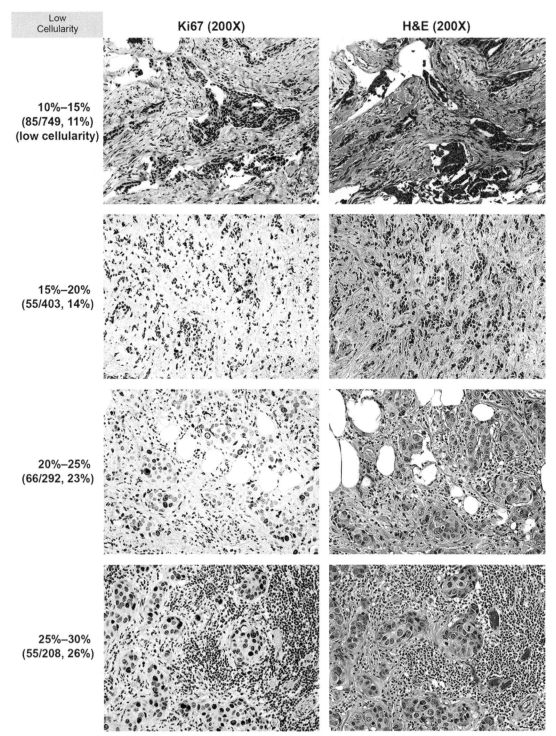

Low Cellularity	Ki67 (200X)	H&E (200X)
10%–15% (85/749, 11%) (low cellularity)		
15%–20% (55/403, 14%)		
20%–25% (66/292, 23%)		
25%–30% (55/208, 26%)		

Fig. 11. Examples of lower cellularity fields of invasive breast cancers with manually counted Ki67 stain results for the field. Examples of well-counted Ki67 fields may help pathologists calibrate their Ki67 estimates.

Panel-based assays

Although most panel-based assays are performed in central commercial laboratories with results reported back to ordering physicians, pathologists still play 2 important roles for these assays: (1) selection of the block for testing, and (2) correlation of results with other findings (see expected vs unexpected results in the next section).[2] For tissue block selection, the most ideal sample for testing should have the largest area of invasive carcinoma available (usually this is done on a surgical excision sample rather than core biopsy) without including large areas of biopsy site changes, inflammation, DCIS, or normal tissue as much as possible. In some cases, these findings cannot be avoided, and it can be helpful to notify the reference laboratory that macrodissection may be required to avoid confounding results. Cases with only microinvasion or blocks from metastatic carcinoma in a lymph node are also generally not appropriate because noncancer tissue is highly likely to influence results in these settings.

Expected Versus Unexpected Results

Ki67

Ki67 is expected to be very high in high-grade, triple-negative cancers (predominately ranging from 30%–80%) and HER2-positive/ER-negative cancers (predominantly ranging from 20%–60%) and results significantly lower than 20% in these case types are not expected. Ki67 scores in ER-positive cancers are much more variable, from less than 5% in very well-differentiated, grade 1, ER-positive cancers, to more than 20% in some higher-grade ER-positive cancers. Therefore, ER-positive cases are more challenging to correlate with Ki67. However, the ends of the spectrum should generally be predictable, such that a grade 1, ER-positive/HER2-negative cancer would not be expected to have a Ki67 rate greater than 20% and an untreated grade 3, ER-positive/HER2-negative cancer would not be expected to have a Ki67 rate less than 10%. This can serve as a useful check on Nottingham grade in this setting. Other factors can influence Ki67 results and be an explanation for seemingly discordant results, for example some reports suggest Ki67 rates are higher in surgical excision samples because of longer tissue ischemic times or as the result of reparative changes after core biopsy.[98] In addition, because Nottingham grade uses mitotic count rather than accounting for all cycling cells (as Ki67 does), these 2 parameters may not always be well correlated.

Oncotype DX

For ER-positive breast cancers, pathologic factors, such as grade, PR levels, and proliferative rate typically correlate well with Oncotype DX RSs at the ends of the pathologic spectrum (cases that are grade 1, PR high, and Ki67 <10% correlate with low RSs, whereas cases that are grade 3, PR low, with Ki67 >10% correlate with high RSs). However, OncotypeDX RS results are not as easily correlated with pathology factors in cases with intermediate-risk factors (for example, grade 2, low PR, 10%–20% Ki67).[99] Although there are multiple multivariate models that attempt to predict RSs, such as the Magee equation, modified-Magee equation, and IHC4 scores, these models are best at predicting high and low RS values.[100–106]

One of the inherent limitations of an assay that is not interpreted in situ (such as IHC and ISH testing) is the possibility that the results may be confounded by the contribution of noncancer tissue. Intermixed inflammation, in situ carcinoma, or desmoplastic stroma may influence results on an individual-case basis.[99,107] Therefore, the results need to be correlated with morphologic findings and taken in the context of other data points about the behavior of the cancer rather than taking any panel-based test results as a new "gold standard."

Further workup should be considered if *major discordance* between standard pathology results and RS is suspected. In particular, if the RS is higher than expected based on grade or proliferation rate and the quantitative ER result is negative or much lower than expected (based on IHC result), then biopsy site changes or intermixed inflammation and normal tissues may have interfered with RS results.[1,108] If such a major discordance is seen, the pathologist should work with the ordering clinician and Genomic Health to troubleshoot results. Consideration for retesting on a core biopsy sample or blocks without biopsy site changes can also be made. **Fig. 12** shows a case with a low-grade invasive ductal carcinoma (H&E on Panels A and B) that had >95%, strong ER expression (Panel C) and a Ki67 proliferative rate <5% by IHC (Panel D). The Oncotype DX RS on this sample was high (35) and the quantitative ER results reported were just above the threshold for positive by quantitative RT-PCR. Because the IHC and RT-PCR ER results were so discordant and the RS was higher than expected in a low-grade cancer, the pathologist contacted Genomic Health to troubleshoot the case. Additional OncotypeDX testing on the initial core needle biopsy sample of the same cancer yielded a low RS (16) and a high quantitative ER result, more in keeping with the other pathologic findings on the case.

Validation

Although there are no CAP guidelines specific to Ki67, its IHC validation should follow the CAP published principles of analytical validation of IHC assays.[109,110] It may also be useful to establish interpretation standards and internal

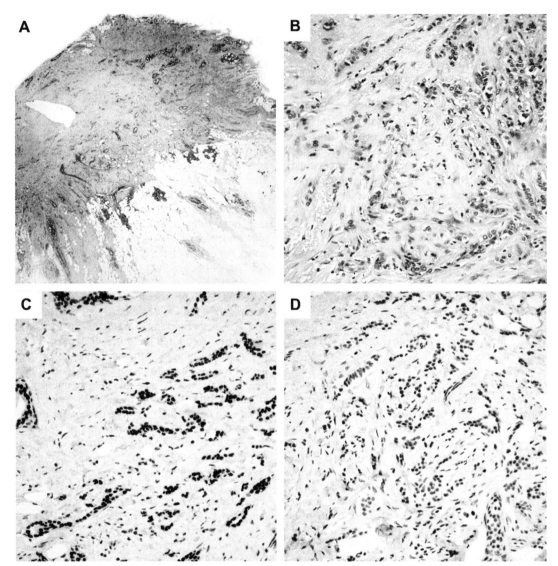

Fig. 12. A case with a low-grade invasive ductal carcinoma ([H&E, original magnification *A*, ×2 *B*, ×200] on *A* and *B*) that had >95%, strong ER expression by IHC (*C*, H&E, original magnification ×200) and a Ki67 proliferative rate <5% by IHC (*D*, H&E, original magnification ×200). The Oncotype DX RS on this postbiopsy surgical sample was high (35) and the quantitative ER results reported were just above the threshold for positive by quantitative RT-PCR. Because the IHC and RT-PCR ER results were so discordant and the RS was higher than expected in a low-grade cancer, the pathologist contacted Genomic Health to troubleshoot the case. Additional OncotypeDX testing on the initial core needle biopsy sample of the same cancer yielded a low RS (16) and a high quantitative ER result, more in keeping with the other pathologic findings on the case.

proficiency testing methods for your laboratory such that interpreters of Ki67 are as standardized as possible.

Validation of OncotypeDX and MammaPrint was initially primarily on large retrospective cohorts using clinical trial data.[111–115] Although studies examining the concordance of multiple gene signatures, including Oncotype DX , MammaPrint, and PAM50 risk of RS have found that each had significant prognostic value, the individual risk assessments were often discordant with one another (Cohen

kappa values ranging from 0.24–0.70).[116–119] Results of large multi-institutional studies including the TAILORx, MINDACT, and ISPY-2 trials have provided some initial 5-year results on the prospective value of these assays.[120–122] The MINDACT trial has released preliminary data on patients with low-risk MammaPrint results and reports a 94.7% 5-year distant metastasis-free survival without chemotherapy, even in the presence of other high-risk clinical factors.[123] Similarly, the TAILORx study has also released data showing cancers with an OncotypeDX RS between 0 and 10 have excellent outcomes with endocrine therapy alone, with the risk of metastatic disease <1% and the risk of any recurrence less than 2% at 5 years.[121]

SUMMARY

Clearly, ancillary testing in breast cancer has changed the way we classify and treat breast cancers, adding predictive and prognostic value to treatment paradigms. The pathologist's role remains central in performing, interpreting, and integrating the increasingly diverse amount of biologic information available on every breast cancer and translating it into clinically relevant information. Pathologists should continue to develop and provide their expertise by consulting on challenging cases in which ancillary test results are unusual or discordant with other clinical and pathologic findings.

REFERENCES

1. Acs G, Esposito NN, Kiluk J, et al. A mitotically active, cellular tumor stroma and/or inflammatory cells associated with tumor cells may contribute to intermediate or high Oncotype DX recurrence scores in low-grade invasive breast carcinomas. Mod Pathol 2012;25(4):556–66.
2. Allison KH. Molecular pathology of breast cancer: what a pathologist needs to know. Am J Clin Pathol 2012;138(6):770–80.
3. Mandong BM. Diagnostic oncology: role of the pathologist in surgical oncology–a review article. Afr J Med Med Sci 2009;38(Suppl 2):81–8.
4. Han HS, Magliocco AM. Molecular testing and the pathologist's role in clinical trials of breast cancer. Clin Breast Cancer 2016;16(3):166–79.
5. Rakha EA, Green AR. Molecular classification of breast cancer: what the pathologist needs to know. Pathology 2017;49(2):111–9.
6. Leong AS, Zhuang Z. The changing role of pathology in breast cancer diagnosis and treatment. Pathobiology 2011;78(2):99–114.
7. Gradishar WJ, Anderson BO, Balassanian R, et al. NCCN guidelines insights: breast cancer, version 1.2017. J Natl Compr Canc Netw 2017;15(4):433–51.
8. Gnant M, Harbeck N, Thomssen C. St. Gallen/Vienna 2017: a brief summary of the consensus discussion about escalation and de-escalation of primary breast cancer treatment. Breast Care (Basel) 2017;12(2):102–7.
9. Goldhirsch A, Winer EP, Coates AS, et al. Personalizing the treatment of women with early breast cancer: highlights of the St Gallen International Expert Consensus on the primary therapy of early breast cancer 2013. Ann Oncol 2013;24(9):2206–23.
10. Harris LN, Ismaila N, McShane LM, et al. Use of biomarkers to guide decisions on adjuvant systemic therapy for women with early-stage invasive breast cancer: American Society of Clinical Oncology clinical practice guideline summary. J Oncol Pract 2016;12(4):384–9.
11. Perou CM, Sorlie T, Eisen MB, et al. Molecular portraits of human breast tumours. Nature 2000; 406(6797):747–52.
12. Sorlie T, Perou CM, Tibshirani R, et al. Gene expression patterns of breast carcinomas distinguish tumor subclasses with clinical implications. Proc Natl Acad Sci U S A 2001;98(19):10869–74.
13. Sorlie T, Tibshirani R, Parker J, et al. Repeated observation of breast tumor subtypes in independent gene expression data sets. Proc Natl Acad Sci U S A 2003;100(14):8418–23.
14. Reis-Filho JS, Pusztai L. Gene expression profiling in breast cancer: classification, prognostication, and prediction. Lancet 2011;378(9805):1812–23.
15. Hu Z, Fan C, Oh DS, et al. The molecular portraits of breast tumors are conserved across microarray platforms. BMC Genomics 2006;7:96.
16. Sotiriou C, Neo SY, McShane LM, et al. Breast cancer classification and prognosis based on gene expression profiles from a population-based study. Proc Natl Acad Sci U S A 2003;100(18):10393–8.
17. Heng YJ, Lester SC, Tse GM, et al. The molecular basis of breast cancer pathological phenotypes. J Pathol 2017;241(3):375–91.
18. Cancer Genome Atlas Network. Comprehensive molecular portraits of human breast tumours. Nature 2012;490(7418):61–70.
19. Prat A, Pineda E, Adamo B, et al. Clinical implications of the intrinsic molecular subtypes of breast cancer. Breast 2015;24(Suppl 2):S26–35.
20. Weigelt B, Mackay A, A'Hern R, et al. Breast cancer molecular profiling with single sample predictors: a retrospective analysis. Lancet Oncol 2010;11(4): 339–49.
21. Mackay A, Weigelt B, Grigoriadis A, et al. Microarray-based class discovery for molecular classification of breast cancer: analysis of interobserver agreement. J Natl Cancer Inst 2011;103(8): 662–73.
22. Fan C, Oh DS, Wessels L, et al. Concordance among gene-expression-based predictors for breast cancer. N Engl J Med 2006;355(6):560–9.
23. Yang Y, Im SA, Keam B, et al. Prognostic impact of AJCC response criteria for neoadjuvant chemotherapy in stage II/III breast cancer patients: breast cancer subtype analyses. BMC Cancer 2016;16:515.
24. Amin MB, Greene FL, Edge SB, et al. The Eighth Edition AJCC Cancer Staging Manual: Continuing to build a bridge from a population-based to a more "personalized" approach to cancer staging. CA Cancer J Clin 2017;67(2):93–9.

25. American Joint Committee on Cancer, Amin MB. AJCC cancer staging manual. 8th edition. New York: Springer; 2017.

26. Harvey JM, Clark GM, Osborne CK, et al. Estrogen receptor status by immunohistochemistry is superior to the ligand-binding assay for predicting response to adjuvant endocrine therapy in breast cancer. J Clin Oncol 1999;17(5):1474–81.

27. Mohsin SK, Weiss H, Havighurst T, et al. Progesterone receptor by immunohistochemistry and clinical outcome in breast cancer: a validation study. Mod Pathol 2004;17(12):1545–54.

28. Elledge RM, Green S, Pugh R, et al. Estrogen receptor (ER) and progesterone receptor (PgR), by ligand-binding assay compared with ER, PgR and pS2, by immuno-histochemistry in predicting response to tamoxifen in metastatic breast cancer: a Southwest Oncology Group Study. Int J Cancer 2000;89(2):111–7.

29. Allison KH. Estrogen receptor expression in breast cancer: we cannot ignore the shades of gray. Am J Clin Pathol 2008;130(6):853–4.

30. Sheffield BS, Kos Z, Asleh-Aburaya K, et al. Molecular subtype profiling of invasive breast cancers weakly positive for estrogen receptor. Breast Cancer Res Treat 2016;155(3):483–90.

31. Hammond ME, Hayes DF, Dowsett M, et al. American Society of Clinical Oncology/College of American Pathologists guideline recommendations for immunohistochemical testing of estrogen and progesterone receptors in breast cancer. Arch Pathol Lab Med 2010;134(6):907–22.

32. Chen T, Zhang N, Moran MS, et al. Borderline ER-positive primary breast cancer gains no significant survival benefit from endocrine therapy: a systematic review and meta-analysis. Clin Breast Cancer 2017, [Epub ahead of print].

33. Gloyeske NC, Dabbs DJ, Bhargava R. Low ER+ breast cancer: Is this a distinct group? Am J Clin Pathol 2014;141(5):697–701.

34. Deyarmin B, Kane JL, Valente AL, et al. Effect of ASCO/CAP guidelines for determining ER status on molecular subtype. Ann Surg Oncol 2013; 20(1):87–93.

35. Slamon DJ, Leyland-Jones B, Shak S, et al. Use of chemotherapy plus a monoclonal antibody against HER2 for metastatic breast cancer that overexpresses HER2. N Engl J Med 2001;344(11):783–92.

36. Goldhirsch A, Gelber RD, Piccart-Gebhart MJ, et al. 2 years versus 1 year of adjuvant trastuzumab for HER2-positive breast cancer (HERA): an open-label, randomised controlled trial. Lancet 2013; 382(9897):1021–8.

37. Perez EA, Romond EH, Suman VJ, et al. Four-year follow-up of trastuzumab plus adjuvant chemotherapy for operable human epidermal growth factor receptor 2-positive breast cancer: joint analysis of data from NCCTG N9831 and NSABP B-31. J Clin Oncol 2011;29(25):3366–73.

38. Swain SM, Kim SB, Cortes J, et al. Pertuzumab, trastuzumab, and docetaxel for HER2-positive metastatic breast cancer (CLEOPATRA study): overall survival results from a randomised, double-blind, placebo-controlled, phase 3 study. Lancet Oncol 2013;14(6):461–71.

39. Baselga J, Bradbury I, Eidtmann H, et al. Lapatinib with trastuzumab for HER2-positive early breast cancer (NeoALTTO): a randomised, open-label, multicentre, phase 3 trial. Lancet 2012;379(9816): 633–40.

40. Verma S, Miles D, Gianni L, et al. Trastuzumab emtansine for HER2-positive advanced breast cancer. N Engl J Med 2012;367(19):1783–91.

41. Wolff AC, Hammond ME, Hicks DG, et al. Recommendations for human epidermal growth factor receptor 2 testing in breast cancer: American Society of Clinical Oncology/College of American Pathologists clinical practice guideline update. J Clin Oncol 2013;31(31):3997–4013.

42. Wolff AC, Hammond ME, Hicks DG, et al. Recommendations for human epidermal growth factor receptor 2 testing in breast cancer: American Society of Clinical Oncology/College of American Pathologists clinical practice guideline update. Arch Pathol Lab Med 2014;138(2):241–56.

43. Wolff AC, Hammond ME, Schwartz JN, et al. American Society of Clinical Oncology/College of American Pathologists guideline recommendations for human epidermal growth factor receptor 2 testing in breast cancer. Arch Pathol Lab Med 2007; 131(1):18–43.

44. Wolff AC, Hammond ME, Schwartz JN, et al. American Society of Clinical Oncology/College of American Pathologists guideline recommendations for human epidermal growth factor receptor 2 testing in breast cancer. J Clin Oncol 2007;25(1):118–45.

45. Varadan V, Sandoval M, Harris LN. Biomarkers for predicting response to anti-HER2 agents. Adv Exp Med Biol 2016;882:155–67.

46. von Minckwitz G, Untch M, Blohmer JU, et al. Definition and impact of pathologic complete response on prognosis after neoadjuvant chemotherapy in various intrinsic breast cancer subtypes. J Clin Oncol 2012;30(15):1796–804.

47. Dunbier AK, Anderson H, Ghazoui Z, et al. Association between breast cancer subtypes and response to neoadjuvant anastrozole. Steroids 2011;76(8): 736–40.

48. Carey LA, Dees EC, Sawyer L, et al. The triple negative paradox: primary tumor chemosensitivity of breast cancer subtypes. Clin Cancer Res 2007; 13(8):2329–34.

49. Cortazar P, Zhang L, Untch M, et al. Pathological complete response and long-term clinical benefit

in breast cancer: the CTNeoBC pooled analysis. Lancet 2014;384(9938):164–72.

50. Liu S, Chapman JA, Burnell MJ, et al. Prognostic and predictive investigation of PAM50 intrinsic subtypes in the NCIC CTG MA.21 phase III chemotherapy trial. Breast Cancer Res Treat 2015; 149(2):439–48.

51. Cui X, Schiff R, Arpino G, et al. Biology of progesterone receptor loss in breast cancer and its implications for endocrine therapy. J Clin Oncol 2005;23(30): 7721–35.

52. Kurozumi S, Matsumoto H, Hayashi Y, et al. Power of PgR expression as a prognostic factor for ER-positive/HER2-negative breast cancer patients at intermediate risk classified by the Ki67 labeling index. BMC Cancer 2017;17(1):354.

53. Troxell ML, Long T, Hornick JL, et al. Comparison of estrogen and progesterone receptor antibody reagents using proficiency testing data. Arch Pathol Lab Med 2017;141(10):1402–12.

54. Muftah AA, Aleskandarany M, Sonbul SN, et al. Further evidence to support bimodality of oestrogen receptor expression in breast cancer. Histopathology 2017;70(3):456–65.

55. Ibrahim M, Dodson A, Barnett S, et al. Potential for false-positive staining with a rabbit monoclonal antibody to progesterone receptor (SP2): findings of the UK National External Quality Assessment Scheme for Immunocytochemistry and FISH highlight the need for correct validation of antibodies on introduction to the laboratory. Am J Clin Pathol 2008;129(3):398–409.

56. Troxell ML. Merkel cell carcinoma, melanoma, metastatic mimics of breast cancer. Semin Diagn Pathol 2017;34(5):479–95.

57. O'Sullivan CC, Swain SM. Pertuzumab: evolving therapeutic strategies in the management of HER2-overexpressing breast cancer. Expert Opin Biol Ther 2013;13(5):779–90.

58. Rakha EA, Starczynski J, Lee AH, et al. The updated ASCO/CAP guideline recommendations for HER2 testing in the management of invasive breast cancer: a critical review of their implications for routine practice. Histopathology 2014;64(5): 609–15.

59. Wolff AC, Hammond ME, Hicks DG, et al. Reply to E.A. Rakha et al. J Clin Oncol 2015;33(11): 1302–4.

60. Rakha EA, Pigera M, Shaaban A, et al. National guidelines and level of evidence: comments on some of the new recommendations in the American Society of Clinical Oncology and the College of American Pathologists human epidermal growth factor receptor 2 guidelines for breast cancer. J Clin Oncol 2015;33(11):1301–2.

61. Grimm EE, Schmidt RA, Swanson PE, et al. Achieving 95% cross-methodological concordance

in HER2 testing: causes and implications of discordant cases. Am J Clin Pathol 2010;134(2):284–92.

62. Ruschoff J, Dietel M, Baretton G, et al. HER2 diagnostics in gastric cancer-guideline validation and development of standardized immunohistochemical testing. Virchows Arch 2010;457(3):299–307.

63. Ruschoff J, Kerr KM, Grote HJ, et al. Reproducibility of immunohistochemical scoring for epidermal growth factor receptor expression in non-small cell lung cancer: round robin test. Arch Pathol Lab Med 2013;137(9):1255–61.

64. Ballard M, Jalikis F, Krings G, et al. 'Non-classical' HER2 FISH results in breast cancer: a multi-institutional study. Mod Pathol 2017;30(2):227–35.

65. Perez EA, Dueck AC, McCullough AE, et al. Predictability of adjuvant trastuzumab benefit in N9831 patients using the ASCO/CAP HER2-positivity criteria. J Natl Cancer Inst 2012;104(2): 159–62.

66. Gulbahce HE, Factor R, Geiersbach K, et al. HER2 immunohistochemistry-guided targeted fluorescence in situ hybridization analysis does not help identify intratumoral heterogeneity in breast cancer. Arch Pathol Lab Med 2016;140(8):741.

67. Perez EA, Press MF, Dueck AC, et al. Immunohistochemistry and fluorescence in situ hybridization assessment of HER2 in clinical trials of adjuvant therapy for breast cancer (NCCTG N9831, BCIRG 006, and BCIRG 005). Breast Cancer Res Treat 2013;138(1):99–108.

68. Shah MV, Wiktor AE, Meyer RG, et al. Change in pattern of HER2 fluorescent in situ hybridization (FISH) results in breast cancers submitted for fish testing: experience of a reference laboratory using US Food and Drug Administration criteria and American Society of Clinical Oncology and College of American Pathologists Guidelines. J Clin Oncol 2016;34(29):3502–10.

69. Press MF, Sauter G, Buyse M, et al. HER2 gene amplification testing by fluorescent in situ hybridization (FISH): comparison of the ASCO-College of American Pathologists Guidelines with FISH scores used for enrollment in Breast Cancer International Research Group Clinical Trials. J Clin Oncol 2016; 34(29):3518–28.

70. Stoss OC, Scheel A, Nagelmeier I, et al. Impact of updated HER2 testing guidelines in breast cancer–re-evaluation of HERA trial fluorescence in situ hybridization data. Mod Pathol 2015;28(12):1528–34.

71. Press MF, Villalobos I, Santiago A, et al. Assessing the New American Society of Clinical Oncology/College of American Pathologists guidelines for HER2 testing by fluorescence in situ hybridization: experience of an academic consultation practice. Arch Pathol Lab Med 2016, [Epub ahead of print].

72. Hanna WM, Ruschoff J, Bilous M, et al. HER2 in situ hybridization in breast cancer: clinical implications

of polysomy 17 and genetic heterogeneity. Mod Pathol 2014;27(1):4–18.

73. Tse CH, Hwang HC, Goldstein LC, et al. Determining true HER2 gene status in breast cancers with polysomy by using alternative chromosome 17 reference genes: implications for anti-HER2 targeted therapy. J Clin Oncol 2011;29(31):4168–74.

74. Troxell ML, Bangs CD, Lawce HJ, et al. Evaluation of Her-2/neu status in carcinomas with amplified chromosome 17 centromere locus. Am J Clin Pathol 2006;126(5):709–16.

75. Moelans CB, de Weger RA, van Diest PJ. Absence of chromosome 17 polysomy in breast cancer: analysis by CEP17 chromogenic in situ hybridization and multiplex ligation-dependent probe amplification. Breast Cancer Res Treat 2010;120(1):1–7.

76. Marchio C, Lambros MB, Gugliotta P, et al. Does chromosome 17 centromere copy number predict polysomy in breast cancer? A fluorescence in situ hybridization and microarray-based CGH analysis. J Pathol 2009;219(1):16–24.

77. Yeh IT, Martin MA, Robetorye RS, et al. Clinical validation of an array CGH test for HER2 status in breast cancer reveals that polysomy 17 is a rare event. Mod Pathol 2009;22(9):1169–75.

78. Vranic S, Teruya B, Repertinger S, et al. Assessment of HER2 gene status in breast carcinomas with polysomy of chromosome 17. Cancer 2011;117(1):48–53.

79. Sneige N, Hess KR, Multani AS, et al. Prognostic significance of equivocal human epidermal growth factor receptor 2 results and clinical utility of alternative chromosome 17 genes in patients with invasive breast cancer: a cohort study. Cancer 2017;123(7):1115–23.

80. Holzschuh MA, Czyz Z, Hauke S, et al. HER2 FISH results in breast cancers with increased CEN17 signals using alternative chromosome 17 probes - reclassifying cases in the equivocal category. Histopathology 2017;71(4):610–25.

81. Petrelli F, Tomasello G, Barni S, et al. Clinical and pathological characterization of HER2 mutations in human breast cancer: a systematic review of the literature. Breast Cancer Res Treat 2017, [Epub ahead of print].

82. Arnedos M, Nerurkar A, Osin P, et al. Discordance between core needle biopsy (CNB) and excisional biopsy (EB) for estrogen receptor (ER), progesterone receptor (PgR) and HER2 status in early breast cancer (EBC). Ann Oncol 2009;20(12):1948–52.

83. Ruschoff J, Lebeau A, Kreipe H, et al. Assessing HER2 testing quality in breast cancer: variables that influence HER2 positivity rate from a large, multicenter, observational study in Germany. Mod Pathol 2017;30(2):217–26.

84. Lin CY, Carneal EE, Lichtensztajn DY, et al. Regional variability in percentage of breast cancers reported as positive for HER2 in California: implications of patient demographics on laboratory benchmarks. Am J Clin Pathol 2017;148(3):199–207.

85. Cheang MC, Chia SK, Voduc D, et al. Ki67 index, HER2 status, and prognosis of patients with luminal B breast cancer. J Natl Cancer Inst 2009;101(10):736–50.

86. Criscitiello C, Disalvatore D, De Laurentiis M, et al. High Ki-67 score is indicative of a greater benefit from adjuvant chemotherapy when added to endocrine therapy in luminal B HER2 negative and node-positive breast cancer. Breast 2014;23(1):69–75.

87. Alba E, Lluch A, Ribelles N, et al. High proliferation predicts pathological complete response to neoadjuvant chemotherapy in early breast cancer. Oncologist 2016;21(2):150–5.

88. von Minckwitz G, Schmitt WD, Loibl S, et al. Ki67 measured after neoadjuvant chemotherapy for primary breast cancer. Clin Cancer Res 2013;19(16):4521–31.

89. Polley MY, Leung SC, McShane LM, et al. An international Ki67 reproducibility study. J Natl Cancer Inst 2013;105(24):1897–906.

90. Polley MY, Leung SC, Gao D, et al. An international study to increase concordance in Ki67 scoring. Mod Pathol 2015;28(6):778–86.

91. Dowsett M, Nielsen TO, A'Hern R, et al. Assessment of Ki67 in breast cancer: recommendations from the International Ki67 in Breast Cancer working group. J Natl Cancer Inst 2011;103(22):1656–64.

92. Laurinavicius A, Plancoulaine B, Rasmusson A, et al. Bimodality of intratumor Ki67 expression is an independent prognostic factor of overall survival in patients with invasive breast carcinoma. Virchows Arch 2016;468(4):493–502.

93. Maeda I, Abe K, Koizumi H, et al. Comparison between Ki67 labeling index determined using image analysis software with virtual slide system and that determined visually in breast cancer. Breast Cancer 2016;23(5):745–51.

94. Zhong F, Bi R, Yu B, et al. A comparison of visual assessment and automated digital image analysis of Ki67 labeling index in breast cancer. PLoS One 2016;11(2):e0150505.

95. Christgen M, von Ahsen S, Christgen H, et al. The region-of-interest size impacts on Ki67 quantification by computer-assisted image analysis in breast cancer. Hum Pathol 2015;46(9):1341–9.

96. Leung SCY, Nielsen TO, Zabaglo L, et al. Analytical validation of a standardized scoring protocol for Ki67: phase 3 of an international multicenter collaboration. NPJ Breast Cancer 2016;2:16014.

97. Denkert C, Budczies J, von Minckwitz G, et al. Strategies for developing Ki67 as a useful biomarker in breast cancer. Breast 2015;24(Suppl 2):S67–72.

98. Chen X, Zhu S, Fei X, et al. Surgery time interval and molecular subtype may influence Ki67 change after core needle biopsy in breast cancer patients. BMC Cancer 2015;15:822.

99. Allison KH, Kandalaft PL, Sitlani CM, et al. Routine pathologic parameters can predict Oncotype DX recurrence scores in subsets of ER positive patients: who does not always need testing? Breast Cancer Res Treat 2012;131(2): 413–24.

100. Farrugia DJ, Landmann A, Zhu L, et al. Magee equation 3 predicts pathologic response to neoadjuvant systemic chemotherapy in estrogen receptor positive, HER2 negative/equivocal breast tumors. Mod Pathol 2017;30(8):1078–85.

101. Flanagan MB, Dabbs DJ, Brufsky AM, et al. Histopathologic variables predict Oncotype DX recurrence score. Mod Pathol 2008;21(10):1255–61.

102. Harowicz MR, Robinson TJ, Dinan MA, et al. Algorithms for prediction of the Oncotype DX recurrence score using clinicopathologic data: a review and comparison using an independent dataset. Breast Cancer Res Treat 2017;162(1): 1–10.

103. Klein ME, Dabbs DJ, Shuai Y, et al. Prediction of the Oncotype DX recurrence score: use of pathology-generated equations derived by linear regression analysis. Mod Pathol 2013;26(5): 658–64.

104. Turner BM, Skinner KA, Tang P, et al. Use of modified Magee equations and histologic criteria to predict the Oncotype DX recurrence score. Mod Pathol 2015;28(7):921–31.

105. Sgroi DC, Sestak I, Cuzick J, et al. Prediction of late distant recurrence in patients with oestrogen-receptor-positive breast cancer: a prospective comparison of the breast-cancer index (BCI) assay, 21-gene recurrence score, and IHC4 in the TransATAC study population. Lancet Oncol 2013; 14(11):1067–76.

106. Cuzick J, Dowsett M, Pineda S, et al. Prognostic value of a combined estrogen receptor, progesterone receptor, Ki-67, and human epidermal growth factor receptor 2 immunohistochemical score and comparison with the Genomic Health recurrence score in early breast cancer. J Clin Oncol 2011; 29(32):4273–8.

107. Massink MP, Kooi IE, van Mil SE, et al. Proper genomic profiling of (BRCA1-mutated) basal-like breast carcinomas requires prior removal of tumor infiltrating lymphocytes. Mol Oncol 2015;9(4):877–88.

108. Acs G, Kiluk J, Loftus L, et al. Comparison of Oncotype DX and Mammostrat risk estimations and correlations with histologic tumor features in low-grade, estrogen receptor-positive invasive breast carcinomas. Mod Pathol 2013;26(11): 1451–60.

109. Goldsmith JD, Fitzgibbons PL, Swanson PE. Principles of analytic validation of clinical immunohistochemistry assays. Adv Anat Pathol 2015;22(6): 384–7.

110. Fitzgibbons PL, Bradley LA, Fatheree LA, et al. Principles of analytic validation of immunohistochemical assays: guideline from the College of American Pathologists Pathology and Laboratory Quality Center. Arch Pathol Lab Med 2014; 138(11):1432–43.

111. Cronin M, Sangli C, Liu ML, et al. Analytical validation of the Oncotype DX genomic diagnostic test for recurrence prognosis and therapeutic response prediction in node-negative, estrogen receptor-positive breast cancer. Clin Chem 2007;53(6): 1084–91.

112. Paik S, Shak S, Tang G, et al. A multigene assay to predict recurrence of tamoxifen-treated, node-negative breast cancer. N Engl J Med 2004; 351(27):2817–26.

113. Bueno-de-Mesquita JM, Linn SC, Keijzer R, et al. Validation of 70-gene prognosis signature in node-negative breast cancer. Breast Cancer Res Treat 2009;117(3):483–95.

114. Bueno-de-Mesquita JM, van Harten WH, Retel VP, et al. Use of 70-gene signature to predict prognosis of patients with node-negative breast cancer: a prospective community-based feasibility study (RASTER). Lancet Oncol 2007;8(12): 1079–87.

115. Knauer M, Mook S, Rutgers EJ, et al. The predictive value of the 70-gene signature for adjuvant chemotherapy in early breast cancer. Breast Cancer Res Treat 2010;120(3):655–61.

116. Iwamoto T, Lee JS, Bianchini G, et al. First generation prognostic gene signatures for breast cancer predict both survival and chemotherapy sensitivity and identify overlapping patient populations. Breast Cancer Res Treat 2011;130(1):155–64.

117. Prat A, Parker JS, Fan C, et al. Concordance among gene expression-based predictors for ER-positive breast cancer treated with adjuvant tamoxifen. Ann Oncol 2012;23(11):2866–73.

118. Kelly CM, Bernard PS, Krishnamurthy S, et al. Agreement in risk prediction between the 21-gene recurrence score assay (Oncotype DX(R)) and the PAM50 breast cancer intrinsic classifier in early-stage estrogen receptor-positive breast cancer. Oncologist 2012;17(4):492–8.

119. Bartlett JM, Bayani J, Marshall A, et al. Comparing breast cancer multiparameter tests in the OPTIMA Prelim Trial: no test is more equal than the others. J Natl Cancer Inst 2016;108(9), [pii:djw050].

120. Slodkowska EA, Ross JS. MammaPrint 70-gene signature: another milestone in personalized medical care for breast cancer patients. Expert Rev Mol Diagn 2009;9(5):417–22.

121. Sparano JA, Gray RJ, Makower DF, et al. Prospective validation of a 21-gene expression assay in breast cancer. N Engl J Med 2015;373(21): 2005–14.

122. Barker AD, Sigman CC, Kelloff GJ, et al. I-SPY 2: an adaptive breast cancer trial design in the setting of neoadjuvant chemotherapy. Clin Pharmacol Ther 2009;86(1):97–100.

123. Cardoso F, van't Veer LJ, Bogaerts J, et al. 70-gene signature as an aid to treatment decisions in early-stage breast cancer. N Engl J Med 2016;375(8): 717–29.

Precursor Lesions of the Low-Grade Breast Neoplasia Pathway

Laura C. Collins, MD

KEYWORDS

- Low-grade breast neoplasia • Flat epithelial atypia • Atypical ductal hyperplasia
- Low-grade ductal carcinoma in situ • Lobular neoplasia • Tubular carcinoma

---

Key points

- Precursor lesions of the low-grade breast neoplasia pathway often coexist.
- This family of lesions shares morphologic, immunophenotypic, and genetic characteristics.
- Loss of 16q is commonly seen.
- Despite the relationship of these lesions to invasive carcinomas, the risk of progression among the earliest lesions is exceedingly low.

ABSTRACT

The nonobligate precursor lesions columnar cell change/hyperplasia and flat epithelial atypia, atypical ductal hyperplasia and atypical lobular hyperplasia, lobular carcinoma in situ, and low-grade ductal carcinoma in situ share morphologic, immunophenotypic, and molecular features supporting the existence of a low-grade breast neoplasia pathway. The practical implication for pathologists is that the identification of one of these lesions should prompt careful search for others. From a clinical management perspective, however, their designation as "precursor lesions" should not be overemphasized, as the risk of progression among the earliest lesions is exceedingly low. Factors determining which lesions will progress remain unknown.

OVERVIEW

It has been several decades since Azzopardi[1] first described a lesion with low-grade cytologic atypia that had initially been overlooked as an area of fibrocystic change, but that on re-review demonstrated dilated acini lined by 2 to 4 layers of atypical epithelial cells showing enlarged, hyperchromatic nuclei, loss of cell polarity, and occasional mitoses. This index case came to Dr Azzopardi's attention because the patient had developed invasive carcinoma with axillary lymph node metastases 8 years after the original biopsy, and subsequently died of disease. Further study of similar lesions led Azzopardi to speculate that these lesions represented a form of well-differentiated ductal carcinoma in situ (DCIS) for which he proposed the term "clinging carcinoma (of the monomorphic type)," given the lack of intraductal proliferation present. This morphologic observation of the relationship between the lesion we now refer to as flat epithelial atypia (FEA) and invasive carcinoma was remarkably prescient. As is discussed in this review, in addition to the morphologic similarities between FEA and low-grade invasive carcinomas, specifically tubular carcinomas, there is now substantial molecular evidence linking these lesions to one another along the low-grade breast neoplasia pathway.[2–6]

Disclosure Statement: No disclosures.
Department of Pathology, Beth Israel Deaconess Medical Center, Harvard Medical School, 330 Brookline Avenue, Boston, MA 02215, USA
E-mail address: lcollins@bidmc.harvard.edu

Surgical Pathology 11 (2018) 177–197
https://doi.org/10.1016/j.path.2017.09.007

COLUMNAR CELL LESIONS

DEFINITION AND MORPHOLOGY

Columnar cell change, columnar cell hyperplasia, and FEA are collectively referred to as columnar cell lesions. This family of lesions is characterized by variable dilatation of the acini of the terminal duct lobular unit, with a single to multilayered epithelial lining, cells with apical snouts, and luminal secretions and calcifications. The epithelial cells of columnar cell change are columnar with elongated nuclei arranged perpendicular to the basement membrane (**Fig. 1**). The epithelial cells of columnar cell hyperplasia are also columnar with elongated nuclei arranged perpendicular to the basement membrane, but there is multilayering of the epithelial cells with tufting of the lining of the acini (**Fig. 2**). However, there should be no true

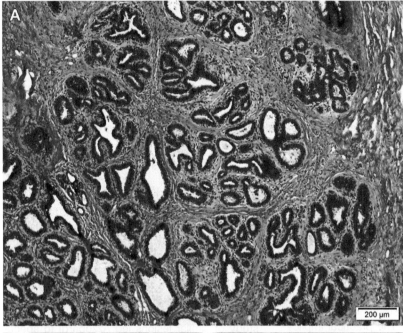

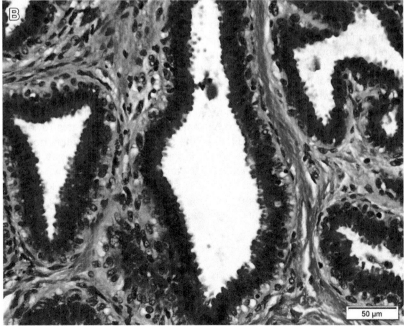

Fig. 1. Columnar cell change. (*A*) Low-power image illustrating the variably dilated acini with irregular contours. (*B*) High-power image demonstrating the regular columnar nuclei arranged perpendicular to the basement membrane.

Fig. 2. Columnar cell hyperplasia. (*A*) Intermediate-power view illustrating dilated acini with multilayered columnar epithelium. (*B*) High-power view detailing tufting of the columnar epithelium without formation of true micropapillae.

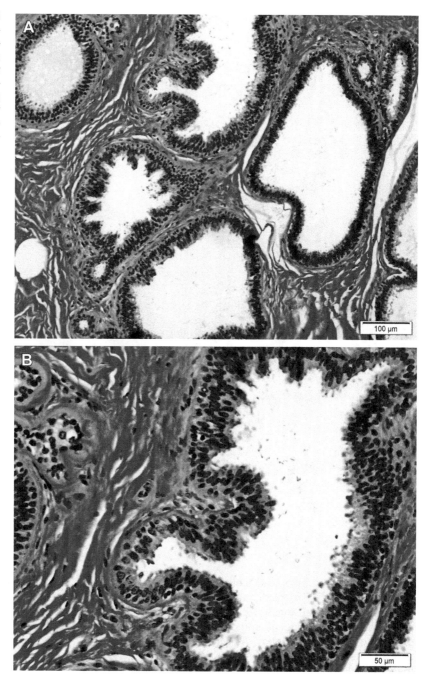

micropapillations. In contrast to these 2 nonatypical columnar cell lesions, FEA is characterized by epithelial cells that are more often cuboidal in nature, with round monomorphic nuclei, akin to those seen in low-grade DCIS, and with loss of polarization with respect to the basement membrane (**Fig. 3**). Often there are 2 to 4 layers of epithelial cells lining the acini, but the lining remains flat with no arcades, bridges, or micropapillations. Another feature distinguishing columnar cell change and hyperplasia from FEA is the more irregular contours of the acini of the former compared with the more rounded and rigid-appearing acini of the latter (**Fig. 4**). **Table 1** summarizes the features distinguishing the columnar cell lesions from one another.

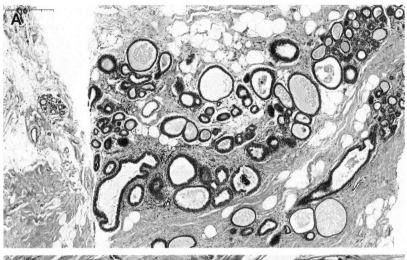

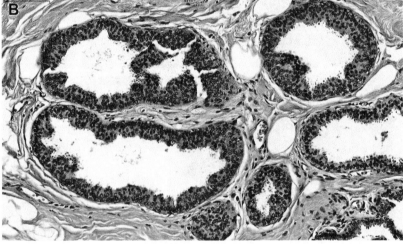

Fig. 3. FEA. (*A*) Low-power image illustrating the rounded contours to the dilated acini, the presence of microcalcifications and secretions, and the relative hyperchromasia of the cells. (*B*) Higher-power image demonstrating the more cuboidal epithelium with round monomorphic nuclei.

PRESENTATION

As mentioned, columnar cell lesions are often associated with microcalcifications, and it is for this reason that these lesions are being detected on screening mammograms, often prompting core needle biopsy. As with all breast core needle biopsy specimens, it is important that radiologic and pathologic findings are correlated.

DIFFERENTIAL DIAGNOSIS

The differential diagnosis of columnar cell lesions and FEA specifically, includes microcysts, apocrine metaplasia and cysts, atypical ductal hyperplasia (ADH) and low-grade DCIS. It is also important to distinguish the nonatypical columnar cell lesions from FEA using the features described previously. Microcysts are differentiated by the attenuated epithelial lining and small nuclear size; apocrine metaplasia is characterized by abundant granular eosinophilic cytoplasm, and although the nuclear features may be a mimic for FEA, the low nuclear-to-cytoplasmic ratio and cytoplasmic features should help rule out FEA (Fig. 5). Cytologically FEA, ADH, and low nuclear grade DCIS resemble one another, but the presence of architectural atypia in the form of bridges, arcades, cribriforming, and micropapillations will enable distinction of ADH and DCIS from FEA. Finally, it is important to remember that there is a form of high nuclear grade DCIS that has a flat growth pattern, "clinging carcinoma," but given the high nuclear grade and frequent presence of comedo necrosis, this pattern of DCIS is readily distinguished from FEA (Fig. 6).

Adjunctive immunostains are not usually required to aid in the aforementioned differential diagnoses, as the cytologic features are

Fig. 4. FEA. Another example of FEA (in a core needle biopsy specimen) illustrating the rounded contours, microcalcifications and hyperchromasia. In this particular example, there is a prominent lymphocytic infiltrate.

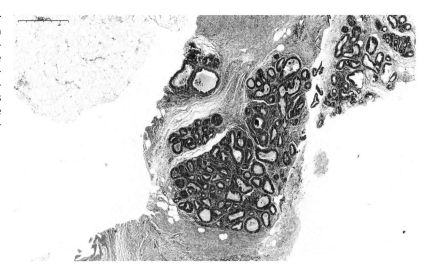

sufficiently distinctive in the benign lesions discussed and the architectural features distinguish FEA from ADH and DCIS. If confirmation is needed, cytokeratin (CK) 5/6 and/or estrogen receptor (ER) can be useful for the benign versus columnar cell lesion differential; CK5/6 is negative in columnar cell lesions and ER is strongly and diffusely positive, irrespective of the presence or absence of atypia.[3,7–12] In microcysts CK5/6 and ER will be variably positive; in apocrine lesions ER is negative. As alluded to previously, these markers do not differentiate the columnar cell lesions from one another, nor from ADH and low-grade DCIS, as all these lesions are CK5/6 negative and strongly ER positive.[13–15]

MANAGEMENT

Excision is not required for columnar cell lesions without atypia diagnosed on core needle biopsy. The management of FEA diagnosed on core needle biopsy is evolving and is discussed more fully

Table 1
Features of columnar cell lesions

Pathologic Feature	Columnar Cell Change	Columnar Cell Hyperplasia	Flat Epithelial Atypia
Features of TDLUs involved	Variable dilatation of the acini Irregular acinar contours	Variable dilatation of the acini Irregular acinar contours	Variable dilatation of the acini Rounded acinar contours
Cytology	Columnar cells arranged perpendicular to the basement membrane Elongated, ovoid nuclei Apical snouts	Columnar cells arranged perpendicular to the basement membrane Elongated, ovoid nuclei Apical snouts, may be pronounced	Cuboidal cells with loss of polarization with respect to basement membrane Rounded, monomorphic nuclei Apical snouts
Epithelial lining	Typically a single epithelial cell layer	Multilayering often seen, with stratification of epithelial cells, and epithelial tufting	Single or multiple epithelial cell layers[2–4] Epithelium remains "flat" with no architectural atypia
Luminal contents	Secretions and microcalcifications	Secretions and microcalcifications, often pronounced	Secretions and microcalcifications, often pronounced

Abbreviation: TDLU, terminal duct lobular unit.

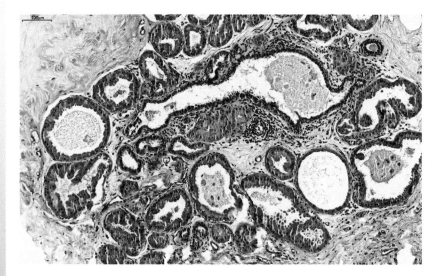

Fig. 5. Apocrine metaplasia/cysts. Apocrine cysts can be a mimic for FEA because of the rounded contour to the cysts and the round, monomorphic nuclei of the apocrine metaplastic cells. However, the abundant granular, eosinophilic cytoplasm readily enables distinction from FEA.

in Benjamin C. Calhoun's article, "Core Needle Biopsy of the Breast: An Evaluation of Contemporary Data," in this issue. In brief, if there are any imaging features of concern (eg, an associated mass or area of distortion) or there are residual calcifications of concern, an excision is warranted.

It should be emphasized that columnar cell lesions are often associated with other lesions on the low-grade breast neoplasia pathway,[3–5,16–18] as such it is critical that examination for any associated "worse" lesion is performed, as management algorithms are more clearly defined for these other lesions.[19]

No further management is necessary for columnar cell lesions with or without atypia when encountered as the most significant pathology in an excision specimen. Importantly, FEA should not be included in measurements reporting the extent of DCIS, nor should margin status be reported for FEA.

OUTCOME

Studies evaluating the subsequent breast cancer risk associated with a diagnosis of columnar cell lesions have shown a very low risk, of the order of that associated with proliferative lesions without atypia or even no elevation of risk, when adjusted for the presence of other proliferative lesions.[20–22] Moreover, the evidence available suggests a very low risk of progression to invasive carcinomas.[23–26] Interestingly, it has been

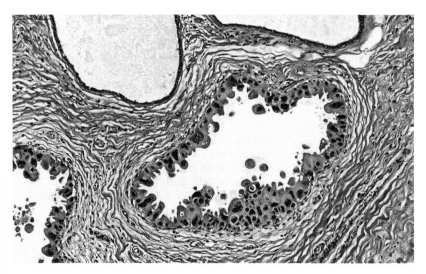

Fig. 6. High nuclear grade DCIS, clinging pattern. Clinging carcinoma can be an "architectural" mimic of FEA, because of the flat epithelial lining in the involved space. However, the nuclei are too atypical for a diagnosis of FEA.

demonstrated that the cancers that do develop in women with a prior history of a columnar cell lesion show no relationship to grade or histologic type,[27] which may be a function of the occurrence of sporadic carcinomas incidental to the original low risk "precursor" lesion. Conversely, as is discussed later, when evaluating low-grade invasive ductal carcinomas, tubular carcinomas and invasive lobular carcinomas, there is a significant association with columnar cell lesions and FEA.[3–5]

ATYPICAL DUCTAL HYPERPLASIA

DEFINITION AND MORPHOLOGY

ADH is defined in terms of its relationship to low nuclear grade DCIS, that is, ADH is characterized by a proliferation of atypical epithelial cells with round monomorphic nuclei with architectural atypia in the form of rigid bridges, arcades, cribriforming, or micropapillations either incompletely involving the affected spaces, or if the spaces are completely involved, that they are fewer than 2 in number or the area is ≤2 mm in extent[28] (Fig. 7).

PRESENTATION

Like columnar cell lesions, ADH is usually detected mammographically because of its association with microcalcifications. When diagnosed on core needle biopsy, excision is recommended to exclude DCIS or invasive carcinoma. There have been many attempts to identify a group of patients who may safely avoid excision following a

diagnosis of ADH; for example, those in whom all the microcalcifications have been removed, or who have limited numbers of microscopic fields of ADH, or who have been sampled using vacuum assisted devices and larger gauge needles. However, no metrics reliably exclude the possibility of finding a worse lesion on excision; this topic is discussed in Benjamin C. Calhoun's article, "Core Needle Biopsy of the Breast: An Evaluation of Contemporary Data," in this issue.

DIFFERENTIAL DIAGNOSIS

The differential diagnosis of ADH is largely with low-grade DCIS for the definitional reasons elaborated up on previously (Table 2).

Collagenous spherulosis is a combined epithelial-myoepithelial proliferation with a cribriform growth pattern that can be a mimic for ADH or DCIS (Fig. 8), particularly if the collagenous spherulosis is involved by lobular carcinoma in situ (LCIS), which confers monomorphism along with the cribriform architecture of the underlying proliferation (Fig. 9). In contradistinction to the polarization of epithelial cells seen around the cribriform spaces in ADH and DCIS, the spaces in collagenous spherulosis are surrounded by myoepithelial cells with spindled nuclei and they contain basement membrane material. If necessary, immunostains can used to confirm the presence of myoepithelial cells surrounding the intraductal spaces (see Fig. 8). An e-cadherin stain can be used to demonstrate involvement of the collagenous spherulosis by LCIS (see Fig. 9); note that

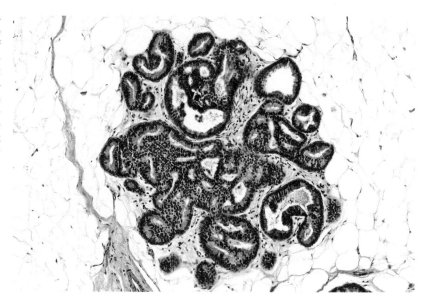

Fig. 7. ADH. Intermediate-power image depicting a focus of ADH. Note the hyperchromatic, monomorphic nuclei and the polarization of epithelial cells around the spaces present. Admixed with the ADH are spaces that alone would qualify for a diagnosis of FEA.

Table 2
Differential diagnoses of atypical ductal hyperplasia and low-grade ductal carcinoma in situ

	Features of Lesion in the DDX	Distinguishing Features of ADH/DCIS
Collagenous spherulosis	Combined epithelial-myoepithelial proliferation with "cribriform-like" spaces and basement membrane material Absence of polarization around spaces May have monomorphic cytology if involved by LCIS CK5/6 positive in UDH and myoepithelial cells within the proliferation; ER variable in UDH; note that the IHC staining pattern will be more similar to ADH when LCIS involves collagenous spherulosis, with the exception of CK5/6 staining of the myoepithelial cells *within* the proliferation	Monomorphic epithelial proliferation Presence of polarization around cribriform spaces CK5/6 negative, ER strongly, diffusely positive
Micropapillary UDH (gynecomastoid hyperplasia)	The micropapillations of UDH have a broad base and narrow pinched tip Nuclei are larger at the base than at the tip CK5/6 positive, ER heterogeneously positive	The micropapillations of ADH/DCIS have a narrow base and a broad bulbous tip Nuclei are enlarged throughout the micropapillation CK5/6 negative, ER strongly and diffusely positive
Adenoid cystic carcinoma, cribriform pattern	Combined epithelial-myoepithelial carcinoma with basement membrane material Infiltrative growth pattern ER negative, myoepithelial cell markers variably positive, c-kit and MYB positive	Monomorphic epithelial proliferation Presence of polarization around cribriform spaces CK5/6 negative, ER strongly, diffusely positive
Invasive cribriform carcinoma	Tumor cell nests with cribriform architecture Irregular contour to some of the tumor cell nests Infiltrative growth pattern Myoepithelial cells absent around tumor cell nests; can be confirmed with IHC if necessary	Tumor cell nests of cribriform pattern DCIS more rounded in contour Infiltrative growth pattern absent Myoepithelial cells present around nests of DCIS
Extensive lymphovascular space invasion	May present as solid or cribriform nests within rounded spaces Presence of normal TDLUs between areas of LVI should be a cue to correct diagnosis D240 can be used to confirm endothelial cell lining to lymphatic spaces; combine with myoepithelial cell marker as cross-reactivity by D240 has been reported	Admixed uninvolved TDLUs not normally seen in areas of DCIS Presence of a myoepithelial cell layer can be confirmed with IHC

Abbreviations: ADH, atypical ductal hyperplasia; CK, cytokeratin; DCIS, ductal carcinoma in situ; DDX, differential diagnosis; ER, estrogen receptor; IHC, immunohistochemistry; LCIS, lobular carcinoma in situ; LVI, lymphovascular space invasion; UDH, usual ductal hyperplasia.

Fig. 8. Collagenous spherulosis. (*A*) Intermediate-power image illustrating the cribriform pattern that is conferred by collagenous spherulosis. Note the spindled myoepithelial cells surrounding the spaces that contain basement membrane material. (*B*) A p63 immunostain highlights the myoepithelial cells.

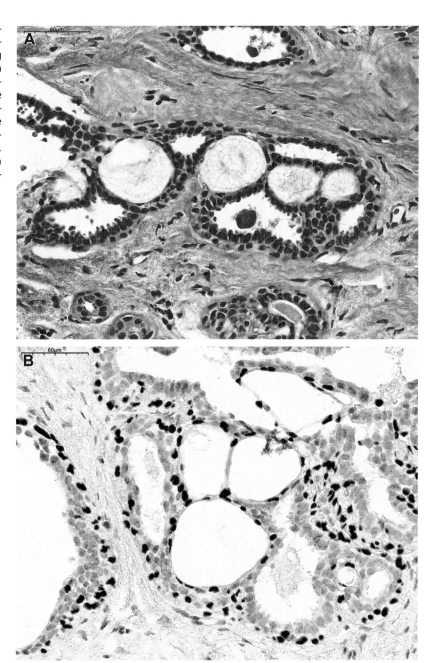

the myoepithelial cells present will retain expression of e-cadherin.

Usual ductal hyperplasia (UDH) with a micropapillary growth pattern (also known as gynecomastoid hyperplasia) can be a mimic for micropapillary ADH and DCIS. Micropapillary ADH and DCIS are characterized by micropapillations with bulbous tips in which the nuclei are enlarged throughout the micropapillations (Fig. 10). In contrast, the micropapillations of gynecomastoid hyperplasia have a broad base with a narrower, pinched tip and the nuclei are larger at the base of the micropapillation and smaller and more pyknotic-appearing at the tip (Fig. 11). In problematic cases, CK5/6 and ER immunohistochemistry can be used to distinguish UDH from atypical ductal proliferations. CK5/6 and ER are heterogeneously positive in UDH whereas CK5/6 is negative and ER strongly and diffusely positive in both ADH and DCIS.[29]

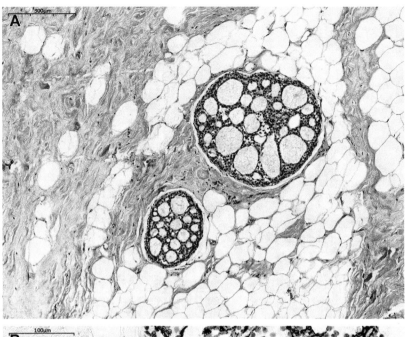

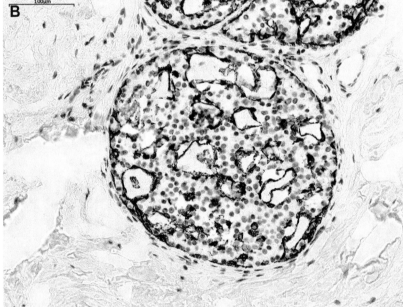

Fig. 9. LCIS involving collagenous spherulosis. (*A*) The cribriform pattern and monomorphic cells present in this example of LCIS involving collagenous spherulosis illustrate how this lesion can be a mimic for ADH and low nuclear grade DCIS. (*B*) An e-cadherin immunostain at higher power. Note the nuclear monomorphism and the absence of e-cadherin staining in the LCIS cells. The myoepithelial cells are highlighted by e-cadherin.

MANAGEMENT

As mentioned previously, excision is recommended for ADH diagnosed on core needle biopsy. When present as the most significant lesion in an excision, no further surgical management is required. At this time there is no recommendation to record the number of foci of ADH, or to report the margin status. Additional levels may be indicated if the focus of ADH is bordering on DCIS (see discussion later in this article), as this may help clarify the diagnosis. Caution should also be exercised if the ADH is exclusively present close to a margin or is bordering on DCIS at a margin, as this may represent the edge of a more significant lesion that has not been adequately sampled. In such cases a note suggesting that reexcision merits consideration may be warranted.

Fig. 10. Micropapillary ADH. Intermediate-power (*A*) and high-power (*B*) images of micropapillary ADH; note the bulbous micropapillations with enlarged monomorphic nuclei present throughout the micropapillations.

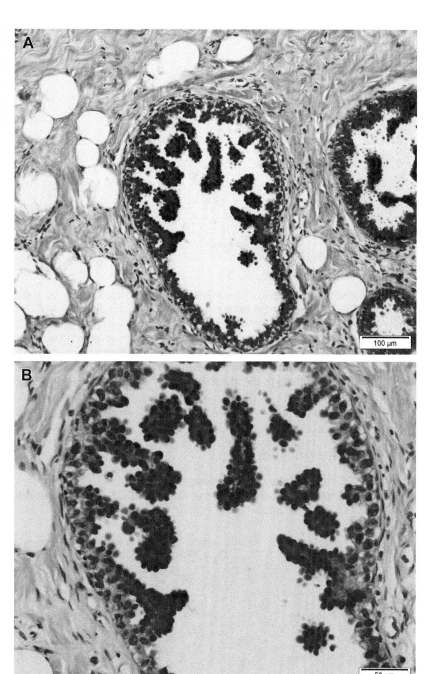

ADH is considered a high-risk lesion with regard to subsequent breast cancer risk, as such patients may be offered risk reducing therapies such as tamoxifen.

OUTCOME

Numerous large, population-based studies have found ADH to be associated with a threefold to fivefold increased risk for the subsequent development of breast cancer.[30–32] An excess of ipsilateral carcinomas is reported, suggesting that ADH has the capacity to behave as a breast cancer precursor.[32,33] However, from a management perspective patients are treated as though ADH is a risk indicator conferring a bilateral increase in breast cancer risk. As with columnar cell lesions,

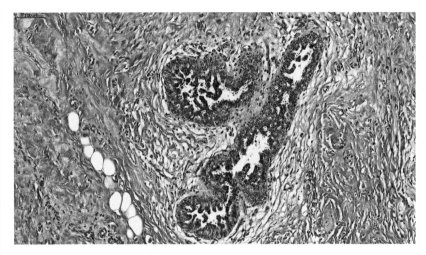

Fig. 11. UDH, gynecomastoid pattern. Compared with the micropapillations in **Fig. 10**, these have broader bases (see particularly lower left of duct) and narrow, pinched tips with smaller, darker nuclei seen at the tips compared with the base of the micropapillation.

the carcinomas that develop in women with a prior history of ADH have been found to be of no particular grade or histologic type.[34] Again, studies that examine the "precursor" lesions associated with low-grade invasive ductal carcinomas and tubular carcinomas do find a preponderance of low-grade DCIS and ADH, in addition to the aforementioned columnar cell lesions.[4]

LOW-GRADE DUCTAL CARCINOMA IN SITU

DEFINITION AND MORPHOLOGY

Low-grade DCIS is defined as a proliferation of neoplastic epithelial cells confined to the ducts and lobules. The atypical proliferation is characterized by round, monomorphic, centrally placed nuclei with amphophilic, eosinophilic or clear cytoplasm. The proliferation completely fills the involved spaces with either a solid, cribriform, micropapillary or papillary growth pattern. Characteristically, there is polarization of the epithelial cells around any cribriform spaces; even within solid pattern DCIS, the epithelial cells attempt to polarize forming microacini and rosettes within the solid proliferation (**Fig. 12**). By definition, low-grade DCIS is >2 mm in extent.

PRESENTATION

DCIS is usually detected mammographically due to its frequent association with microcalcifications.

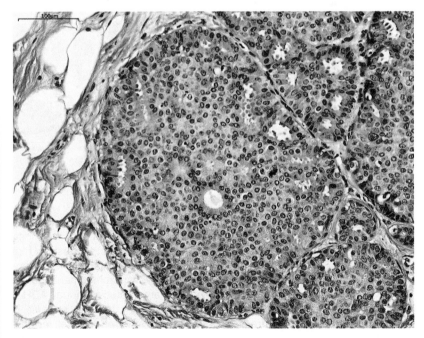

Fig. 12. DCIS, low nuclear grade. Intermediate-power image illustrating the round, monomorphic nuclei characteristic of low-grade DCIS. Notice also the polarization of cells around the lumens and the formation of "rosettes" even in the more solid parts of the proliferation.

Occasionally, it can be an MRI-detected non-mass-like enhancing lesion, or more rarely it may present as a mass lesion, due to its involvement of a preexisting benign structure, such as a papilloma.

DIFFERENTIAL DIAGNOSIS

The differential diagnosis includes those entities discussed previously for ADH. In addition,

invasive cribriform carcinoma and adenoid cystic carcinoma enter the differential diagnosis for cribriform pattern DCIS (see Table 2). Morphologic features favoring a diagnosis of invasive cribriform carcinoma include irregular contours to the cribriform nests and an infiltrative growth pattern (Fig. 13). Immunostains for myoepithelial cells can be helpful in difficult cases, or if help is needed determining the extent of the invasive

Fig. 13. Invasive cribriform carcinoma. (A) At low power, the irregular contour of the nests and the infiltrative growth pattern are readily appreciated. (B) At higher power, the cribriform architecture and monomorphic nuclei might suggest cribriform pattern DCIS, but the absence of a myoepithelial cell layer (as well as the infiltrative growth pattern appreciated on low power) support the diagnosis of an invasive carcinoma.

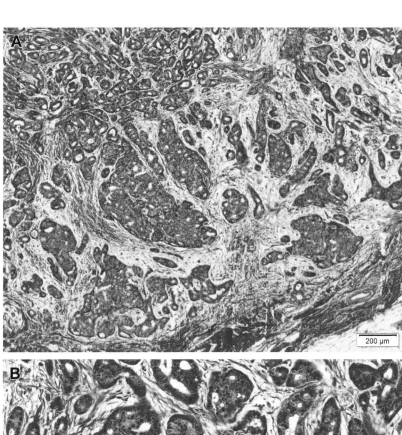

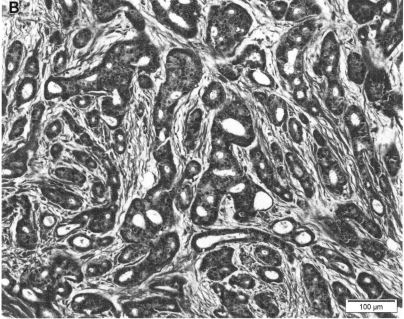

versus in situ component. Adenoid cystic carcinoma can also have a cribriform growth pattern, but it is a combined epithelial-myoepithelial carcinoma in which there is production of basement membrane material. A further distinguishing feature is that there are 2 types of "cribriform spaces" in adenoid cystic carcinoma, those produced by epithelial cells, in which polarization may be appreciated, but the more readily recognizable spaces are produced by the myoepithelial cells which have their nuclei arranged parallel to the spaces containing the basement membrane material (Fig. 14). Usually DCIS and adenoid cystic carcinoma can be distinguished on hematoxylin-eosin–stained sections, but if necessary immunostains for myoepithelial cells can be used to highlight the biphasic nature of the carcinoma. CK7 and c-kit may also be of value in highlighting the various components of adenoid cystic carcinoma; strong, diffuse nuclear staining with MYB has been shown to be both a sensitive and

specific marker.[35] Rarely, extensive lymphovascular space invasion can be a mimic for DCIS. Clues to the correct diagnosis are the presence of intervening normal terminal duct lobular units and the location of the involved spaces adjacent to other vascular structures. D240 and myoepithelial cell markers will be helpful in this differential diagnosis, with D240 staining the endothelial cells and myoepithelial cell markers being used as a positive stain for DCIS. Note that D240 can cross react with myoepithelial cells, hence the importance of having a confirmatory myoepithelial cell marker.[36]

MANAGEMENT

The diagnosis of DCIS on a core needle biopsy should prompt an excision. When present in an excision specimen or mastectomy, the report should include documentation of the nuclear grade, the presence or absence of comedo

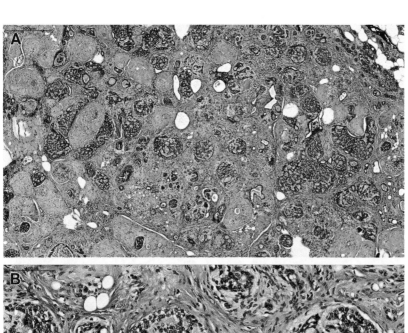

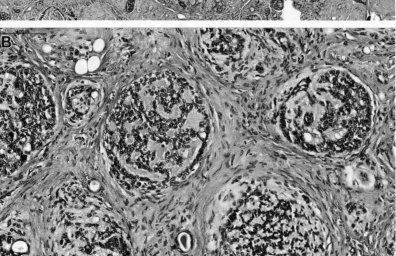

Fig. 14. Adenoid cystic carcinoma. (A) At low power, the cribriform growth pattern of some adenoid cystic carcinomas might raise the possibility of DCIS. (B) At higher power, the "cribriform" spaces are seen to contain basement membrane material and are surrounded by myoepithelial cells which do not polarize around the lumens. "True" lumens formed by the epithelial component of this mixed tumor can be harder to appreciate.

necrosis, the architectural pattern and some esti-mate of the extent or volume of DCIS, as well as a report of the margin status. A recent meta-analysis and consensus statement indicated that for patients with pure DCIS undergoing whole breast irradiation, a margin of 2 mm or greater be considered adequate.[37,38] Patients with foci of DCIS <2 mm from an inked specimen margin may require reexcision; but multiple other patient and tumor-related factors may play into the deci-sion to perform further surgery which is beyond the scope of this review.

Following complete surgical excision of the DCIS, many, but not all, patients receive radiation therapy, a therapeutic option that results in extremely low recurrence rates.[39–42] Efforts to identify a group of patients for whom radiation therapy does not add substantial benefit are ongoing; studies to date continue to show a benefit for radiation even among the lowest risk patients, though whether the added risk is justified in this group is a matter of debate.[43–46]

ER testing should be performed on all DCIS cases. This can be performed on either the core needle biopsy or the excision. Given that a propor-tion of DCIS cases diagnosed on core needle bi-opsy are upgraded to invasive carcinoma on excision, there is an economical argument to be made to perform ER testing on the excision spec-imen, once it is known whether or not there is an invasive component.[47] Anti-estrogen therapy (eg, tamoxifen or an aromatase inhibitor) may be offered to patients with ER-positive DCIS.

OUTCOME

Patients with DCIS, particularly low-grade DCIS, have a very good outcome. The risk of recurrence or progression to invasive carcinoma is approxi-mately 2% per year for women treated with exci-sion alone, and this risk is halved in patients receiving radiation therapy, with a further reduc-tion seen among women using tamoxifen.[39–42] Pa-tients with low-grade DCIS have a more protracted time to progression than those with high-grade le-sions; so prolonged follow-up is indicated in this group.

LOBULAR NEOPLASIA

Atypical lobular hyperplasia (ALH) and classic LCIS are characterized by a monotonous prolifer-ation of dyshesive, neoplastic epithelial cells. The cells often have clear cytoplasm. The nuclei are round, centrally or slightly eccentrically placed, with even chromatin (Fig. 15). ALH is distinguished from LCIS in that it is quantitatively lesser in extent.

LCIS is the subject of Hannah Y. Wen's article, "Lobular Carcinoma In Situ," in this issue, as such it will be discussed further here only in the context of its relationship to the other precursor le-sions of the low-grade breast neoplasia pathway (see later in this article).

INVASIVE CARCINOMAS

Tubular, low-grade invasive ductal and invasive lobular carcinomas are the invasive cancers most commonly found in association with the aforemen-tioned nonobligate precursor lesions.[3–5,18,48] Tubular carcinoma shares cytologic features with FEA, ADH, and low-grade DCIS with all lesions be-ing characterized by cells with moderate amounts of cytoplasm and round, monomorphic centrally placed nuclei (Fig. 16). On occasion, cells within the tubules of tubular carcinoma display apical snouts similar to those seen in FEA. ALH, LCIS, and invasive lobular carcinoma share their charac-teristic cytologic features of cellular dyshesion, intracytoplasmic vacuoles, and small, round monomorphic nuclei; the latter feature overlapping with the atypical ductal proliferations and tubular carcinoma. Like their precursors, all of these inva-sive carcinomas show strong, diffuse staining with ER; invasive lobular carcinomas additionally demonstrate loss of e-cadherin expression. All of these observations contributed to the proposal of a low-grade breast neoplasia pathway.

THE LOW-GRADE BREAST NEOPLASIA PATHWAY

As can be appreciated from the previous des-criptions of FEA, ADH, and low-grade DCIS, the lesions bear great morphologic and immunophe-notypic similarity to one another. ALH and LCIS share some of these characteristics, but have in addition, cytologic dyshesion as a defining feature. To evaluate the molecular relationship of columnar cell lesions to DCIS and invasive cancers, Simp-son and colleagues[3] conducted very elegant experiments using high-resolution–comparative genomic hybridization. The investigators microdis-sected areas of columnar cell lesions (with and without atypia), ADH/DCIS, lobular neoplasia, and invasive carcinoma from 3 different cases and cataloged the chromosomal losses and gains in the various lesions and their relationship to one another in the 3 separate cases. Interestingly, chromosomal copy number gains and losses were seen across the spectrum of columnar cell lesions with the relative level of genetic instability mirroring the morphologic classification scheme (ie, fewer aberrations seen in columnar cell change and

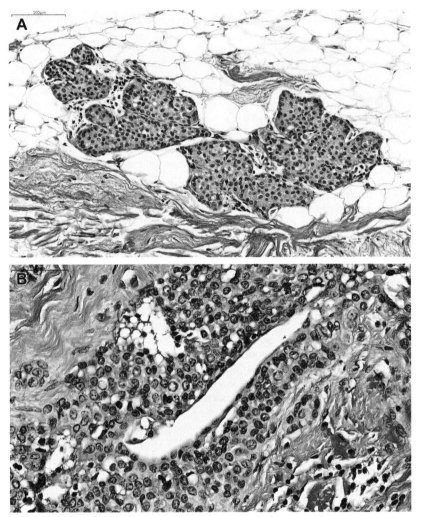

Fig. 15. LCIS. (*A*) LCIS involving a lobule. Note the round, monomorphic nuclei and the presence of intracytoplasmic vacuoles. (*B*) High-power image of LCIS involving a duct in a pagetoid fashion.

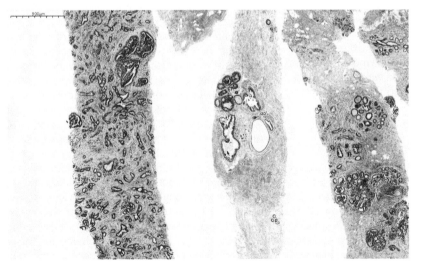

Fig. 16. Tubular carcinoma. Low-power image of a core needle biopsy samples with tubular carcinoma and its associated precursor lesions. The left-hand core biopsy has the greatest expanse of tubular carcinoma, characterized by angular glands and tubules infiltrating through a desmoplastic stroma in a haphazard pattern. The middle core of tissue has areas of FEA and ADH, and the right-hand core of tissue has more of the tubular carcinoma, some FEA and ADH.

greater numbers of chromosomal alterations being seen in FEA). Further, the genetic complexity of alterations identified increased with the architectural complexity of the lesions evaluated. Low numbers of chromosomal alterations were found among the columnar cell lesions analyzed, more losses than gains were observed, and recurrent loss of 16q was seen[3]; features that have been characterized as the genetic hallmarks of low-grade DCIS and invasive carcinomas.[49] This molecular evidence led the investigators to propose that FEA was the missing link in the progression from normal breast epithelium to atypical hyperplasia.[3] Numerous studies have now documented the presence of 16q loss in all the lesions under discussion, and accumulation of additional genetic alterations, such as 1q gain, with progression along the pathway toward invasive carcinoma.[3,16,50–55]

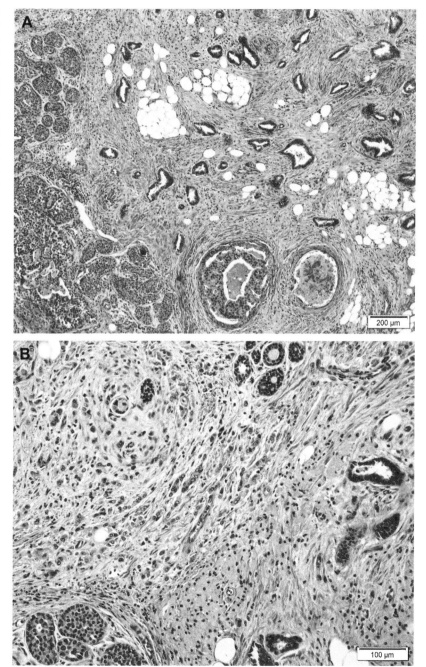

Fig. 17. Lesions of the low-grade breast neoplasia pathway. (*A*) Low-power image illustrating the constellation of tubular carcinoma, LCIS and ADH/DCIS (lower, center of field). (*B*) High-power image of the same case showing an area of invasive lobular carcinoma adjacent to the tubular carcinoma as well as ALH/LCIS.

200 µm

100 µm

Lobular lesions harbor similar chromosomal alterations and have additional aberrations of the *CDH1* (E-cadherin) gene.[56–59] The genetics of LCIS is discussed in greater detail in Hannah Y. Wen's article, "Lobular Carcinoma In Situ," in this issue.

As further evidence of the relationship among the lesions under discussion, Abdel-Fatah and colleagues[4,5] reviewed a series of cases of low-grade invasive ductal carcinomas, tubular carcinomas and lobular carcinomas and documented the presence of any concurrent lesions. These investigators found a significant increase in the presence of columnar cell lesions, ADH and low-grade DCIS among patients with low-grade invasive ductal and tubular carcinomas and similarly, among patients with invasive lobular carcinomas, there was a significant increase in the likelihood of finding columnar cell lesions, ALH, and LCIS.[4,5] Others have also documented the coexistence of this group of precursor lesions (**Fig. 17**).[18,48] In fact, the term "Rosen Triad" has been given to the constellation of columnar cell lesions, lobular neoplasia, and tubular carcinoma in tribute to Dr Peter Paul Rosen[48] who first reported this association in 1999.

Given the previously described morphologic, immunophenotypic, geographic, and genetic associations, the existence of a low-grade breast neoplasia pathway, which begins with columnar cell lesions, progresses through ADH to low-grade DCIS and low-grade invasive ductal carcinomas is now firmly established.[3–5] A branch point at FEA may alternatively lead to the development of lobular lesions and invasive lobular carcinoma.[60] More recent work has demonstrated gene copy number alterations in several breast cancer–related genes even in the earliest lesions on the low-grade breast neoplasia pathway[61]; specifically copy number gains in *CCND1* and *ESR1* and copy number losses in *CDH1* were identified in columnar cell lesions, which is of particular interest given the location of this latter gene on the long arm of chromosome 16 and the role of *CDH1* in lobular neoplasia and by extension the role of FEA as a precursor lesion.[61] Gains of *CCND1* and losses of *CDH1* have also been reported in DCIS, albeit of varying grades.[62]

It is important to emphasize that although these lesions are morphologically and genetically precursor lesions, there is a very low rate of progression along the pathway, at least with the earliest lesions (FEA and atypical hyperplasias).[23,25,63] In fact, it may be that the risk of progression is so low that the development of incident carcinomas unrelated to these particular precursor lesions predominates. This hypothesis is supported by the finding that cancers that do develop in women with a history of columnar cell lesions or atypical hyperplasias can be either ipsilateral or contralateral, of any histologic type and grade, and that a preponderance of low-grade invasive carcinomas is not seen.[27,33,34]

SUMMARY

In summary, there is morphologic, immunophenotypic, and molecular evidence to support the existence of a low-grade breast neoplasia pathway for which the nonobligate precursor lesions, columnar cell change/hyperplasia and FEA, ADH and ALH, and LCIS and low-grade DCIS are found, and commonly coexist with low-grade invasive ductal, tubular, or lobular carcinomas. The practical implications of this observation for pathologists are that the identification of one of these lesions should prompt careful search for others. From a clinical management perspective, however, the designation as "precursor lesions" should not be overemphasized, as the risk of progression among the earliest lesions is exceedingly low. Factors determining which lesions will progress remain unknown.

REFERENCES

1. Azzopardi JG. Problems in breast pathology. Philadelphia: WB Saunders; 1979.
2. Eusebi V, Foschini MP, Cook MG, et al. Long-term follow-up of in situ carcinoma of the breast with special emphasis on clinging carcinoma. Semin Diagn Pathol 1989;6(2):165–73.
3. Simpson PT, Gale T, Reis-Filho JS, et al. Columnar cell lesions of the breast: the missing link in breast cancer progression? A morphological and molecular analysis. Am J Surg Pathol 2005;29(6):734–46.
4. Abdel-Fatah TM, Powe DG, Hodi Z, et al. High frequency of coexistence of columnar cell lesions, lobular neoplasia, and low grade ductal carcinoma in situ with invasive tubular carcinoma and invasive lobular carcinoma. Am J Surg Pathol 2007;31(3):417–26.
5. Abdel-Fatah TM, Powe DG, Hodi Z, et al. Morphologic and molecular evolutionary pathways of low nuclear grade invasive breast cancers and their putative precursor lesions: further evidence to support the concept of low nuclear grade breast neoplasia family. Am J Surg Pathol 2008;32(4):513–23.

6. Moinfar F. Flat ductal intraepithelial neoplasia of the breast: evolution of Azzopardi's "clinging" concept. Semin Diagn Pathol 2010;27(1):37–48.

7. Oyama T, Iijima K, Takei H, et al. Atypical cystic lobule of the breast: an early stage of low-grade ductal carcinoma in-situ. Breast Cancer 2000;7(4): 326–31.

8. Fraser J, Raza S, Chorny K, et al. Immunophenotype of columnar alteration with prominent apical snouts and secretions (CAPSS). Lab Invest 2000; 80:21A.

9. Allred DC, Mohsin SK, Fuqua SA. Histological and biological evolution of human premalignant breast disease. Endocr Relat Cancer 2001;8(1):47–61.

10. Dabbs DJ, Kessinger RL, McManus K, et al. Biology of columnar cell lesions in core biopsies of the breast. Mod Pathol 2003;16:26A.

11. Tremblay G, Deschenes J, Alpert L, et al. Overexpression of estrogen receptors in columnar cell change and in unfolding breast lobules. Breast J 2005;11(5):326–32.

12. Lee S, Mohsin SK, Mao S, et al. Hormones, receptors, and growth in hyperplastic enlarged lobular units: early potential precursors of breast cancer. Breast Cancer Res 2006;8(1):R6.

13. Otterbach F, Bankfalvi A, Bergner S, et al. Cytokeratin 5/6 immunohistochemistry assists the differential diagnosis of atypical proliferations of the breast. Histopathology 2000;37(3):232–40.

14. Carlo V, Fraser J, Pliss N, et al. Can absence of high molecular weight cytokeratin expression be used as a marker of atypia in columnar cell lesions of the breast? Mod Pathol 2003;16:24A.

15. Moinfar F, Man YG, Lininger RA, et al. Use of keratin 35betaE12 as an adjunct in the diagnosis of mammary intraepithelial neoplasia-ductal type–benign and malignant intraductal proliferations. Am J Surg Pathol 1999;23(9):1048–58.

16. Dabbs DJ, Carter G, Fudge M, et al. Molecular alterations in columnar cell lesions of the breast. Mod Pathol 2006;19(3):344–9.

17. Brogi E, Oyama T, Koerner FC. Atypical cystic lobules in patients with lobular neoplasia. Int J Surg Pathol 2001;9(3):201–6.

18. Brandt SM, Young GQ, Hoda SA. The "Rosen triad": tubular carcinoma, lobular carcinoma in situ, and columnar cell lesions. Adv Anat Pathol 2008;15(3): 140–6.

19. Calhoun BC, Collins LC. Recommendations for excision following core needle biopsy of the breast: a contemporary evaluation of the literature. Histopathology 2016;68(1):138–51.

20. Boulos FI, Dupont WD, Simpson JF, et al. Histologic associations and long-term cancer risk in columnar cell lesions of the breast: a retrospective cohort and a nested case-control study. Cancer 2008; 113(9):2415–21.

21. Aroner SA, Collins LC, Schnitt SJ, et al. Columnar cell lesions and subsequent breast cancer risk: a nested case-control study. Breast Cancer Res 2010;12(4):R61.

22. Said SM, Visscher DW, Nassar A, et al. Flat epithelial atypia and risk of breast cancer: a Mayo cohort study. Cancer 2015;121(10):1548–55.

23. Eusebi V, Feudale E, Foschini MP, et al. Long-term follow-up of in situ carcinoma of the breast. Semin Diagn Pathol 1994;11(3):223–35.

24. Bijker N, Peterse JL, Duchateau L, et al. Risk factors for recurrence and metastasis after breast-conserving therapy for ductal carcinoma-in-situ: analysis of European Organization for Research and Treatment of Cancer trial 10853. J Clin Oncol 2001;19(8):2263–71.

25. de Mascarel I, MacGrogan G, Picot V, et al. Results of a long term follow-up study of 115 patients with flat epithelial atypia. Lab Invest 2006; 86(suppl 1):25A.

26. Schnitt SJ. Clinging carcinoma: an American perspective. Semin Diagn Pathol 2010;27(1):31–6.

27. Boulos FI, Dupont WD, Schuyler PA, et al. Clinicopathologic characteristics of carcinomas that develop after a biopsy containing columnar cell lesions: evidence against a precursor role. Cancer 2012;118(9):2372–7.

28. Simpson J, Schnitt S, Visscher D, et al. Atypical ductal hyperplasia. In: Lakhani S, Ellis IO, Schnitt SJ, et al, editors. WHO classification of tumours of the breast. Lyon (France): IARC press; 2012. p. 88–9.

29. Lerwill MF. Current practical applications of diagnostic immunohistochemistry in breast pathology. Am J Surg Pathol 2004;28(8):1076–91.

30. Dupont WD, Page DL. Risk factors for breast cancer in women with proliferative breast disease. N Engl J Med 1985;312(3):146–51.

31. London SJ, Connolly JL, Schnitt SJ, et al. A prospective study of benign breast disease and the risk of breast cancer. JAMA 1992;267(7):941–4.

32. Hartmann LC, Sellers TA, Frost MH, et al. Benign breast disease and the risk of breast cancer. N Engl J Med 2005;353(3):229–37.

33. Collins LC, Baer HJ, Tamimi RM, et al. Magnitude and laterality of breast cancer risk according to histologic type of atypical hyperplasia: results from the Nurses' Health Study. Cancer 2007;109(2):180–7.

34. Jacobs TW, Byrne C, Colditz G, et al. Pathologic features of breast cancers in women with previous benign breast disease. Am J Clin Pathol 2001; 115(3):362–9.

35. Poling J, Yonescu R, Sharma R, et al. MYB labeling by immunohistochemistry is more sensitive and specific for breast adenoid cystic carcinoma than MYB labeling by FISH. Am J Surg Pathol 2017;41(7): 973–9.

36. Rabban JT, Chen YY. D2-40 expression by breast myoepithelium: potential pitfalls in distinguishing intralymphatic carcinoma from in situ carcinoma. Hum Pathol 2008;39(2):175–83.

37. Marinovich ML, Azizi L, Macaskill P, et al. The association of surgical margins and local recurrence in women with ductal carcinoma in situ treated with breast-conserving therapy: a meta-analysis. Ann Surg Oncol 2016;23(12):3811–21.

38. Morrow M, Van Zee KJ, Solin LJ, et al. Society of Surgical Oncology-American Society for Radiation Oncology-American Society of Clinical Oncology consensus guideline on margins for breast-conserving surgery with whole-breast irradiation in ductal carcinoma in situ. Ann Surg Oncol 2016; 23(12):3801–10.

39. Fisher B, Costantino J, Redmond C, et al. Lumpectomy compared with lumpectomy and radiation therapy for the treatment of intraductal breast cancer. N Engl J Med 1993;328(22):1581–6.

40. Bijker N, Meijnen P, Peterse JL, et al. Breast-conserving treatment with or without radiotherapy in ductal carcinoma-in-situ: ten-year results of European Organisation for Research and Treatment of Cancer randomized phase III trial 10853–a study by the EORTC Breast Cancer Cooperative Group and EORTC Radiotherapy Group. J Clin Oncol 2006;24(21):3381–7.

41. Fisher B, Land S, Mamounas E, et al. Prevention of invasive breast cancer in women with ductal carcinoma in situ: an update of the national surgical adjuvant breast and bowel project experience. Semin Oncol 2001;28(4):400–18.

42. Houghton J, George WD, Cuzick J, et al. Radiotherapy and tamoxifen in women with completely excised ductal carcinoma in situ of the breast in the UK, Australia, and New Zealand: randomised controlled trial. Lancet 2003; 362(9378):95–102.

43. Wong JS, Chen YH, Gadd MA, et al. Eight-year update of a prospective study of wide excision alone for small low- or intermediate-grade ductal carcinoma in situ (DCIS). Breast Cancer Res Treat 2014;143(2):343–50.

44. Wong JS, Kaelin CM, Troyan SL, et al. Prospective study of wide excision alone for ductal carcinoma in situ of the breast. J Clin Oncol 2006;24(7):1031–6.

45. Hughes LL, Wang M, Page DL, et al. Local excision alone without irradiation for ductal carcinoma in situ of the breast: a trial of the Eastern Cooperative Oncology Group. J Clin Oncol 2009;27(32): 5319–24.

46. Solin LJ, Gray R, Hughes LL, et al. Surgical excision without radiation for ductal carcinoma in situ of the breast: 12-year results from the ECOG-ACRIN E5194 study. J Clin Oncol 2015;33(33): 3938–44.

47. VandenBussche CJ, Cimino-Mathews A, Park BH, et al. Reflex estrogen receptor (ER) and progesterone receptor (PR) analysis of ductal carcinoma in situ (DCIS) in breast needle core biopsy specimens: an unnecessary exercise that costs the United States $35 million/y. Am J Surg Pathol 2016;40(8): 1090–9.

48. Rosen PP. Columnar cell hyperplasia is associated with lobular carcinoma in situ and tubular carcinoma. Am J Surg Pathol 1999;23(12):1561.

49. Buerger H, Otterbach F, Simon R, et al. Comparative genomic hybridization of ductal carcinoma in situ of the breast-evidence of multiple genetic pathways. J Pathol 1999;187(4):396–402.

50. Moinfar F, Man YG, Bratthauer GL, et al. Genetic abnormalities in mammary ductal intraepithelial neoplasia-flat type ("clinging ductal carcinoma in situ"): a simulator of normal mammary epithelium. Cancer 2000;88(9):2072–81.

51. Aulmann S, Braun L, Mietzsch F, et al. Transitions between flat epithelial atypia and low-grade ductal carcinoma in situ of the breast. Am J Surg Pathol 2012;36(8):1247–52.

52. Aulmann S, Elsawaf Z, Penzel R, et al. Invasive tubular carcinoma of the breast frequently is clonally related to flat epithelial atypia and low-grade ductal carcinoma in situ. Am J Surg Pathol 2009;33(11): 1646–53.

53. Gong G, DeVries S, Chew KL, et al. Genetic changes in paired atypical and usual ductal hyperplasia of the breast by comparative genomic hybridization. Clin Cancer Res 2001; 7(8):2410–4.

54. Lakhani SR. Molecular genetics of solid tumours: translating research into clinical practice. What we could do now: breast cancer. Mol Pathol 2001; 54(5):281–4.

55. Lakhani SR, Collins N, Stratton MR, et al. Atypical ductal hyperplasia of the breast: clonal proliferation with loss of heterozygosity on chromosomes 16q and 17p. J Clin Pathol 1995;48(7):611–5.

56. Vos CB, Cleton-Jansen AM, Berx G, et al. E-cadherin inactivation in lobular carcinoma in situ of the breast: an early event in tumorigenesis. Br J Cancer 1997;76(9):1131–3.

57. Sarrio D, Moreno-Bueno G, Hardisson D, et al. Epigenetic and genetic alterations of APC and CDH1 genes in lobular breast cancer: relationships with abnormal E-cadherin and catenin expression and microsatellite instability. Int J Cancer 2003; 106(2):208–15.

58. Buerger H, Simon R, Schafer KL, et al. Genetic relation of lobular carcinoma in situ, ductal carcinoma in situ, and associated invasive carcinoma of the breast. Mol Pathol 2000;53(3):118–21.

59. Lu YJ, Osin P, Lakhani SR, et al. Comparative genomic hybridization analysis of lobular

carcinoma in situ and atypical lobular hyperplasia and potential roles for gains and losses of genetic material in breast neoplasia. Cancer Res 1998; 58(20):4721–7.

60. Ellis IO. Intraductal proliferative lesions of the breast: morphology, associated risk and molecular biology. Mod Pathol 2010;23(Suppl 2): S1–7.

61. Verschuur-Maes AH, Moelans CB, de Bruin PC, et al. Analysis of gene copy number alterations by multiplex ligation-dependent probe amplification in columnar cell lesions of the breast. Cell Oncol (Dordr) 2014;37(2):147–54.

62. Pang JB, Savas P, Fellowes AP, et al. Breast ductal carcinoma in situ carry mutational driver events representative of invasive breast cancer. Mod Pathol 2017;30(7):952–63.

63. Bijker N, Rutgers EJ, Peterse JL, et al. Variations in diagnostic and therapeutic procedures in a multi-centre, randomized clinical trial (EORTC 10853) investigating breast-conserving treatment for DCIS. Eur J Surg Oncol 2001;27(2):135–40.

Genotype-Phenotype Correlations in Breast Cancer

Jonathan D. Marotti, MD[a,b], Stuart J. Schnitt, MD[c,*]

KEYWORDS

- Genotype-phenotype • Breast cancer • Molecular • IDH2

Key points

- Of the many breast cancer histologic subtypes recognized by WHO, only a few harbor known recurrent genetic alterations associated with a specific morphology.

- Secretory carcinoma, adenoid cystic carcinoma, invasive lobular carcinoma, and the recently defined solid papillary carcinoma with reverse polarity have unique morphologic features and exhibit characteristic recurrent genetic abnormalities.

- Identifying the genetic underpinnings of breast cancer subtypes permits more accurate diagnosis and may provide new therapeutic targets.

ABSTRACT

Only a few breast cancer histologic subtypes harbor distinct genetic alterations that are associated with a specific morphology (genotype-phenotype correlation). Secretory carcinomas and adenoid cystic carcinomas are each characterized by recurrent translocations, and invasive lobular carcinomas frequently have *CDH1* mutations. Solid papillary carcinoma with reverse polarity is a rare breast cancer subtype with a distinctive morphology and recently identified *IDH2* mutations. We review the clinical and pathologic features and underlying genetic alterations of those breast cancer subtypes with established genotype-phenotype correlations and discuss the phenotypes associated with germline mutations in genes associated with hereditary breast cancer.

OVERVIEW

Genotype-phenotype correlation (ie, a recurrent genetic abnormality associated with a specific morphology) is relatively common in some tumor types. For example, nearly half of the diagnostic entities described in the most recent edition of the *WHO Classification of Tumors of Soft Tissue and Bone* are associated with recurrent cytogenetic and/or molecular alterations.[1,2] Many hematopoietic and lymphoid neoplasms also have genetic abnormalities associated with a specific morphology, such as the *PML-RARA* fusion gene defining acute promyelocytic leukemia.[3]

In contrast, of the 21 breast cancer histologic subtypes defined by the World Health Organization (WHO),[4] few are known to harbor distinct recurrent genetic alterations. Secretory carcinomas and adenoid cystic carcinomas (ACCs) are characterized by recurrent *ETV6-NTRK3* and

---

The authors have no financial disclosures.

[a] Department of Pathology and Laboratory Medicine, Dartmouth-Hitchcock Medical Center, One Medical Center Drive, Lebanon, NH 03756, USA; [b] Department of Pathology and Laboratory Medicine, Geisel School of Medicine at Dartmouth, One Rope Ferry Road, Hanover, NH 03755-1404, USA; [c] Department of Pathology, Brigham and Women's Hospital, Dana-Farber Cancer Institute, Harvard Medical School, 75 Francis Street, Boston, MA 02115, USA
* Corresponding author.
E-mail address: sschnitt@bwh.harvard.edu

MYB-NFIB fusion genes, respectively,[5,6] and invasive lobular carcinomas commonly have somatic *CDH1* mutations.[7] Recently, a rare breast cancer subtype, solid papillary carcinoma with reverse polarity (SPCRP), was more fully defined.[8] These tumors display a unique morphology and are associated with a high frequency of *IDH2* R172 hotspot mutations.[8] Finally, breast cancers associated with germline mutations in some breast cancer susceptibility genes, particularly *BRCA1*, have a characteristic constellation of histologic findings in many cases.[9,10]

Here we provide an updated review of those breast cancer subtypes with established genotype-phenotype correlations. Special emphasis is placed on the newly described molecular features of SPCRP. We also discuss the phenotypes associated with germline mutations in genes associated with hereditary breast cancer.

SECRETORY CARCINOMA

Secretory carcinoma is an exceptionally rare special subtype that represents fewer than 0.02% of all breast cancers.[4] It was first described by McDivitt and Stewart[11] in 1966 as a distinct tumor occurring in children and, therefore, was originally named "juvenile carcinoma." After this initial case series, multiple reports of the tumor occurring in adults were described, prompting a change in terminology to secretory carcinoma.[12] Recent analyses from larger population-based databases including the National Cancer Data Base and the National Cancer Institute's Survival, Epidemiology, and End Results program have shown that secretory carcinoma largely affects older patients with a median age of approximately 53 to 54 years[13,14]; however, when compared with invasive ductal carcinoma of no special type (IDC), a greater proportion of younger women are diagnosed with secretory carcinoma.[14] Cases of secretory carcinoma arising in men also have been reported.[15,16]

The architecture of secretory carcinoma is typically microcystic (honeycomb), solid, or tubular, with many tumors containing a mixture of all 3 patterns. Some tumors display a peripheral papillary architecture, and central sclerosis is often observed. The edges of the cancer are often well-circumscribed with pushing borders, but more infiltrative areas may be seen. The tumor cells are polygonal with granular to foamy amphophilic cytoplasm, small bland nuclei, and few mitoses (**Fig. 1**). The histologic hallmark of secretory carcinoma is the presence of intracellular and extracellular eosinophilic secretions that are periodic acid-Schiff (PAS)-positive and diastase-resistant.

Secretory carcinoma typically lacks estrogen receptor (ER) and progesterone receptor (PR) expression, and is negative for human epidermal growth factor 2 (HER2) overexpression and amplification and is thus a "triple-negative" breast cancer. Jacob and colleagues[14] suggested that contrary to prior reports, up to 64% of secretory carcinomas may be positive for ER. However, major limitations of this study include the lack of both central histologic review and molecular status to confirm the diagnosis of secretory carcinoma. Furthermore, most ER-positive secretory carcinomas are reported to display only focal, weak ER immunoreactivity. Based on variable immunoreactivity with the basal cytokeratins (CK) 5/6 and/or CK14, as well as CD117 and epidermal growth factor receptor (EGFR), secretory carcinoma can be considered a basal-like carcinoma.[17] S100 protein and α-lactalbumin are consistently positive, although the latter stain is not used in current clinical practice. The tumor cells also show expression of mammaglobin, GATA3, and STAT5a, and are usually negative for

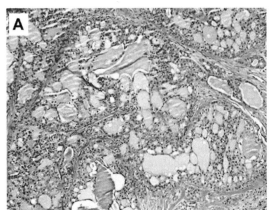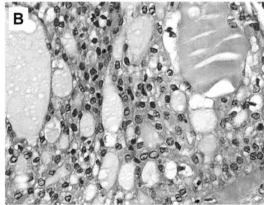

Fig. 1. Secretory carcinoma. (*A*) This tumor is composed of cribriform islands of cells with numerous glandular spaces containing eosinophilic secretions. (*B*) At higher power, the tumor cells have foamy cytoplasm and relatively uniform nuclei with variably prominent nucleoli.

gross cystic disease fluid protein (GCDFP) and monoclonal carcinoembryonic antigen.

The differential diagnosis of secretory carcinoma includes several other rare special types of breast cancer, such as lipid-rich carcinoma, glycogen-rich carcinoma, and acinic cell carcinoma, as well as the more common IDC and invasive lobular carcinoma (ILC). Whereas secretory carcinomas contain PAS-positive, diastase-resistant secretions, lipid-rich carcinomas demonstrate oil red O-positive cytoplasmic vacuoles and glycogen-rich clear cell carcinomas have PAS-positive, diastase-sensitive secretions. In a small series of breast cancers initially classified as secretory carcinoma, 3 of the 19 cases were determined to be acinic cell carcinoma on review.[18] These 2 tumor types share morphologic and immunohistochemical staining patterns, yet acinic cell carcinoma has yet to be confirmed in either young (prepubertal) or male patients and they do not harbor the characteristic translocation of secretory carcinoma discussed below.[19] Likewise, ILCs, which may contain prominent intracytoplasmic mucin, and IDCs, which may have focal secretory histologic features, also consistently lack the specific translocation. Last, several benign entities, such as lactational change, collagenous spherulosis, cystic hypersecretory change and cystic hypersecretory hyperplasia, as well as cystic hypersecretory ductal carcinoma in situ (DCIS), may also resemble secretory carcinoma. In all instances, an appropriate panel of myoepithelial cell immunostains will confirm the presence of a myoepithelial cell layer surrounding the glands of these lesions, although rare cases of cystic hypersecretory DCIS have been reported to lack a surrounding myoepithelial cell layer.[20]

Secretory carcinomas are characterized by a recurrent translocation, t(12;15) (p13;q25). This translocation, which results in a fusion of the ETS variant gene 6 (*ETV6*) and the neurotrophic tyrosine kinase receptor 3 gene (*NTRK3*), was first demonstrated in secretory carcinoma by Tognon and colleagues[5] in 2002. The *ETV6* gene on chromosome 12 encodes an E26 transformation-specific transcription factor and the *NTRK3* gene on chromosome 15 encodes a membrane receptor tyrosine kinase. The resulting ETV6-NTRK3 fusion product is a chimeric tyrosine kinase that has the ability to transform ductal epithelial cells via the Ras-MAP kinase and phosphatidyl inositol-3-kinase-Akt (PI3K-Akt) pathways.[21] The t(12;15) translocation was first identified in the pediatric mesenchymal tumors, congenital fibrosarcoma and congenital cellular mesoblastic nephroma. ETV6 dual-color break-apart fluorescence in situ hybridization (FISH) probes are now commercially available for detection of ETV6 alterations (Fig. 2).

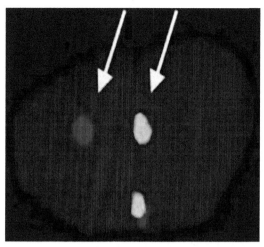

Fig. 2. Dual-color break-apart FISH probes for *ETV6* in a secretory carcinoma. There is 1 pair of adjacent green and red signals at the bottom of the nucleus representing the non-rearranged locus at chromosome 12 and 1 pair of separated green and red signals in the center of the nucleus representing the translocation (*arrows*).

In 2010, Skálová and colleagues[22] described a salivary gland tumor with morphology similar to secretory carcinoma of the breast and that also contained the t(12;15) translocation. Initially referred to as mammary analogue secretory carcinoma, this salivary gland tumor is regarded as a low-grade malignancy with overall favorable prognosis compared with other salivary gland carcinomas, but with occasional reported cases demonstrating a more aggressive course.[23] Rare cases in the salivary gland have also been shown to harbor *ETV6* fusions with non-*NTRK3* genes (eg, *ETV6*-X fusion)[24,25]; such fusions have yet to be fully evaluated in secretory carcinoma of the breast. The salivary gland tumor is not as rare as initially perceived, and recent updates to the WHO classification of salivary gland tumors recommend using the term, "secretory carcinoma" to standardize nomenclature across organ sites.[23,26]

Secretory carcinoma of the breast is usually associated with a better prognosis than IDC[13,14]; only rare cases with distant metastases have been reported.[15] Treatment for secretory carcinoma includes at least a wide excision with negative margins. Lymph node sampling is usually recommended, but the benefit of adjuvant radiation therapy and chemotherapy is uncertain given the limited number of reported cases.[19] The relatively indolent clinical course of secretory carcinoma despite its triple-negative, basal-like phenotype highlights the heterogeneity of triple-negative breast cancer and provides support for the view that there are low-grade, triple-negative neoplasms. Secretory carcinomas lack the complex genomic alterations seen in conventional triple-negative breast cancers and in particular do not contain *TP53* mutations.[27,28] The *ETV6-NTRK3* translocation of secretory carcinoma may serve as a potential therapeutic target for those cases that are more aggressive. For example, entrectinib (RXDX-101) and larotrectinib (LOXO-101), agents that selectively inhibit tyrosine receptor kinases encoded by the *NTRK* genes, are currently under clinical investigation.[29,30]

ADENOID CYSTIC CARCINOMA

ACC of the breast is also a rare type, accounting for fewer than 0.1% of breast cancers.[4] Although morphologically similar to ACCs that arise in other sites, most commonly salivary glands, lung, and skin, and that tend to have an aggressive clinical course, ACC of the breast is generally considered a carcinoma of low malignant potential. ACC is composed of a proliferation of both epithelial and myoepithelial/basaloid cells, most often

arranged in tubular, cribriform, or trabecular patterns. A solid variant with predominantly basaloid morphology can occasionally be seen (**Fig. 3**). The utility of grading ACC of the breast using criteria accepted for salivary gland ACC remains unclear.[4] Although one group was able to identify prognostic differences between grades,[31] other studies were not able to confirm these results.[32,33]

The lesional cells of ACC form 2 types of spaces: true glandular lumina and pseudolumina. True glandular lumina are surrounded by luminal epithelial cells with variably abundant eosinophilic cytoplasm and often contain PAS-positive mucin. These glandular lumina can be difficult to discern, especially in solid ACC with basaloid features. In contrast, pseudolumina are surrounded by myoepithelial cells, are usually larger than true glandular lumina, and typically contain dense, eosinophilic basement membrane material or a myxoid stromal substance.

ACC of the breast, like secretory carcinoma, is usually a triple-negative breast cancer lacking ER, PR, and HER2 overexpression/amplification. However, in a series of 28 ACC cases, 46% of tumors (without

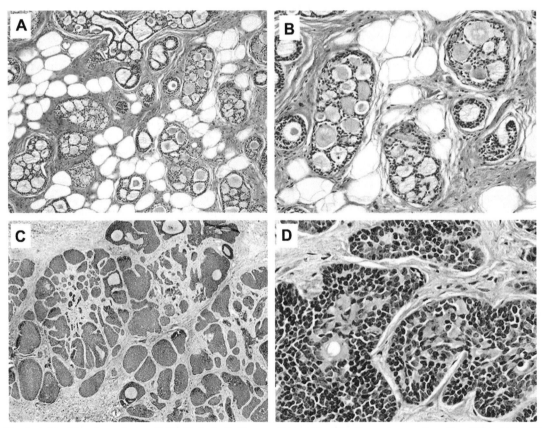

Fig. 3. Adenoid cystic carcinoma (ACC). Typical cribriform pattern adenoid cystic carcinoma at medium (*A*) and high (*B*) power. (*C, D*) Solid ACC with basaloid features. Low-power view (*C*) shows irregular nests of basaloid tumor cells. At high power (*D*), foci of eosinophilic, basement membrane material are present in association with the basaloid cells.

molecular testing) were reported to be ER-positive.[34] The dual cell population of ACC can best be highlighted by using CK7, p63, and CD117 (c-kit) immunostains. The luminal epithelial cells are most often CK7 and CD117 positive and p63 negative, whereas the myoepithelial cells express p63, but lack CK7 and CD117 expression. This distinctive staining pattern permits differentiation from most other malignant cribriform lesions, particularly invasive cribriform carcinoma and cribriform pattern DCIS, in which the neoplastic cells are typically all CK7-positive and lack staining for CD117 and p63. It should be noted, however, that in some cases, the neoplastic cells of ACC do not display the expected patterns of reactivity. We have seen cases in which both luminal epithelial cells and cells resembling myoepithelial/basaloid cells express CK7 and CD117, and cases in which the myoepithelial/basaloid cells show little or no staining for p63. Further, we have also observed staining for basal cytokeratins such as CK5/6 in both luminal epithelial cells and myoepithelial/basaloid cells. Collagenous spherulosis, a benign myoepithelial cell proliferation, can mimic ACC with a nearly identical low-power "sievelike" pattern. Rabban and colleagues[35] proposed using an expanded immunohistochemical panel to distinguish between these 2 lesions. They demonstrated that whereas the luminal epithelial cells of ACC were consistently positive for CD117, the lesional cells of collagenous spherulosis were negative for CD117. Furthermore, due to p63 positivity in both ACC and collagenous spherulosis, they suggested also performing calponin and smooth muscle myosin heavy chain, as these makers were found to be uniformly positive in collagenous spherulosis, but negative in ACC.[35]

After secretory carcinoma, ACC was the second special-type breast cancer found to harbor a unique genetic translocation. Persson and colleagues[6] first reported the presence of a t(6;9) (q22–23;p23–24) translocation in head and neck ACC and breast ACC, resulting in a MYB-NFIB fusion gene. This fusion gene has since been reported to occur in 23% to 100% of breast ACCs,[36] and in most cases, results in overexpression of c-MYB at the mRNA and protein levels. The c-MYB protein is a transcription factor that regulates progenitor cells and is involved in breast cancer development.[37] Molecular analyses have shown that in addition to this characteristic translocation, ACCs of the breast also have a higher frequency of mutations of genes involved in chromatin remodeling, cellular adhesion and cell signaling pathways, including BRAF, FBXW7, FGFR2, and MTOR.[36] Notably, ACCs appear to lack the TP53 and PIK3CA mutations that are often present in the more common triple-negative ductal carcinomas.[36] Occasionally, ACC may progress to high-grade triple-negative ductal cancers, and

evaluation of both components has demonstrated the presence of the MYB-NFIB fusion gene in each; progression likely occurs through clonal selection and/or development of additional genetic alterations.[38] Alternative fusions have been recently identified in salivary gland ACC including MYBL1 to NFIB and MYBL1 to RAD51B.[39,40] The MYBL1 gene, located on chromosome 8q, encodes the A-MYB protein. This protein is closely related to c-MYB, as they both bind and activate similar reporter genes, but appear to regulate different gene targets in human cells.[39] The role of MYBL1 and A-MYB in breast ACC has yet to be determined.

Evaluation of MYB overexpression using immunohistochemistry (IHC) or detection of the MYB-NFIB translocation by FISH can assist in diagnosing ACC in cases with histologic uncertainty (Fig. 4). Dual break-apart FISH probes are commonly used to identify MYB rearrangements, and current next-generation sequencing platforms can also detect MYB fusions. Poling and colleagues[41] recently suggested that IHC is more sensitive and specific than FISH for the diagnosis of breast ACC. They reported that MYB IHC showed diffuse and strong nuclear immunoreactivity of primarily the myoepithelial cells in 100% of breast ACC (11/11) compared with detection of MYB rearrangement in 8 (89%) of 9 evaluable cases.[41] Only weak and focal MYB staining was seen in mimics of ACC including basal-like triple-negative breast cancer, microglandular adenosis, and collagenous spherulosis.[41] In a series of solid ACCs with basaloid features, a variant of ACC with a potentially more aggressive clinical course, fewer tumors

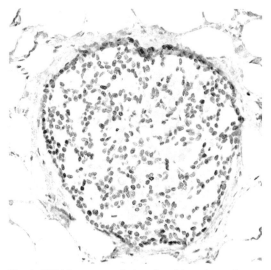

Fig. 4. MYB immunostain in adenoid cystic carcinoma showing strong nuclear staining of many of the tumor cells.

were found to contain the *MYB-NFIB* fusion gene (2/16, 12%).[42] Two patients with the solid ACC variant had axillary lymph node metastases, 1 patient developed distant metastasis, and 1 patient had a local recurrence.[42]

ACC of the breast has a very favorable outcome with 5-year and 10-year survival rates of greater than 95% and 90%, respectively.[4,43] The additional benefit of lymph node sampling, chemotherapy, and radiation for the treatment of early-stage, "low-grade" ACC of the breast remains questionable.[44] Standard targeted therapy for ACC currently does not exist; however, trials investigating downstream effectors of MYB, such as vascular endothelial growth factor A (VEGFA) and fibroblast growth factor 2 (FGF2) are underway.[30] Despite overexpression of CD117 (c-kit) in ACC, it is now clear that ACCs lack c-KIT mutations[36,45] and therefore, targeting c-kit with imatinib appears to be largely ineffective.[45]

INVASIVE LOBULAR CARCINOMA

ILC is the second most common histologic type of breast cancer, accounting for 5% to 15% of invasive breast cancers.[4] The histologic features of ILC are well known to pathologists. These tumors are composed of relatively small, dyshesive epithelial cells, some with intracytoplasmic lumens, infiltrating the stroma in a single-file pattern with minimal stromal reaction (Fig. 5). Several variants of ILC have been described, including solid, alveolar, histiocytoid, and pleomorphic types. Most ILCs are of low to intermediate histologic grade, express ER and PR, and are negative for HER2 overexpression or amplification. A few unusual entities may mimic ILC, such as metastatic signet ring cell carcinoma, sclerosing epithelioid fibrosarcoma, myeloid sarcoma, and plasma cell dyscrasias; the differentiation between these lesions has been discussed elsewhere.[46]

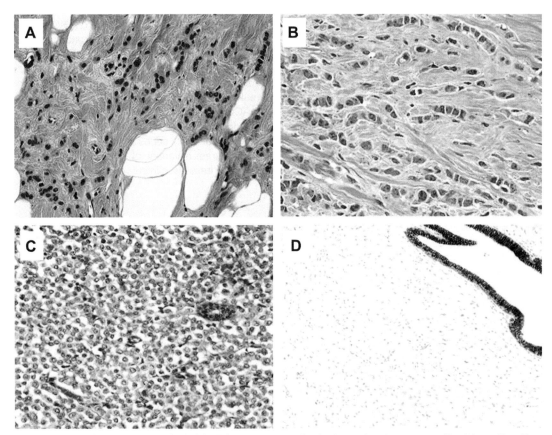

Fig. 5. Invasive lobular carcinoma (ILC). (*A*) High-power view of a classic ILC showing tumor cells with small, uniform nuclei infiltrating fibroadipose tissue as single cells and linear strands, and with no desmoplastic stromal reaction. (*B*) In this pleomorphic variant of ILC, the nuclei show more variation in size and shape than in classical ILC shown in Fig. 5A. (*C*) Solid variant of ILC with striking cellular dyshesion. (*D*) E-cadherin immunostain of a classic ILC demonstrates lack of membrane staining of the tumor cells. In contrast, normal ductal epithelium in the upper right part of the field shows strong membrane staining for E-cadherin.

The molecular hallmark of all forms of lobular neoplasia (including ILC, lobular carcinoma in situ, and atypical lobular hyperplasia), and which largely accounts for its dyshesive phenotype, is decreased or absent expression of E-cadherin on the cell membranes[47,48] (see Fig. 5). Loss of E-cadherin expression has been observed in approximately 90% of ILCs,[48] and IHC evaluation of E-cadherin can be used to distinguish ductal from lobular neoplasms, albeit with some caveats.[49] E-cadherin, encoded by the *CDH1* gene, is a cell-cell adhesion glycoprotein and a key component of the cadherin-catenin complex present at the junction between adjacent epithelial cells.[50] In addition to its role in cell-cell adhesion, E-cadherin also has important signaling activity via regulation of p120 catenin and β-catenin; sequestration of these proteins by E-cadherin results in decreased transcriptional activity.[50] Therefore, loss of E-cadherin (a tumor suppressor) assists tumor proliferation and contributes to increased invasiveness and development of metastases.

The most comprehensive molecular analysis of ILC to date confirmed a high percentage of E-cadherin alterations.[7] Nearly all of the ILCs analyzed (95%) had E-cadherin loss, either at the DNA, mRNA, or protein level.[7] Most *CDH1* mutations were truncating mutations and they almost always occurred in combination with chromosome 16q loss, which is the location of the *CDH1* gene.[7] Mutations in *PTEN*, *TBX3*, and *FOXA1* were enriched in ILCs as well, and when compared with other breast cancer subtypes, ILC also had the highest level of Akt phosphorylation.[7] This latter finding, likely due to associated PTEN loss, reinforces the possibility of targeting the PI3K/Akt pathway as a viable therapeutic approach in ILC.

The prognosis of patients with ILC, as compared with IDC, remains controversial.[4] ILCs are more likely to be of larger size, more advanced stage, and have a higher frequency of lymph node involvement.[4] Furthermore, the metastatic pattern of ILC is substantially different from that of IDC. In particular, ILC has a greater propensity for metastasizing to the gastrointestinal tract, gynecologic organs, meninges, and peritoneal surfaces than IDC.[4]

Germline mutations in the *CDH1* gene were first described nearly 20 years ago in families with a propensity for developing diffuse gastric cancer,[51] an epithelial malignancy demonstrating considerable cytomorphologic overlap with ILC. *CDH1* mutations have since been shown to be the genetic cause of hereditary diffuse gastric cancer (HDGC) in up to 40% of cases.[52] Not surprisingly, ILC is relatively more common in families with HDGC,

and germline *CDH1* mutations have been identified in families with increased incidence of ILC, but without evidence of diffuse gastric cancer.[53] Recent clinical guidelines suggest considering *CDH1* testing in patients with bilateral or familial lobular breast cancer before the age of 50, and recommend annual breast cancer surveillance using MRI beginning at age 30 for those patients with confirmed pathogenic *CDH1* mutations.[54]

SOLID PAPILLARY CARCINOMA WITH REVERSE POLARITY

SPCRP is the recently proposed name for a distinctive histologic type of breast cancer not recognized in the most recent WHO classification of tumors of the breast.[8] Due to cytomorphologic overlap with papillary thyroid carcinoma, including the variable presence of nuclear grooves and intranuclear cytoplasmic inclusions, these tumors were initially described as "breast tumor resembling the tall cell variant of papillary thyroid carcinoma" and, more recently, as "solid papillary carcinoma resembling the tall cell variant of papillary thyroid carcinoma."[55–57]

SPCRP are seen primarily in older women. Among the cases reported to date, the median age was 64 years (range: 45–85 years); 61% of patients were older than 60.[56,57] These tumors also tend to be small, with a median reported tumor size of 1.5 cm (range: 0.6–5.0 cm); 64% of tumors were smaller than 2 cm.[56,57]

These tumors are characterized by solid, circumscribed nodules of columnar epithelial cells, often with a rounded contour but occasionally exhibiting a geographic, jigsawlike growth pattern. The nodules are distributed haphazardly throughout the breast stroma and extend around and between normal ductal lobular structures. The stroma is typically composed of dense fibrous connective tissue without desmoplasia; some nodules extend into adipose tissue without an associated stromal reaction. Many nodules contained fibrovascular cores, some of which contain foamy histiocytes. The columnar epithelium is often present as a double-layer. Taken together, these features result in a solid papillary appearance. In occasional cases, nodules with true papillations can be seen. The cells in many nodules appear back-to-back and, in particular, the nuclei are often present at the apical rather than basal pole of the cells, creating the impression of reverse polarity. These tumor nodules invariably lack a surrounding myoepithelial cell layer supporting the invasive nature of these lesions[8] (Fig. 6).

The cells comprising SPCRP show strong cytoplasmic expression of low molecular weight

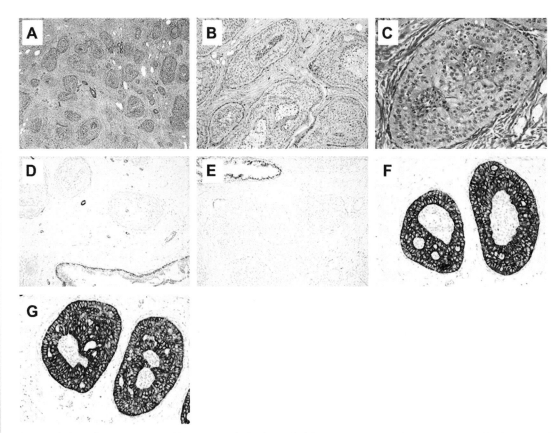

Fig. 6. Solid papillary carcinoma with reverse polarity (SPCRP). (*A*) Low-power view showing circumscribed tumor cell nests distributed haphazardly through the breast stroma. A few normal ducts are present in-between the tumor cell nests. (*B*) Medium-power view demonstrates that some of the nests have central fibrovascular cores, some with foamy histiocytes. The nuclei of many of the tumor cells are at the apical rather than the basal pole of the cells. (*C*) High-power view better demonstrates the apparent reversal of cell polarity with nuclei at the apical pole of the cells. (*D*) Smooth muscle myosin heavy chain immunostain demonstrates absence of myoepithelial cells around the tumor cell nests (myoepithelial cells are present around the normal duct in the lower part of the field). (*E*) ER immunostain showing absence of staining in the tumor cells (epithelial cells of the normal duct at the top of the field show ER staining and serve as an internal positive control). The tumor cells show strong cytoplasmic staining for both luminal keratins as shown in a CK7 immunostain (*F*) and basal cytokeratins as shown in a CK5/6 immunostain (*G*).

cytokeratins (as demonstrated on CK7 immunostains), but also strongly express high-molecular weight/basal cytokeratins CK5/6 and CK34βE12. GCDFP-15 and mammaglobin expression are seen in slightly more than half of the cases, supporting the breast origin of the tumors, whereas thyroglobulin and TTF-1 are consistently negative. In one recent study, the tumor cells were entirely ER-negative in 62% of cases; ER expression was seen in 1% to 10% of cells in the remaining tumors.[8] PR expression was seen in 15% of cases, and all cases studied were negative for HER2 protein overexpression. Androgen receptor (AR) was focally positive in only 1 case. In 2 cases studied, the Ki67 proliferation rate was low (<5%). E-cadherin staining revealed strong lateral membrane expression with absent apical or basal expression, suggesting that the epithelium is polarized. Mucin 1 (MUC1) staining, which highlights the apical membranes of columnar epithelial cells, was identified at the end of the tumor cell closest to the nucleus, further implying that the nuclei were in an abnormal location (ie, apical rather than basal).[8]

Given some histologic similarity of SPCRP to papillary thyroid carcinoma, metastatic papillary thyroid carcinoma to the breast is often considered in the differential diagnosis, but can usually be excluded after thorough clinical and radiologic correlation, as well as consistently negative immunoreactivity in SPCRP for the thyroid markers TTF-1 and thyroglobulin. SPCRP must also be differentiated from other primary papillary lesions of the breast, particularly conventional forms of solid papillary carcinoma. Whereas the usual type of solid papillary carcinoma is strongly positive for ER and negative for CK5 or CK5/6, the tumor cells of SPCRP are usually negative or weakly positive for ER and positive for CK5/6. It should also be noted that the reverse nuclear polarity of SPCRP is different from the "inside-out" pattern of invasive micropapillary carcinoma first described by Peterse in 1993.[58] The tumor cell clusters of invasive micropapillary carcinoma lack fibrovascular cores, and although cell orientation is inverted, the nuclei remain in the basal pole. This "inside-out" orientation is best highlighted by epithelial membrane antigen or MUC1 IHC; strong immunoreactivity for each is seen along the outer edges of the tumor cell clusters.[59,60]

To identify potential molecular alterations responsible for the distinctive morphology of SPCRPs, Chiang and colleagues[8] performed whole-exome, targeted, and Sanger sequencing on a series of 13 previously unreported cases. Interestingly, most (77%) of the SPRCPs were found to contain mutations at R172H of the isocitrate dehydrogenase (NADP+), mitochondrial (IDH2) gene. Eight of these tumors also harbored PI3K pathway mutations. One tumor with wild-type IDH2 contained a TET2 Q548-truncating mutation, coupled with a PI3KCA hotspot mutation. Bhargava and colleagues[56] subsequently reported IDH2 and ATM mutations in 2 of 3 additional cases, and a PIK3CA mutation in 1 of their 3 cases. This is the first histologic type of breast cancer associated with IDH mutations, which are more commonly found in glioma, acute myeloid leukemia, chondrosarcoma, and cholangiocarcinoma.[61] The concurrent functional studies performed by Chiang and colleagues[8] demonstrated that the IDH2 and PI3KCA mutations are likely drivers of tumor development and contribute to the unique phenotype of SPCRP. Specifically, by using a 3-dimensional model system, they demonstrated that expression of IDH2[R172S] in a breast cancer cell line resulted in an increased number of cells displaying reversed nuclear polarity.[8]

Review of the available cases with limited follow-up suggests a generally favorable prognosis of SPCRP with only a few cases containing regional nodal involvement or distant metastases.[8,56,57] As with the previously discussed rare special types of breast cancer, negative surgical margins should be sought; however, the need for lymph node sampling, radiation, and/or systemic therapy remains unknown. The IDH2 mutation may provide an opportunity for targeted therapy in more aggressive cases. Phase I trials evaluating IDH inhibitors in glioma and acute myeloid leukemia are ongoing.[62]

PHENOTYPIC CORRELATES OF MOLECULAR SUBTYPES AND HEREDITARY BREAST CANCERS

It has been nearly 2 decades since the seminal studies using gene expression profiling identified multiple molecular (intrinsic) subtypes of breast cancer.[63,64] The most common molecular subtypes (luminal A, luminal B, HER2-enriched, basal-like) have been studied extensively. Although these subtypes differ with regard to their patterns of gene expression, clinical course and response to various forms of systemic therapy, phenotypic correlations are problematic because most of the breast cancers in each of these subtypes are IDCs of no special type. Although molecular subtype is sometimes inferred by using ER, PR, and HER2 status, often in combination with histologic grade, these features alone are insufficient to reliably predict the underlying molecular subtype in an individual case.[65] However, basal-like cancers demonstrate a fairly high degree of correlation between histologic features and molecular subtype. Tumors that are basal-like by transcriptional profiling are most often characterized histologically by solid sheets of tumor cells with high-grade nuclei and numerous mitoses, pushing borders, a prominent lymphocytic infiltrate, and central zones of necrosis or fibrosis.[66] They commonly demonstrate EGFR overexpression or amplification and express the basal cytokeratins CK 5/6 and/or 14. These tumors are most often negative for ER and PR expression and lack HER2 overexpression and gene amplification ("triple-negative"). However, it should be noted that not all tumors that are basal-like by gene expression analysis are triple-negative, and not all tumors that are clinically triple-negative are basal-like at the transcriptome level.[65]

Most tumors arising in patients with germline BRCA1 mutations display basal-like histologic features, and sporadic basal-like breast cancers often have a dysfunctional BRCA pathway.[9,67] The BRCA1 gene, located on chromosome 17q, is involved in multiple cellular processes, including DNA repair, X chromosome inactivation, transcriptional regulation, and ER signaling. Conditional mouse models with inactivated Brca1 and Trp53 genes, a genotype frequently present in human basal-like cancers, consistently develop tumors with histologic and IHC features similar to human basal-like tumors.[68] It should be emphasized that most basal-like breast cancers are not associated with germline BRCA mutations, and these sporadic tumors are essentially identical in appearance to their hereditary counterparts.[9] Therefore, our ability as pathologists to accurately predict germline BRCA mutations based on the presence of a basal-like morphology alone remains limited; the addition of basal markers, ER status, and family history increases sensitivity and specificity.[67] A

Table 1
Genotype-phenotype correlation in breast cancer

Histologic Type	Genotype	Ancillary Assay(s)	Potential Targeted Therapies
Secretory carcinoma	t(12;15) (p13;q25) translocation resulting in *ETV6-NTRK3* fusion gene	*ETV6* dual break-apart FISH	TRK inhibitors
Adenoid cystic carcinoma	t(6;9) (q22–23;p23–24) translocation resulting in *MYB-NFIB* fusion gene	MYB IHC[a] *MYB* dual break-apart FISH	Inhibitors of downstream effectors of MYB (VEGFA, FGF2)
Invasive lobular carcinoma	*CDH1* mutations	E-cadherin IHC[b]	PI3K/Akt inhibitors
Solid papillary carcinoma with reverse polarity	*IDH2* mutations (often in association with *PIK3CA* mutations)	NGS	PI3K inhibitors IDH2 inhibitors

Abbreviations: FGF2, fibroblast growth factor 2; FISH, fluorescence in situ hybridization; IHC, immunohistochemistry; NGS, next-generation sequencing; TRK, tropomyosin receptor kinase; VEGFA, vascular endothelial growth factor A.

[a] MYB IHC has been shown to be more sensitive and specific than FISH for evaluation of ACC[41]; however, focal, weak immunostaining can be seen in ACC mimics.

[b] Aberrant E-cadherin immunostaining has been reported to occur in up to 24% of ILCs.[49]

specific phenotype that consistently identifies *BRCA2*-associated tumors has yet to be identified, although these tumors tend to be high grade and ER-positive.[69] Although most luminal A-type cancers are IDCs of no special type, some special-type tumors, such as tubular carcinomas, mucinous carcinomas, and carcinomas with neuroendocrine features are invariably of luminal A molecular subtype, whereas ACCs, secretory carcinomas, and carcinomas with medullary features typically cluster in the basal-like group.[70]

For non-*BRCA* hereditary breast cancers, other than the familial lobular breast cancers associated with *CDH1* mutations discussed previously, genotype-phenotype correlations are less well-defined. It has been suggested that breast cancers arising in the setting of Lynch syndrome or hereditary nonpolyposis colorectal cancer syndrome with germline mutations in the mismatch repair genes (*MLH1, MSH2, MSH6, PMS2*) may have a dense lymphocytic infiltrate and are more likely to be ER and PR negative.[10] Conversely, breast cancers associated with Cowden syndrome (resulting from germline *PTEN* mutations) are usually luminal-type (ER-positive), low-grade to intermediate-grade IDCs.[10] In a series of 12 patients with Li-Fraumeni syndrome (due to germline *TP53* mutations), HER2 overexpression or amplification was reported to be present in most (83%) breast cancers.[71] Last, distinctive morphologies have not yet been definitively identified in patients with ataxia-telangiectasia (*ATM* mutations), Fanconi anemia pathway (*FANCD1, FANCN/PALB2, FANCJ/BRIP1,* or

FANCC mutations), and Fanconi anemialike disorder (*RAD51C* mutations).[10]

SUMMARY

A few special-type breast cancers are now known to be underpinned by recurrent genetic alterations that are associated with their unique morphology and clinical features. These include secretory carcinoma, adenoid cystic carcinoma, ILC, and SPCRP (**Table 1**). The mechanistic relationship between genetic alteration and histologic appearance has been determined for ILC (*CDH1* mutations), and recently, it was discovered that *IDH2* mutations likely account for the distinctive reverse nuclear polarity of SPCRP. In the future, advances in molecular methods may result in the identification of genotype-phenotype correlations in other subtypes of breast cancer.

REFERENCES

1. Bridge JA. The role of cytogenetics and molecular diagnostics in the diagnosis of soft-tissue tumors. Mod Pathol 2014;27:S80–97.
2. Fletcher CDM, Bridge JA, Hogendoorn PCW, et al. In: WHO classification of tumours of soft tissue and bone. Lyon (France): IARC; 2013.
3. Swerdlow SH, Campo E, Harris NL, et al. In: WHO classification of tumours of haematopoietic and lymphoid tissues. Lyon (France): IARC; 2008.
4. Lakhani SR, Ellis IO, Schnitt SJ, et al. In: WHO classification of tumours of the breast. Lyon (France): IARC; 2012.

5. Tognon C, Knezevich SR, Huntsman D, et al. Expression of the ETV6-NTRK3 gene fusion as a primary event in human secretory breast carcinoma. Cancer Cell 2002;2:367–76.

6. Persson M, Andren Y, Mark J, et al. Recurrent fusion of MYB and NFIB transcription factor genes in carcinomas of the breast and head and neck. Proc Natl Acad Sci U S A 2009;106:18740–4.

7. Ciriello G, Gatza ML, Beck AH, et al. Comprehensive molecular portraits of invasive lobular breast cancer. Cell 2015;163:506–19.

8. Chiang S, Weigelt B, Wen HC, et al. IDH2 mutations define a unique subtype of breast cancer with altered nuclear polarity. Cancer Res 2016;76:7118–29.

9. Turner NC, Reis-Filho JS. Basal-like breast cancer and the BRCA1 phenotype. Oncogene 2006;25:5846–53.

10. Vargas AC, Reis-Filho JS, Lakhani SR. Phenotype-genotype correlation in familial breast cancer. J Mammary Gland Biol Neoplasia 2011;16:27–40.

11. McDivitt RW, Stewart FW. Breast carcinoma in children. JAMA 1966;195:388–90.

12. Tavassoli FA, Norris HJ. Secretory carcinoma of the breast. Cancer 1980;45:2404–13.

13. Horowitz DP, Sharma CS, Connolly E, et al. Secretory carcinoma of the breast: results from the survival, epidemiology and end results database. Breast 2012;21:350–3.

14. Jacob JD, Hodge C, Franko J, et al. Rare breast cancers: 246 invasive secretory carcinomas from the national cancer data base. J Surg Oncol 2016;113:721–5.

15. Arce C, Cortes-Padilla D, Huntsman DG, et al. Secretory carcinoma of the breast containing the ETV6-NTRK3 fusion gene in a male: case report and review of the literature. World J Surg Oncol 2005;3:35.

16. Li D, Xiao X, Yang W, et al. Secretory breast carcinoma: a clinicopathological and immunophenotypic study of 15 cases with a review of the literature. Mod Pathol 2012;25:567–75.

17. Laé M, Fréneaux P, Sastre-Garau X, et al. Secretory breast carcinomas with ETV6-NTRK3 fusion gene belong to the basal-like carcinoma spectrum. Mod Pathol 2009;22:291–8.

18. Osako T, Takeuchi K, Horii R, et al. Secretory carcinoma of the breast and its histopathological mimics: value of markers for differential diagnosis. Histopathology 2013;63:509–19.

19. Geyer FC, Lacroix-Triki M, Reis-Filho JS. Rare breast carcinomas: adenoid cystic carcinoma, neuroendocrine carcinoma, secretory carcinoma, carcinoma with osteoclast-like giant cells, lipid-rich carcinoma, and glycogen-rich clear cell carcinoma. In: Dabbs DJ, editor. Breast pathology. Philadelphia: Elsevier Saunders; 2012. p. 573–95.

20. D'Alfonso TM, Ginter PS, Liu YF, et al. Cystic hypersecretory (in situ) carcinoma of the breast: a clinicopathologic and immunohistochemical characterization of 10 cases with clinical follow-up. Am J Surg Pathol 2014;38:45–53.

21. Tognon C, Garnett M, Kenward E, et al. The chimeric protein tyrosine kinase ETV6-NTRK3 requires both Ras-Erk1/2 and PI3-kinase-Akt signaling for fibroblast transformation. Cancer Res 2001;61:8909–16.

22. Skálová A, Vanecek T, Sima R, et al. Mammary analogue secretory carcinoma of salivary glands containing the ETV6-NTRK3 fusion gene: a hitherto undescribed salivary gland tumor entity. Am J Surg Pathol 2010;34:599–608.

23. Stevens TM, Parekh V. Mammary analogue secretory carcinoma. Arch Pathol Lab Med 2016;140:997–1001.

24. Ito Y, Ishibashi K, Masaki A, et al. Mammary analogue secretory carcinoma of salivary glands: a clinicopathologic and molecular study including 2 cases harboring ETV6-X fusion. Am J Surg Pathol 2015;39:601–10.

25. Skálová A, Vanecek T, Simpson RH, et al. Mammary analogue secretory carcinoma of salivary glands: molecular analysis of 25 ETV6 gene rearranged tumors with lack of detection of classical ETV6-NTRK3 fusion transcript by RT-PCR: report of 4 cases harboring ETV6-X gene fusion. Am J Surg Pathol 2016;40:3–13.

26. Seethala RR, Stenman G. Update from the 4th edition of the World Health Organization classification of head and neck tumours: tumors of the salivary gland. Head Neck Pathol 2017;11:55–67.

27. Krings G, Joseph NM, Bean GR, et al. Genomic profiling of breast secretory carcinomas reveals distinct genetics from other breast cancers and similarity to mammary analog secretory carcinomas. Mod Pathol 2017;30:1086–99.

28. Del Castillo M, Chibon F, Arnould L, et al. Secretory breast carcinoma: a histopathologic and genomic spectrum characterized by a joint specific ETV6-NTRK3 gene fusion. Am J Surg Pathol 2015;39:1458–67.

29. Drilon A, Li G, Dogan S, et al. What hides behind the MASC: clinical response and acquired resistance to entrectinib after ETV6-NTRK3 identification in a mammary analogue secretory carcinoma (MASC). Ann Oncol 2016;27:920–6.

30. Available at: https://clinicaltrials.gov/. Accessed June 27, 2017.

31. Roy JY, Silva EG, Gallager HS. Adenoid cystic carcinoma of the breast. Hum Pathol 1987;18:1276–81.

32. Kleer CG, Oberman HA. Adenoid cystic carcinoma of the breast: value of histologic grading and proliferative activity. Am J Surg Pathol 1998;22:569–75.

33. Lamovec J, Us-Krasovec M, Zidar A, et al. Adenoid cystic carcinoma of the breast: a histologic,

cytologic, and immunohistochemical study. Semin Diagn Pathol 1989;6:153–64.

34. Arpino G, Clark GM, Mohsin S, et al. Adenoid cystic carcinoma of the breast: molecular markers, treatment, and clinical outcome. Cancer 2002;94:2119–27.

35. Rabban JT, Swain RS, Zaloudek CJ, et al. Immunophenotypic overlap between adenoid cystic carcinoma and collagenous spherulosis of the breast: potential diagnostic pitfalls using myoepithelial markers. Mod Pathol 2006;19:1351–7.

36. Martelotto LG, De Filippo MR, Ng CK, et al. Genomic landscape of adenoid cystic carcinoma of the breast. J Pathol 2015;237:179–89.

37. Miao RY, Drabsch Y, Cross RS, et al. MYB is essential for mammary tumorigenesis. Cancer Res 2011; 71:7029–37.

38. Fusco N, Geyer FC, De Filippo MR, et al. Genetic events in the progression of adenoid cystic carcinoma of the breast to high-grade triple-negative breast cancer. Mod Pathol 2016;29:1292–305.

39. Brayer KJ, Frerich CA, Kang H, et al. Recurrent fusions in MYB and MYBL1 define a common, transcription factor-driven oncogenic pathway in salivary gland adenoid cystic carcinoma. Cancer Discov 2016;6:176–87.

40. Fujii K, Murase T, Beppu S, et al. MYB, MYBL1, MYBL2, and NFIB gene alterations and MYC overexpression in salivary gland adenoid cystic carcinoma. Histopathology 2017;71:823–34.

41. Poling JS, Yonescu R, Subhawong AP, et al. MYB labeling by immunohistochemistry is more sensitive and specific for breast adenoid cystic carcinoma than MYB labeling by FISH. Am J Surg Pathol 2017;41:973–9.

42. D'Alfonso TW, Mosquera JM, MacDonald TY, et al. MYB-NFIB gene fusion in adenoid cystic carcinoma of the breast with special focus paid to the solid variant with basaloid features. Hum Pathol 2014; 45:2270–80.

43. Kulkarni N, Pezzi CM, Greif JM, et al. Rare breast cancer: 933 adenoid cystic carcinomas from the national cancer data base. Ann Surg Oncol 2013;20: 2236–41.

44. Treitl D, Radkani P, Rizer M, et al. Adenoid cystic carcinoma of the breast, 20 years of experience in a single center with review of the literature. Breast Cancer 2017, [Epub ahead of print].

45. Dillon PM, Chakraborty S, Moskaluk CA, et al. Adenoid cystic carcinoma: a review of recent advances, molecular targets, and clinical trials. Head Neck 2016;38:620–7.

46. Ishikawa MK, Pinsky RW, Smith LD, et al. Morphologic mimics of invasive lobular carcinoma. Arch Pathol Lab Med 2015;139:1253–7.

47. Morrogh M, Andrade VP, Giri D, et al. Cadherin-catenin complex dissociation in lobular neoplasia

of the breast. Breast Cancer Res Treat 2012;132: 641–52.

48. McCart Reed AE, Kutasovic JR, Lakhani SR, et al. Invasive lobular carcinoma of the breast: morphology, biomarkers and 'omics. Breast Cancer Res 2015;17:12.

49. Canas-Marques R, Schnitt SJ. E-cadherin immunohistochemistry in breast pathology: uses and pitfalls. Histopathology 2016;68:57–69.

50. van Roy F, Berx G. The cell-cell adhesion molecule e-cadherin. Cell Mol Life Sci 2008;65:3756–88.

51. Guilford P, Hopkins J, Harraway J, et al. E-cadherin germline mutation in familial gastric cancer. Nature 1998;392:402–5.

52. Hansford S, Kaurah P, Li-Chang H, et al. Hereditary diffuse gastric cancer syndrome: CDH1 mutations and beyond. JAMA Oncol 2015;1:23–32.

53. Corso G, Intra M, Trentin C, et al. CDH1 mutations and hereditary lobular breast cancer. Fam Cancer 2016;15:215–9.

54. van der Post RS, Vogelaar IP, Carneiro F, et al. Hereditary diffuse gastric cancer: updated clinical guidelines with an emphasis on germline CDH1 mutation carriers. J Med Genet 2015;52:361–74.

55. Eusebi V, Damiani S, Ellis IO, et al. Breast tumor resembling the tall cell variant of papillary thyroid carcinoma: report of 5 cases. Am J Surg Pathol 2003;27:1114–8.

56. Bhargava R, Florea AV, Pelmus M, et al. Breast tumor resembling tall cell variant of papillary thyroid carcinoma. Am J Clin Pathol 2017;147:399–410.

57. Foschini MP, Asioli S, Foreid S, et al. Solid papillary breast carcinomas resembling the tall cell variant of papillary thyroid neoplasms: a unique invasive tumor with indolent behavior. Am J Surg Pathol 2017;41: 887–95.

58. Peterse JL. Breast carcinomas with an unexpected inside out growth pattern. Rotation of polarization associated with angioinvasion, [abstract]. Pathol Res Pract 1993;189:780.

59. Luna-More S, Gonzalez B, Acedo C, et al. Invasive micropapillary carcinoma of the breast. A new special type of invasive mammary carcinoma. Pathol Res Pract 1994;190:668–74.

60. Nassar H, Pansare V, Zhang H, et al. Pathogenesis of invasive micropapillary carcinoma: role of MUC1 glycoprotein. Mod Pathol 2004;17:1045–50.

61. Clark O, Yen K, Mellinghoff IK. Molecular pathways: isocitrate dehydrogenase mutations in cancer. Clin Cancer Res 2016;22:1837–42.

62. Dang L, Yen K, Attar EC. IDH mutations in cancer and progress toward development of targeted therapeutics. Ann Oncol 2016;27:599–608.

63. Perou CM, Sorlie T, Eisen MB, et al. Molecular portraits of human breast tumours. Nature 2000;406: 747–52.

64. Sorlie T, Perou CM, Tibshirani R, et al. Gene expression patterns of breast carcinomas distinguish tumor subclasses with clinical implications. Proc Natl Acad Sci USA 2001;98:10869–74.

65. Cheang MC, Martin M, Nielsen TO, et al. Defining breast cancer intrinsic subtypes by quantitative receptor expression. Oncologist 2015;5:474–82.

66. Livasy CA, Karaca G, Nanda R, et al. Phenotypic evaluation of the basal-like subtype of invasive breast carcinoma. Mod Pathol 2006;19:264–71.

67. Badve S, Dabbs DJ, Schnitt SJ, et al. Basal-like and triple-negative breast cancers: a critical review with an emphasis on the implications for pathologists and oncologists. Mod Pathol 2011;24:157–67.

68. Weigelt B, Geyer FC, Reis-Filho JS. Histologic types of breast cancer: how special are they? Mol Oncol 2010;4:192–208.

69. Bane AL, Beck JC, Bleiwess I, et al. BRCA2 mutation-associated breast cancers exhibit a distinguishing phenotype based on morphology and molecular profiles from tissue microarrays. Am J Surg Pathol 2007;31:121–8.

70. Dieci MV, Orvieto E, Dominici M, et al. Rare breast cancer subtypes: histological, molecular and clinical peculiarities. Oncologist 2014;19:805–13.

71. Wilson JR, Bateman AC, Hanson H, et al. A novel HER2-positive breast cancer phenotype arising from germline TP53 mutations. J Med Genet 2010;47:771–4.

Processing and Reporting of Breast Specimens in the Neoadjuvant Setting

Veerle Bossuyt, MD

KEYWORDS

- Breast cancer • Neoadjuvant • Pathology • Response to treatment • Residual disease • pCR
- Sampling • Cellularity

Key points

- Post-neoadjuvant surgical breast cancer specimens are challenging. Systematic sampling of the correct area of the breast with correlation of gross and microscopic findings allows efficient and accurate reporting.

- Specimens should be clearly identified, as neoadjuvant, and the location and size of the tumor pretreatment must be known. Equipment to photograph or radiograph sliced specimens and create a map of the gross findings and the sections submitted is essential.

- Pathologic complete response (pCR), residual cancer burden (RCB), and yAJCC (American Joint Commission on Cancer) stage are recommended measures of residual disease.

- Patients with a pCR (ypT0/is ypN0 or ypT0ypN0) have an excellent prognosis regardless of breast cancer subtype and of the type of neoadjuvant systemic therapy received. RCB is prognostic overall, in breast cancer subtypes, and within stage groups.

- The processing approach and elements needed in the report for quantification of residual disease in the breast and lymph nodes will likely be the same regardless of the addition of other prognostic factors and irrespective of breast cancer subtype or type of treatment received.

ABSTRACT

Standardization of quantification of residual disease in the breast and lymph nodes with routine pathologic macroscopic and microscopic evaluation leads to accurate and reproducible measures of response to neoadjuvant treatment. Multidisciplinary collaboration and correlation of clinical, imaging, gross and microscopic findings is essential. The processing approach to post-neoadjuvant breast cancer surgical specimens and the elements needed in the pathology report are the same regardless of breast cancer subtype or type of neoadjuvant treatment. The residual cancer burden incorporates response in the breast and in the lymph nodes into a score that can be combined with other emerging prognostic factors.

NEOADJUVANT TREATMENT OF BREAST CANCER

Although many patients with breast cancer may be cured by surgery alone, adjuvant systemic chemotherapy, endocrine therapy, and/or anti-HER2 therapy reduce the risk of recurrence and mortality for selected patients. With more than 15 years of follow-up, we know that survival is the same whether the adjuvant chemotherapy is given before (neoadjuvant) or after surgery (adjuvant).[1] Systemic neoadjuvant treatment is increasingly

---

Disclosures: None.
Department of Pathology, Yale University, PO Box 208023, 310 Cedar Street, New Haven, CT 06520-8023, USA
E-mail address: veerle.bossuyt@yale.edu

Surgical Pathology 11 (2018) 213–230
https://doi.org/10.1016/j.path.2017.09.010

used for locally advanced breast cancer, for downstaging tumors to facilitate breast-conserving surgery, and for early stage high-risk breast cancer. Systemic neoadjuvant treatment can be considered any time it is known before the surgery that the patient will require systemic (neo)adjuvant treatment. A discussion of the pros and cons of systemic neoadjuvant treatment and which patients might benefit the most from the different types of systemic neoadjuvant treatment are beyond the scope of this article. **Fig. 1** summarizes how neoadjuvant systemic treatment affects some aspects of the care of patients with breast cancer. When treatment is given before surgery, response to treatment can be evaluated. For individual

patients with a poor response to neoadjuvant treatment there is an opportunity to change or add treatment after surgery. Neoadjuvant clinical trials are an opportunity to accelerate the development of new therapeutic agents and biomarkers. Clinical response to systemic neoadjuvant treatment does not correlate well with pathologic response. Accurate and reproducible pathologic evaluation of the post-neoadjuvant surgical breast cancer specimen is crucial.

MULTIDISCIPLINARY COLLABORATION

Neoadjuvant treatment of breast cancer introduces challenges for each discipline involved.

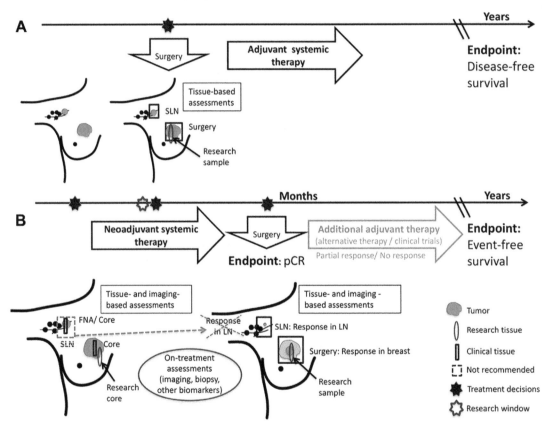

Fig. 1. Clinical and research tissue sampling and indicators of treatment effectiveness in the traditional setting (A) and in the neoadjuvant setting (B). In the setting of *adjuvant therapy* (A), the pathologist has the opportunity to evaluate the lymph nodes and the primary tumor unaltered by systemic therapy. The first available endpoint for clinical trials of adjuvant systemic therapy is generally disease-free survival after a many years. In contrast, in the setting of *neoadjuvant systemic therapy* (B), stage (tumor size and lymph node status) is determined by physical examination and imaging. Tumor grade and type as well as ER, PR, HER2, Ki67, and multigene assays are performed on a representative core needle biopsy sample. Research samples can be obtained at different time points. The surgical specimen provides the opportunity to evaluate the response to therapy in both the lymph node and the breast. If pretreatment SLN biopsy was performed, the opportunity to evaluate the response in the lymph nodes is lost. For patients with residual disease, there is an opportunity for additional therapy or to change to an alternative therapy after months rather than years. pCR provides a short-term, after months rather than years, endpoint for clinical trials. FNA, fine needle aspiration; LN, lymph node; SLN, sentinel lymph node. Note that disease-free survival and/or event-free survival (EFS) are the preferred survival endpoints (the FDA recommended EFS).

Generous multidisciplinary collaboration is essential. For example, some changes in workflow may be required in the pathology laboratory to make available in a timely manner all information necessary to determine whether neoadjuvant treatment would be appropriate and if so what type of treatment is indicated. Conversely, pathologists depend on information from the radiologist and surgeon to provide efficient and accurate reporting of the post-neoadjuvant surgical specimen. An international multidisciplinary working group convened by the Breast International Group–North American Breast Cancer Group (BIG-NABCG) collaboration published practical methods for standardizing pathology for clinical trials in patients receiving neoadjuvant systemic treatment.[2,3] These methods emphasize the need for communication and multidisciplinary collaboration and can be used for all patients regardless of whether they are on a clinical trial or not. The standardized approach recommended in these publications makes it easier and more efficient to process the post-neoadjuvant surgical specimen and to provide accurate and complete information in the pathology report. The elements recommended for the surgical pathology report of the post-neoadjuvant surgical specimen are summarized in **Table 1**.

ROLE OF PATHOLOGY BEFORE NEOADJUVANT TREATMENT

INITIAL DIAGNOSIS

A core needle biopsy is strongly recommended. An unequivocal diagnosis of invasive breast carcinoma and assessment of tumor type, tumor grade, estrogen receptor (ER), progesterone receptor (PR), and human epidermal growth factor receptor 2 (HER2) and any other ancillary tests used to select treatment are required before neoadjuvant treatment can be considered. Pretreatment stage is determined by imaging and clinical findings.

It is important to provide the ER, PR, and HER2 results on the core biopsy in a timely fashion to make sure that patients who might benefit from neoadjuvant treatment can be identified and that consultation with a medical oncologist can take place in the multidisciplinary setting so all options for timing of adjuvant treatment can be considered as appropriate. To emphasize the obvious: the diagnosis of invasive carcinoma must be certain. Most institutions require review of relevant outside pathology before any treatment can be started. Initially medical oncologists may not be as familiar with such policies or with common nuances in breast core biopsy pathology reports. Good communication with surgeons, medical oncologists, and radiologists is essential to ensure that any uncertainty about the diagnosis, need for additional tissue for ancillary testing, or questions about the size of the primary tumor are addressed. For example, additional sampling or surgery first may be more appropriate for a patient with predominantly in situ carcinoma or a papillary carcinoma on core biopsy even in the presence of a large lesion on imaging. If the amount of invasive carcinoma on the core biopsy is very small additional sampling to assess ER, PR, HER2, and other tests (for example multigene assays) to help determine treatment may be helpful. An excisional biopsy or oversampling precludes assessment of response after treatment.

EVALUATION OF THE AXILLA

Knowledge of axillary lymph node status before neoadjuvant treatment determines prognosis and informs treatment decisions–: (neoadjuvant) systemic therapy, completion axillary dissection, and radiation therapy. Response in the lymph nodes may be so pronounced that previously involved lymph nodes appear unremarkable on pathologic evaluation after neoadjuvant treatment. Removing a positive lymph node with a sentinel lymph node biopsy before neoadjuvant treatment precludes assessment of response in the lymph node. Response in the lymph nodes is an important determinant of prognosis.[4]

Therefore routine axillary ultrasound with fine needle aspiration or core needle biopsy of lymph nodes, that are abnormal by clinical or ultrasound examination, is recommended. By this means, positive lymph nodes are documented and response after neoadjuvant treatment can still be assessed because the positive lymph nodes have not been removed. At the moment, there are limited data to make subsequent radiation therapy choices in this setting.[5]

CLIPS

Clip placement in the primary tumor and in any biopsied lymph node is recommended. If the response to neoadjuvant treatment is good it may not be possible to identify the correct area of the breast for surgery or for pathology sampling without placement of a clip. Clip placement is therefore advised even when mastectomy is planned. Clip placement in the axillary lymph node with localization and removal of the clipped lymph node improves the accuracy of post-neoadjuvant treatment sentinel lymph node biopsy.[6]

Table 1
The elements recommended in the surgical pathology report of the post-neoadjuvant surgical specimen (in addition to the elements recommended for non–post-neoadjuvant specimens)

		Individual Elements	
1.	Size	• Size for AJCC staging (AJCC size)	Size of largest contiguous focus of residual tumor excluding treatment-related fibrosis adjacent to residual invasive carcinoma
		• Size to calculate the RCB score (RCB size)	Size in 2 dimensions of the largest cross-section of the residual invasive carcinoma bed (or "residual tumor bed"); that is, the largest cross-section that contains possibly scattered residual invasive carcinoma
2.	Cellularity	• Qualitative statement • Compared with pretreatment cellularity (if available) • Average invasive cancer cellularity in % across the largest cross-section that contains residual invasive carcinoma	Average invasive cancer cellularity in the residual invasive carcinoma bed
3.	Tumor bed	• Identified or not	
4.	Lymph node metastasis	• Size of largest lymph node metastasis for AJCC staging	Largest focus of residual tumor excluding treatment-related fibrosis adjacent to nodal tumor deposits
		• Size of largest lymph node metastasis for calculating the RCB score	Largest extent of lymph node involvement by tumor cells including intervening treatment-related fibrosis
5.	Treatment effect	• Treatment effect in the breast • Number of lymph nodes with possible treatment effect	Describe involvement by tumor and presence of possible treatment effect, biopsy site changes, and/or clip

Information about size, cellularity, and lymph node metastasis is required for quantification of residual disease.

	Suggested Notes
AJCC staging note in cases with scattered residual tumor cells	Multiple foci of residual invasive carcinoma are present in a single fibrotic tumor bed. The largest contiguous focus measures — mm. This dimension is used for AJCC staging.
Note for reporting RCB	The largest cross-sectional area of residual invasive carcinoma bed (represented in cassettes — per diagram) measures — mm × — mm. The overall cancer cellularity in this area (as percentage of area) is — %, with — % in situ. — Axillary lymph nodes are positive for carcinoma (largest focus — mm). The residual cancer burden is — corresponding to a RCB class of —.
Note documenting blocks of interest if RCB is not reported	Largest cross-section of residual invasive carcinoma bed represented in blocks: — (for example, "G through F")

Recommended Methods of Quantifying Residual Disease	
AJCC stage	y prefix
pCR (if applicable)	Including definition used (ypT0/is ypN0 or ypT0 ypN0)
RCB	RCB score and class

Abbreviations: AJCC, American Joint Committee on Cancer; pCR, pathologic complete response; RCB, residual cancer burden.

ROLE OF PATHOLOGY AFTER NEOADJUVANT TREATMENT

Post-neoadjuvant surgical specimens are challenging for pathologists. In cases with an excellent response it can be very difficult to find the correct area of the breast to sample. Tumor response is most often heterogeneous. Microscopic disease is often present without macroscopic findings. Systematic sampling of the correct area of the breast with correlation of gross and microscopic findings allows efficient and accurate reporting. Specimens should be clearly identified, as neoadjuvant, and the location and size of the tumor pretreatment must be known. Equipment to photograph or radiograph sliced specimens and annotate these images with the sections submitted for histologic evaluation (ie, to create a map of the gross findings and the sections submitted)

make correlation of microscopic and gross findings considerably easier.

The principles of processing that permit appropriate fixation and correlation of gross and microscopic findings are the same as for non-neoadjuvant specimens. Strategies particular to the neoadjuvant situation are discussed here.

PROCESSING OF POST-NEOADJUVANT BREAST CANCER SPECIMENS

Table 2 summarizes sampling recommendations for post-neoadjuvant surgical specimens.

Post-neoadjuvant Sentinel Lymph Node Biopsy and Axillary Dissection Specimens

The processing is the same as for non-neoadjuvant sentinel lymph node and axillary dissection specimens. All lymph nodes should be sectioned at

Table 2
Summary of sampling recommendations

Sentinel lymph nodes and axillary lymph node dissections	Same as for non-neoadjuvant specimens. • Section all lymph nodes at 2-mm intervals along the long axis of the lymph node and submit them entirely for histologic evaluation • For grossly involved lymph nodes, representative section(s) documenting the largest focus of metastatic carcinoma and any extracapsular extension are sufficient
Small lumpectomy	Same as for non-neoadjuvant specimens. • Often entirely submitted • A map/description to allow reconstruction at the time of microscopic evaluation
Large lumpectomy and mastectomy specimens	• Submit representative sections • A map/description to allow reconstruction at the time of microscopic evaluation *Residual carcinoma present:* Document 1 largest cross-section of residual tumor to assess tumor size and cellularity for AJCC staging and calculation of the RCB score.[7–9] • Usually 1 full-face section of largest area of suspected tumor is sufficient • Often several similar full-face sections 1-cm apart are submitted to investigate the extent of the lesion • For very large tumors, 5 representative sections per full face are sufficient • Sampling beyond the visible lesion to document microscopic extent is prudent • Sampling should cover the pretreatment tumor size *No residual carcinoma:* More sampling is required One full-face section of the area suspected of tumor involvement pretreatment per 1 cm (or for very large tumors, 5 representative sections per full face for every 1–2 cm) of pretreatment size up to a total maximum of about 25 blocks
Multiple clinically and grossly separate lesions	Each lesion should be handled as above. In addition, sections documenting the tissue in-between the lesions should be submitted.

Abbreviations: AJCC, American Joint Committee on Cancer; RCB, residual cancer burden.

2-mm intervals along the long axis of the lymph node and entirely submitted for histologic evaluation. It is important to note if a clip was placed in a previously biopsied lymph node and to locate the clip in the specimen with the help of a specimen radiograph, if necessary. For grossly involved lymph nodes representative section(s) documenting the largest focus of metastatic carcinoma and any extracapsular extension are sufficient.

Small Lumpectomy Specimens

The processing is the same as for non-neoadjuvant small lumpectomy specimens. Small lumpectomy specimens are inked according to their orientation then sliced at 3-mm to 5-mm intervals and often entirely submitted. A map or description is needed to allow reconstruction of the specimen at the time of microscopic evaluation for correlation of gross and microscopic findings. The presence of a clip should be documented. Grossly visible tumor bed and/or tumor should be described.

Large Lumpectomy Specimens

The processing is the same as for non-neoadjuvant large lumpectomy specimens. Large lumpectomy specimens are inked according to their orientation then sliced at 3-mm to 5-mm intervals. Preferably a radiograph or photograph of the sliced specimen is used to document the sections submitted for histologic evaluation and to allow reconstruction of the specimen at the time of microscopic evaluation for correlation of gross and microscopic findings. A diagram or, more cumbersome, a description can be used as well. Representative sections are submitted including sections documenting the specimen margins. The presence of a clip should be documented. Grossly visible tumor bed and/or tumor should be described.

Mastectomy Specimens

The processing is the same as for non-neoadjuvant mastectomy specimens. Appropriate margins are inked. It is very helpful when the surgeon identifies the location of the tumor with a stitch on the specimen. All location information (from communication with the surgeon, imaging, previous biopsy reports, and/or clip location) is used to identify the location of the tumor. The specimen is sliced at 0.5-cm to 1.0-cm intervals. The presence and location of clips should be documented. Grossly visible tumor bed and/or tumor should be described.

A diagram and preferably a radiograph or photograph of relevant slices are used to document the sections submitted for histologic evaluation and to allow correlation of gross and microscopic findings. Representative sections are submitted, including the usual representative sections of uninvolved nipple and breast tissue as well as sections documenting extension of tumor to nipple and/or skin as well as the deep margin.

Extent of Sampling for Large Lumpectomy and Mastectomy Specimens

When residual carcinoma is present, 1 large cross-section of residual tumor needs to be submitted to assess and document tumor size and cellularity for American Joint Committee on Cancer (AJCC) staging and calculation of the residual cancer burden (RCB) score.[7–9] Usually submitting 1 full-face section of the slice with the largest area suspected of involvement by tumor for histologic evaluation is sufficient. Often several similar full-face sections of slices 1 cm apart are submitted to investigate the extent of the lesion and investigate areas that appear to have more or less tumor on gross examination. For very large tumors, 5 representative sections of such a full-face are sufficient. As is usually done in gross examination it is good to sample just beyond the visible lesion to see if microscopic extent is greater. Sampling should cover the pretreatment size of the tumor. If no residual invasive carcinoma is seen on the initial sections submitted or if microscopic findings do not correspond to the gross impression, it may be necessary to submit additional sections.

When no residual carcinoma is present, extensive sampling may be required. It is difficult to document the absence of something. Again it is the pretreatment size of the tumor that determines the extent of sampling. Systematic sampling of the correct area of the breast, which is best identified by careful clinical and imaging correlation, is more important than exhaustive sampling of any visible fibrotic area or than blindly submitting a required number of blocks. When no invasive carcinoma is identified, a pragmatic approach is to submit 1 full-face (or for very large tumors, 5 representative sections of 1 full face) of the cross-section of the pretreatment area of involvement per 1 cm (or for very large tumors per 1–2 cm) of pretreatment size up to a total maximum of approximately 25 blocks. The US Food and Drug Administration (FDA) has recommended submitting "a minimum of 1 block per cm of pretreatment tumor size or at least 10 blocks in total whichever is greater."[10]

When multiple clinically and grossly separate lesions are present, each lesion should be handled as described previously. In addition, sections documenting the tissue in-between the lesions should be submitted.

Submitting Samples for Research

The BIG-NABCG publications suggest ways to submit samples for research that do not interfere with the assessments required for clinical care.[2,3] Many patients treated with neoadjuvant therapy participate in clinical trials. We owe it to these patients who deal with the extra risks and inconveniences of participating in a clinical trial that not only their clinical care should not be compromised, but also that whenever possible without compromising their clinical care, the information gained from their participation in the clinical trial is maximized. One of the promises of neoadjuvant clinical trials is to be able to evaluate tumor tissues at different time points (before treatment, on treatment, after treatment) to gain insights into predictive markers, into resistance mechanisms and into the way treatments work, possibly leading to novel treatments. If many of these patients are willing to undergo a research biopsy then I personally think we owe it to them to be flexible and inventive to maximize how we use the tissue from the post-neoadjuvant surgical specimen to make tissue available for research. Submission of the entire tumor bed for pathologic evaluation is not required. For most patients, samples can be obtained for research without interfering with assessment of pathologic response.

MICROSCOPIC EVALUATION

In a previous issue of *Surgical Pathology Clinics*, Sahoo and Lester[11] described the morphologic findings in post-neoadjuvant breast cancer specimens in detail. Here practical considerations are discussed related to reporting tumor type and grade, tumor size and extent, tumor cellularity, lymphovascular invasion, margins, lymph node status, pathologic complete response (pCR), RCB, and yAJCC stage.

Tumor Type and Grade

Criteria used to determine tumor type and grade are the same as for non-neoadjuvant specimens. It is important to compare findings with pretreatment biopsies before assuming they are treatment related. For example, necrosis may be present before or after treatment. Of course, because the sample obtained of the pretreatment tumor is limited it is impossible to be sure if a finding is treatment related even after comparison to the pretreatment biopsy; that is, some prognostic information is lost when patients are treated with neoadjuvant treatment. However, after neoadjuvant treatment, we have the opportunity to evaluate treatment response, which is likely one of the most important prognostic factors. Tumor grade after neoadjuvant treatment correlates with survival.[12]

It is important to report areas of tumor with a different morphology or grade than the previous biopsy. This is especially useful if that morphology or grade is not usually associated with a good response to the chosen neoadjuvant therapy. In such areas, repeat assessment of ER, PR, and HER2 may be indicated.

Size and Extent

The AJCC eighth edition staging manual[7] states that ypT size should be estimated based on the best combination of imaging, gross, and microscopic findings. When the size is not apparent by imaging or gross examination, it states the size can be estimated by carefully measuring and recording the relative positions of tissue samples submitted for microscopic evaluation and determining which contain invasive cancer. This is made easier by mapping gross findings and the sections submitted for histologic evaluation, as suggested previously.

Assessments of tumor size are prone to interobserver variability in the post-neoadjuvant surgical specimen because many tumors respond to neoadjuvant treatment heterogeneously and are present as scattered foci of invasive carcinoma in a fibrous tumor bed. Several different measurements may be relevant (**Fig. 2, Table 3**). Similar to the seventh edition,[13] the summary of changes to the new AJCC staging manual eighth edition[7] states that the ypT category is based on the largest contiguous focus of residual tumor excluding treatment-related fibrosis adjacent to residual invasive carcinoma (this is referred to as the AJCC size). The (m) modifier is included when multiple foci of residual tumor are present. The new manual also states that the pathology report should include a description of the extent of residual tumor explaining the basis for the ypT categorization when possible, as this may assist the clinician in estimating the extent of residual disease. When possible, the pretreatment cT category should also be documented. The elements in **Table 1** (size in 2 dimensions of the largest cross-section of the "residual tumor bed"; ie, the largest cross-section that contains [possibly] scattered residual invasive carcinoma, and the average invasive cancer cellularity in % across the largest cross-section that contains residual invasive carcinoma) are suggested by the BIG-NABCG residual disease characterization working group. Of note, the sixth edition of the AJCC staging manual[14] considered the largest extent of residual cancer

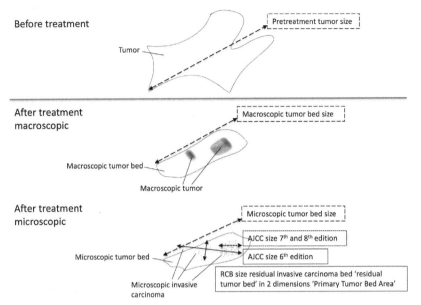

Fig. 2. Several different measurements of the tumor may be relevant. See also Table 2. The macroscopic and microscopic tumor bed (the grossly or microscopically abnormal tissue in the location of the original tumor before treatment with or without residual carcinoma) are usually not the same.

Table 3
Possible measurements of the tumor

AJCC ypT size 7th and 8th edition[7,13]	Size of largest contiguous focus.
AJCC ypT size 6th edition[14]	Largest extent of residual cancer allowing for intervening fibrosis.
Tumor bed size	Size of usually fibrotic tumor bed recognizable as abnormal tissue grossly or microscopically in the location of the original tumor before treatment with or without residual carcinoma. Not necessarily corresponding to the size of the original tumor pretreatment.
RCB size[8,9,a] (analogous to the AJCC ypT size 6th edition[14])	= "Primary tumor bed area" in RCB calculator. Residual invasive carcinoma bed: The entire area involved by possibly scattered residual invasive tumor foci.
Reduction in tumor size	Comparing the pretreatment and posttreatment tumor size. The size of the original tumor by imaging pretreatment is probably the most reliable measure of pretreatment tumor size.
Number of foci of invasive carcinoma	
Average cancer cellularity[a]	= Overall cancer cellularity (as percentage of area) in RCB calculator. Average cellularity over 1 entire largest cross-section of the residual invasive carcinoma bed explicitly including areas with low cellularity or no invasive carcinoma.
Reduction in cellularity	As compared with pretreatment biopsy.

Abbreviations: AJCC, American Joint Committee on Cancer; RCB, residual cancer burden.
  [a] Most meaningful and reproducible measurements.

allowing for intervening fibrosis. This sixth edition measurement was used in the publications that correlated prognosis to the ypTNM system[15,16] and is analogous to the measurements used to calculate the RCB score. The largest cross-section of the "residual tumor bed" in 2 dimensions is used to calculate the RCB score, as discussed later in this article.[8,9] The term "residual tumor bed,"' as used by the MD Anderson group, refers to the part of the tumor bed involved by residual invasive carcinoma (henceforth referred to as the residual invasive carcinoma bed or the RCB size).

The pretreatment burden of disease influences prognosis particularly in hormone receptor–positive disease.[16,17] A measure of the reduction in tumor burden after treatment could be calculated by comparing the pretreatment and posttreatment burden of disease. The size of the original tumor by imaging is probably a more reliable measure of pretreatment burden of disease than the size of the tumor bed (entire tumor bed with or without invasive carcinoma) in the posttreatment surgical specimen.

When clearly distinct tumors are seen that are confirmed microscopically to have intervening areas of normal breast tissue, and that presented as separate tumors before treatment, the dimension of the largest tumor is used for staging, and the dimensions of the largest residual invasive carcinoma bed (RCB size) are used for calculation of the RCB score. It may also be useful to calculate the RCB score for the smaller tumors if they are more highly cellular and may yield a higher RCB score or if they are a different more aggressive breast cancer subtype.

Cellularity

In addition to decreasing tumor size, systemic neoadjuvant treatment often changes tumor cellularity. The Miller-Payne score compares pretreatment and posttreatment cellularity and predicts survival after neoadjuvant chemotherapy.[18] Before developing the RCB score Dr Symmans' group demonstrated that cellularity of breast tumors after neoadjuvant therapy varies within T categories and that after neoadjuvant treatment the product of tumor size and cellularity showed a different distribution than size alone in their cohort.[19] They also showed that in a cohort of untreated tumors, the distribution of tumor size and of the product of tumor size and cellularity was similar. This suggests that it is of limited value to look at cellularity in addition to tumor size in nontreated tumors, but that after treatment cellularity adds crucial information.

Cellularity after neoadjuvant treatment often varies throughout the residual tumor. It is also important to remember that the cellularity of the pretreatment biopsy may not be representative of the entire tumor. Although it is tempting to assess only the most cellular areas of the residual tumor, the RCB system deals with heterogeneity of cellularity after treatment by standardizing sampling and by assessing the average cellularity over 1 entire largest cross-section of the residual invasive carcinoma bed explicitly *including* those areas within the residual invasive carcinoma bed with low cellularity or no invasive carcinoma.[8,9]

Lymphovascular Invasion

Lymphovascular invasion is associated with worse survival.[12] Sometimes residual carcinoma after neoadjuvant therapy is present in the breast as lymphovascular invasion only, usually with involvement of axillary lymph nodes. Even in the rare cases in which there is no disease in the axillary lymph nodes, lymphovascular invasion only without other invasive carcinoma in the breast should not be considered pCR.[3]

Margins

Surgical resection of the entirety of the tissue involved by the original tumor pretreatment is not necessarily performed. The significance of tumor bed at the margin in the absence of invasive carcinoma at the margin is unclear. As such, except perhaps in a rare extraordinary situation, a reexcision is not performed in this situation.

Lymph Node Status

The number of positive lymph nodes, size of the largest metastasis, number with macrometastases, with micrometastases, and number of lymph nodes with isolated tumor cells should be recorded. The presence of possible treatment effect, biopsy site changes and/or a clip associated with the previous findings should be documented. Changes associated with neoadjuvant systemic treatment cannot necessarily be distinguished from biopsy site changes or reactive changes in lymph nodes that may be unrelated to treatment. Furthermore, previously involved lymph nodes can look histologically unremarkable after neoadjuvant treatment.

The ypN categories are the same as for specimens that are not post-neoadjuvant. The summary of changes to the new AJCC staging manual eighth edition[7] clarifies that the largest focus of residual tumor in the lymph nodes is used for ypN categorization, excluding treatment-related fibrosis adjacent to residual nodal tumor deposits. For the purpose of calculating the RCB score the largest extent of lymph node involvement by tumor cells *including* intervening treatment-related fibrosis is used as the diameter of largest metastasis.[20]

The presence of lymph node metastases confers a worse prognosis regardless of the response in the breast.[4] Isolated tumor cells and micrometastases predict a worse survival after neoadjuvant treatment compared to the same finding in the non-neoadjuvant setting.[21] The presence of treatment effect in the lymph nodes may provide additional prognostic information and should be recorded.[22] Clinical management of the axilla after neoadjuvant treatment is evolving.[5,23]

PUTTING IT ALL TOGETHER

Complete Pathologic Response

In the best-case scenario, there is a pCR to neoadjuvant systemic treatment. We know from the large meta-analysis including thousands of patients and more than 15 years of follow-up published in 2014 that patients with a pCR defined as no disease in the breast (ypT0/is or ypT0) and no disease in the lymph nodes (ypN0) have an excellent prognosis regardless of breast cancer subtype and of the type of neoadjuvant systemic therapy received.[24] However, the relationship between pCR rates and event-free survival on a clinical trial level is complex.[25] Gains in pCR rates in clinical trials do not necessarily translate into gains in survival rates. The US FDA proposed the use of pCR as an endpoint for the accelerated preliminary approval of new agents for neoadjuvant treatment for high-risk early-stage breast cancer and approved Pertuzumab on this basis in 2013.[26,27] However, improved event-free survival remains the endpoint for full approval. In this context standardization of the pathologic determination of pCR is critical.

Pathologic assessment of pCR requires adequate sampling of the correct area of the breast with correlation of clinical, imaging, gross, and microscopic findings.[2,3] Suggestions for the extent of sampling have been outlined previously. The significance of residual ductal carcinoma in situ alone is not clear.[2] Adding pT0 or pT0/is to pCR clarifies the pCR definition used. Lobular carcinoma in situ is considered pCR.[2,3] Lymphovascular invasion only without other invasive carcinoma in the breast or lymph nodes is not considered pCR.[2,3] Isolated tumor cells in lymph nodes are not considered pCR.[2,3,7] Necrosis only

is considered pCR.[7] However it is difficult to be certain whether tumor cells are nonviable. Recognizable tumor cells in necrosis should be interpreted with caution. Mucin only is considered pCR.[7] **Box 1** and **Table 4** summarize the recommendations for pathologic assessment of pCR by the BIG-NABCG residual disease characterization working group.[2]

Residual Disease

If we just look at pCR, we lose a lot of information. Most patients will not achieve a pCR. Patients may not need to have achieved a pCR to benefit from the treatment. In addition to AJCC stage, the most commonly used measure of residual disease is the RCB. The RCB index score is a continuous number calculated from the size in 2 dimensions and the average cellularity of the largest cross-section of "residual tumor bed" (reflecting the amount of residual invasive carcinoma in the breast) and the number of involved lymph nodes and the size of the largest lymph node metastasis (reflecting the residual axillary involvement).[8] pCR (stage ypT0/is ypN0) corresponds to RCB 0. The other RCB classes are RCB I minimal, RCB II moderate, and RCB III extensive residual disease on the basis of predefined cut points of index scores.[8] The RCB calculator and teaching materials are available at http://www3.mdanderson.org/app/medcalc/index.cfm?pagename=jsconvert3.[9] **Tables 5** and **6** summarize common pitfalls in assessing RCB and suggested approaches to uncommon situations encountered when calculating the RCB score. **Figs. 3** and **4** show an example of assessment of RCB. RCB index and classes are prognostic. They are prognostic overall, in breast cancer subtypes (triple-negative disease, hormone receptor–positive HER2-negative disease, and in HER2-positive disease), and within stage groups. This has been shown in multiple, different institutional cohorts with up to 18 years of follow-up in the original validation cohort.[8,12,17,28–32] The distribution of RCB index in clinical trials may be more informative than the pCR rate alone.[17,33,34] RCB and yAJCC stage help identify patients at highest risk of recurrence. In the I-SPY1 Trial, yAJCC and RCB were discrepant in 34% of patients, suggesting there is value in reporting both measures.[29]

Multiple different groups have reported excellent reproducibility among different pathologists who learned the RCB method from published and Web-based teaching materials.[35–37] In most patients in these reports, RCB was

Box 1
Recommendations for pathologic assessment of pCR from the BIG-NABCG residual disease characterization working group

Pathologic complete response (pCR) = No residual invasive carcinoma in the breast and in all sampled lymph nodes (ypT0/is ypN0 or ypT0 ypN0)[24,27]

Accurate and reliable pathologic assessment of pCR requires:

- For the breast specimen:
  - Systematic sampling of the correct area of the breast with mapping of the specimen to correlate clinical, imaging, gross, and microscopic findings rather than overly exhaustive sampling.
  - Systematic sampling should include macroscopically visible tumor bed and immediately adjacent tissue or tissue surrounding the clip to represent the area suspected of involvement by carcinoma before treatment. Additional sampling may be needed after reviewing the initial sections.
  - An entire cross-section of the area suspected of involvement by carcinoma before treatment per 1 cm of pretreatment size or, for very large tumors, 5 representative sections of a cross-section of the area suspected of involvement by carcinoma before treatment per 1 to 2 cm of pretreatment size up to a total maximum of approximately 25 sections should be sufficient provided a tumor bed or clip is identified.[a]
  - Immunohistochemistry is not routinely required but may be helpful. Tumor cells are regarded as present whether they are identified by hematoxylin and eosin stain or by immunohistochemistry.
- For the lymph nodes:
  - All surgically removed lymph nodes must be entirely submitted for histologic evaluation, sectioned at 2-mm intervals. (Additional levels and immunohistochemistry are not routinely required. Tumor cells are regarded the same whether they are identified by hematoxylin and eosin stain or by immunohistochemistry.)

[a] The US Food and Drug Administration recommended a minimum of 1 block per centimeter of pretreatment tumor size or at least 10 blocks in total, whichever is greater.[10]
Data from Bossuyt V, Provenzano E, Symmans WF, et al. Recommendations for standardized pathological characterization of residual disease for neoadjuvant clinical trials of breast cancer by the BIG-NABCG collaboration. Ann Oncol 2015;26(7):1280–91; and Provenzano E, Bossuyt V, Viale G, et al. Standardization of pathologic evaluation and reporting of postneoadjuvant specimens in clinical trials of breast cancer: recommendations from an international working group. Mod Pathol 2015;28(9):1185–201.

Table 4
Recommendations for occasionally controversial elements in determining pathologic complete response (pCR)

Finding	pCR	Reference
Ductal carcinoma in situ (DCIS)	Y or N[a]	Bossuyt et al,[2] 2015; Cortazar et al,[24] 2014
Lobular carcinoma in situ (LCIS)	Y	Bossuyt et al,[2] 2015
Lymphovascular invasion (LVI)	N	Bossuyt et al,[2] 2015; Provenzano et al,[3] 2015
Micrometastasis and macrometastasis in lymph node(s) (pN1mic and above)	N	Bossuyt et al,[2] 2015; Provenzano et al,[3] 2015; American Joint Committee on Cancer,[7] 2017
Isolated tumor cells in lymph node(s) (pN0i+)	N	Bossuyt et al,[2] 2015; Provenzano et al,[3] 2015; American Joint Committee on Cancer,[7] 2017
Necrosis only	Y	American Joint Committee on Cancer,[7] 2017
Mucin only	Y	American Joint Committee on Cancer,[7] 2017

[a] Depending on the residual disease classification system used.

calculated retrospectively without standardized processing of the specimen and/or access to pathology reports, gross descriptions, and/or tissue maps. Standardized processing is an important part of the RCB system.[9] In the I-SPY 1 trial pCR rates dropped by almost 10% after training in the RCB system and prospectively implementing a standardized approach to processing of neoadjuvant specimens, including mapping of gross and microscopic findings.[2] Furthermore, pathologic evaluation of the elements needed to calculate the RCB score is more easily performed prospectively than on retrospective review. It is to be expected that prospectively implementing the standardized RCB protocol would lead to even better reproducibility and even more meaningful prognostic information. Naidoo and colleagues[36] and Thomas and colleagues[37] documented some potential differences in interpretation of pathology findings when calculating RCB scores. Tables 5 and 6 summarize practical suggestions to address some of these differences.

Other Prognostic Factors

Other prognostic factors, in addition to measures quantifying the amount of residual disease

---

Table 5
Common pitfalls assessing RCB

Residual invasive carcinoma bed (residual tumor bed)	The size of the residual invasive carcinoma bed (residual tumor bed) may be different from the size of the (fibrous) tumor bed, grossly identified tumor bed, or the size used for AJCC staging 8th edition (largest contiguous focus of residual invasive carcinoma, excluding surrounding areas of fibrosis).[7] The "residual tumor bed" may include scattered tumor deposits within a fibrous area.[9]
The microscopic extent of the residual invasive carcinoma bed does not correlate with the gross estimated measurement of the "residual tumor bed"	The residual invasive carcinoma bed (residual tumor bed) dimensions are to be revised according to the microscopic findings.[9] The gross estimated measurement of the "residual tumor bed" might be larger than the actual residual invasive tumor bed. Conversely, microscopic residual cancer may also extend beyond the confines of the macroscopic tumor bed so the gross estimated measurement may be smaller than the residual invasive carcinoma bed. See also Fig. 5.
Areas with low cellularity or no tumor should be explicitly included in the average overall cancer cellularity	Practical approach: Dot the perimeter of cancer in each slide to measure and help reconstruct the residual invasive carcinoma bed (residual tumor bed) across multiple slides. Go from field to field in each slide to estimate the cancer cellularity (eg, left to right then top to bottom) in increments of 10% or as 1% and 5% for very low cellularity fields or 0% for fields with no cancer, specifically including areas with very little or no cancer. Then calculate average of the fields (sum of % in each field/number of fields).[9]
Ductal carcinoma in situ (DCIS) component	The important number is the % cellularity invasive carcinoma. In some cases ignoring (excluding) the DCIS component when assessing cancer cellularity and simply entering 0 for percentage of cancer that is in situ disease may be easier than assessing both invasive and in situ cellularity. In other cases, it may be easier to assess overall cellularity and then adjusting for the DCIS cellularity as recommended in the RCB methods.[9]
Multiple separate tumors	The size of the RCB measurements are from the largest residual invasive carcinoma bed.[9] It may be useful to also calculate the RCB score for the smaller tumors if they are more highly cellular and may yield a higher RCB score or if they are a different more aggressive breast cancer subtype.

Abbreviations: AJCC, American Joint Committee on Cancer; RCB, residual cancer burden.

Table 6
Suggested approaches to some less common situations encountered when calculating the RCB score

Isolated tumor cells (ITC) only in lymph nodes	Number of Positive Lymph Nodes: Number of nodes with ITC. Diameter of Largest Metastasis: Size of largest ITC focus as a number <1 (for example, 0.01 mm would be a 10-μm cell).
Very low cellularity tumors	A number smaller than 1 can be entered for the invasive cancer cellularity. For example, with two 0.1-mm clusters 2 cm apart: Primary Tumor Bed Area: 20 mm × 0.1 mm Overall Cancer Cellularity (as percentage of area): 0.01%
Involvement of intramammary lymph nodes	Counted as positive nodes.
Involvement of internal mammary lymph nodes	Counted as positive nodes.[9]
Lymphovascular invasion (LVI) only	Primary Tumor Bed Area: Measure area of the breast involved by LVI in 2 dimensions. Overall Cancer Cellularity (as percentage of area): Appropriate estimated cellularity with LVI considered as invasive disease.
RCB score after pretreatment sentinel lymph node biopsy (SLNB)	If all sentinel lymph nodes were negative before treatment the RCB score is not affected.[9] If a positive lymph node was removed by the SLNB only a range of RCB score and class can be given. The range assumes that either none of the previously positive lymph nodes responded and would all still be positive with the same largest dimension as before treatment or that all of the previously positive lymph nodes responded and would be negative after treatment. Suggested note: X axillary lymph nodes are positive for carcinoma (largest focus x mm). A SLNB was performed before neoadjuvant treatment. (Before neoadjuvant therapy Y sentinel lymph nodes were positive for carcinoma [largest focus y mm]) The residual cancer burden is — (X + Y positive lymph nodes, largest focus largest of x or y mm) to — (X positive lymph nodes, largest focus x mm), corresponding to a residual cancer burden Class of — (to —).

in the breast and lymph nodes, are important. Particularly in hormone receptor–positive breast cancer, factors such as pretreatment disease burden and Ki67 index after treatment have been shown to predict survival.[17,31] Different classification systems incorporating such factors have been developed. For example, Clinical-Pathologic stage + Estrogen-Grade[16] combines pathologic stage after neoadjuvant treatment with clinical stage before neoadjuvant treatment, nuclear grade, and ER status. The preoperative endocrine prognostic index combines posttreatment ypT stage, posttreatment ypN stage, posttreatment Ki67, and posttreatment ER expression.[38] The residual proliferative cancer burden combines the RCB score with posttreatment ki67 index.[31] Dr Penault-Llorca and Radosevic-Robin reviewed biomarker candidates in residual disease.[39]

Future Directions

We know that ER, PR, and HER2-defined breast cancer subsets respond very differently to neoadjuvant treatment. pCR rates for HER2-positive and triple-negative patients are high with the newest treatment regimens. Patients

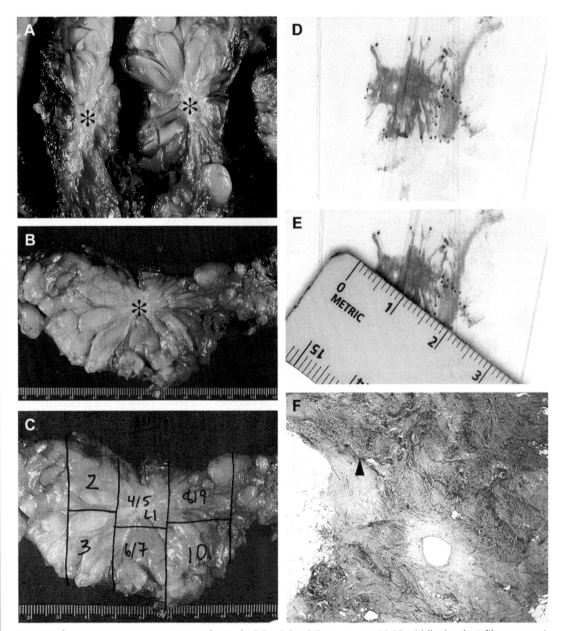

Fig. 3. Before treatment a mammogram showed a 3.2 × 2.3 × 2.7-cm mass at 11:00 middle depth. A fibrous area in that location is identified after slicing the mastectomy (*A*). A representative slice is photographed (*B*). This photograph is used to document the sections submitted for histologic evaluation (*C*). On microscopic review, invasive carcinoma is marked on the slide with dots (*D*). The 2 slides are put together as they relate to each other per the diagram in (*C*). A measurement of the residual invasive carcinoma bed in 2 dimensions (23 mm and 17 mm) is obtained (*E*). The invasive carcinoma cellularity varies across the residual invasive carcinoma bed (*F*). Star indicates fibrous area in (*A*), (*B*), and (*C*). Solid arrow indicates invasive carcinoma in (*F*) [H&E, original magnification].

with hormone receptor–positive disease have less reduction in disease burden after neoadjuvant chemotherapy and/or endocrine therapy. However, use of neoadjuvant endocrine therapy is increasing. Other measures that detect the cytostatic effect of anti-endocrine therapy (such as posttreatment and on treatment Ki67 index) show promise in this setting.[38,40] In the article reporting the long-term prognosis related to RCB, the investigators suggested refined cut

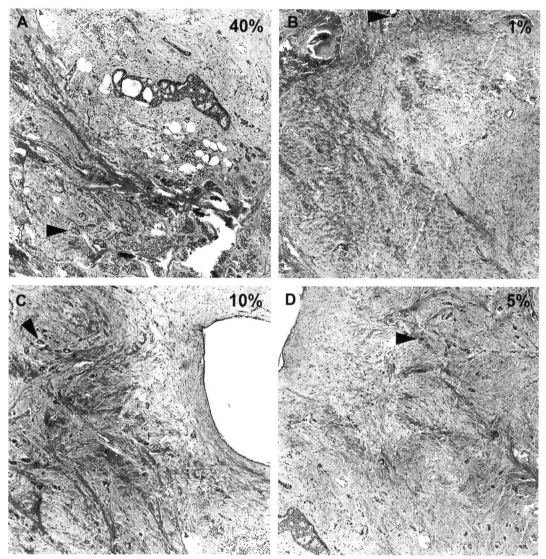

Fig. 4. The invasive carcinoma cellularity is assessed in each microscopic field moving from one side to the other across the residual invasive carcinoma bed. The average invasive carcinoma cellularity across the residual invasive carcinoma bed is estimated from these microscopic fields. It is calculated as (40% [A] + 1% [B] + 10% [C] + 5% [D] + 10% [E] + 70% [F] + 30% [G])/7 (number of fields). It is approximately 25%. The 2 dimensions of the residual invasive carcinoma bed from Fig. 3 (23 mm and 17 mm) are entered as the "Primary Tumor Bed Area" in the RCB calculator (H). The average invasive carcinoma cellularity across the residual invasive carcinoma bed (25%) is entered as "Overall Cancer Cellularity" (as percentage of area) in the RCB calculator. The in situ carcinoma did not interfere with estimating the cellularity in this example, therefore the "Percentage of Cancer That Is In Situ Disease" is entered as 0% in the RCB calculator. There were no positive lymph nodes in this example. The value 0 is entered for the "Number of Positive Lymph Nodes" and for the "Diameter of Largest Metastasis" in the RCB calculator. The residual cancer burden is 1.837. The residual cancer burden Class is II. Solid arrow indicates invasive carcinoma [H&E, original magnification].

points for the RCB classes and a rebalanced RCB index for each breast cancer subset may be useful.[17] It makes sense to search for and validate biomarkers in the neoadjuvant setting for each breast cancer subset and for each (newly developed) therapy. However, there is value in optimizing quantification of the amount of residual disease in the breast and lymph

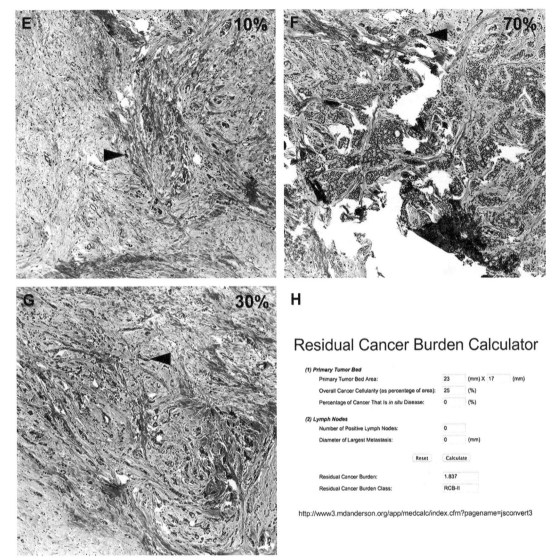

Fig. 4. (continued).

nodes with routine pathologic macroscopic and microscopic evaluation. This can be achieved through systematic sampling of the correct area of the breast and with standardized measurements of size and cellularity of invasive carcinoma in the breast and of lymph node involvement. The amount of residual disease in the breast and lymph nodes can be expressed as a single meaningful number in the form of the RCB score. Other prognostic factors can be added to the RCB score. The processing approach and elements needed in the report for quantification of residual disease in the breast and lymph nodes will likely be the same regardless of future refinements in the RCB calculation, regardless of the addition of other prognostic factors and biomarkers, and regardless of breast cancer subset or type of treatment.

SUMMARY

Standardization of quantification of residual disease in the breast and lymph nodes with routine pathologic macroscopic and microscopic evaluation leads to accurate and reproducible measures of response to neoadjuvant treatment. pCR, RCB, and yAJCC stage are recommended measures of residual disease. The RCB incorporates response in the breast and in the lymph nodes into a prognostic score that can be combined with other emerging prognostic factors.

A Macroscopic tumor bed

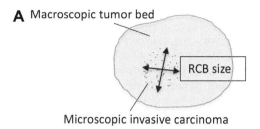

Microscopic invasive carcinoma

B Macroscopic tumor bed

Microscopic invasive carcinoma

C

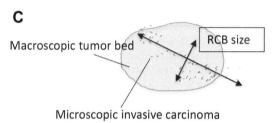

Macroscopic tumor bed

Microscopic invasive carcinoma

Fig. 5. Examples of how the residual invasive carcinoma bed dimensions may differ from the dimensions of the macroscopic tumor bed. In the first example there is uniform shrinking of the tumor. The dimensions of the residual invasive carcinoma bed are smaller than the dimensions of the macroscopic tumor bed (*A*). In the second example, the reduction in tumor size and cellularity is heterogeneous. The dimensions of the residual invasive carcinoma bed are again smaller than the dimensions of the macroscopic tumor bed (*B*). Microscopic residual cancer may extend beyond the macroscopic tumor bed as in the third example (*C*).

REFERENCES

1. Rastogi P, Anderson SJ, Bear HD, et al. Preoperative chemotherapy: updates of National Surgical Adjuvant Breast and Bowel Project Protocols B-18 and B-27. J Clin Oncol 2008;26(5):778–85.
2. Bossuyt V, Provenzano E, Symmans WF, et al. Recommendations for standardized pathological characterization of residual disease for neoadjuvant clinical trials of breast cancer by the BIG-NABCG collaboration. Ann Oncol 2015;26(7):1280–91.
3. Provenzano E, Bossuyt V, Viale G, et al. Standardization of pathologic evaluation and reporting of post-neoadjuvant specimens in clinical trials of breast cancer: recommendations from an international working group. Mod Pathol 2015;28(9):1185–201.
4. Mamounas EP, Anderson SJ, Dignam JJ, et al. Predictors of locoregional recurrence after neoadjuvant chemotherapy: results from combined analysis of National Surgical Adjuvant Breast and Bowel Project B-18 and B-27. J Clin Oncol 2012;30(32):3960–6.
5. Pilewskie M, Morrow M. Axillary nodal management following neoadjuvant chemotherapy: a review. JAMA Oncol 2017;3(4):549–55.
6. Caudle AS, Yang WT, Krishnamurthy S, et al. Improved axillary evaluation following neoadjuvant therapy for patients with node-positive breast cancer using selective evaluation of clipped nodes: implementation of targeted axillary dissection. J Clin Oncol 2016;34(10):1072–8.
7. Amin MB, Edge SB, Byrd DR, et al, editors. American Joint Committee on Cancer. 8th edition. American Joint Committee on Cancer (AJCC) cancer staging manual, vol. I. Springer; 2017.
8. Symmans WF, Peintinger F, Hatzis C, et al. Measurement of residual breast cancer burden to predict survival after neoadjuvant chemotherapy. J Clin Oncol 2007;25(28):4414–22.
9. Residual Cancer Burden calculator and associated documents [guide for measuring cancer cellularity, examples of gross & microscopic evaluation, pathology protocol for macroscopic and microscopic assessment of RCB]. Available at: http://www3.mdanderson.org/app/medcalc/index.cfm?pagename=jsconvert3. Accessed on October 26, 2017.
10. Guidance for industry: pathological complete response in neoadjuvant treatment fo High-Risk Early-STAGe BReast Cancer: use as an endpoint to support accelerated approval. In: Administration. USFaD, editor. 2014. Available at: http://www.fda.gov/downloads/Drugs/GuidanceComplianceRegulatoryInformation/Guidances/UCM305501.pdf. Accessed on October 25, 2017.
11. Sahoo S, Lester SC. Pathology considerations in patients treated with neoadjuvant chemotherapy. Surg Pathol Clin 2012;5(3):749–74.
12. Choi M, Park YH, Ahn JS, et al. Assessment of pathologic response and long-term outcome in locally advanced breast cancers after neoadjuvant chemotherapy: comparison of pathologic classification systems. Breast Cancer Res Treat 2016;160(3):475–89.
13. Edge SB, Byrd DR, Compton CC, et al, editors. American Joint Committee on Cancer (AJCC) cancer staging manual. 7th edition. Springer; 2009.
14. Greene FL, Page DL, Fleming ID, et al, editors. American Joint Committee on Cancer (AJCC) cancer staging manual. 6th edition. Springer-Verlag; 2002.
15. Carey LA, Metzger R, Dees EC, et al. American Joint Committee on Cancer tumor-node-metastasis stage after neoadjuvant chemotherapy and breast cancer outcome. J Natl Cancer Inst 2005;97(15):1137–42.
16. Mittendorf EA, Jeruss JS, Tucker SL, et al. Validation of a novel staging system for disease-specific

survival in patients with breast cancer treated with neoadjuvant chemotherapy. J Clin Oncol 2011; 29(15):1956–62.

17. Symmans WF, Wei C, Gould R, et al. Long-term prognostic risk after neoadjuvant chemotherapy associated with residual cancer burden and breast cancer subtype. J Clin Oncol 2017;35(10):1049–60.

18. Ogston KN, Miller ID, Payne S, et al. A new histological grading system to assess response of breast cancers to primary chemotherapy: prognostic significance and survival. Breast 2003;12(5):320–7.

19. Rajan R, Poniecka A, Smith TL, et al. Change in tumor cellularity of breast carcinoma after neoadjuvant chemotherapy as a variable in the pathologic assessment of response. Cancer 2004;100(7):1365–73.

20. Bossuyt V, Symmans WF. Standardizing of pathology in patients receiving neoadjuvant chemotherapy. Ann Surg Oncol 2016;23(10):3153–61.

21. Fisher ER, Wang J, Bryant J, et al. Pathobiology of preoperative chemotherapy: findings from the National Surgical Adjuvant Breast and Bowel (NSABP) protocol B-18. Cancer 2002;95(4):681–95.

22. Newman LA, Pernick NL, Adsay V, et al. Histopathologic evidence of tumor regression in the axillary lymph nodes of patients treated with preoperative chemotherapy correlates with breast cancer outcome. Ann Surg Oncol 2003;10(7):734–9.

23. Ollila DW, Cirrincione CT, Berry DA, et al. Axillary management of stage II/III breast cancer in patients treated with neoadjuvant systemic therapy: results of CALGB 40601 (HER2-positive) and CALGB 40603 (triple-negative). J Am Coll Surg 2017;224(4):688–94.

24. Cortazar P, Zhang L, Untch M, et al. Pathological complete response and long-term clinical benefit in breast cancer: the CTNeoBC pooled analysis. Lancet 2014;384(9938):164–72.

25. Bossuyt V, Hatzis C. The neoadjuvant model and complete pathologic response in breast cancer: all or nothing? JAMA Oncol 2016;2(6):760–1.

26. U.S. Food and Drug Administration News Release. FDA approves Perjeta for neoadjuvant breast cancer treatment: first drug approved for use in preoperative breast cancer. 2013. Available at: http://www.fda.gov/newsevents/newsroom/pressannouncements/ucm370393.htm. Accessed November 15, 2013.

27. U.S. Food and Drug Administration. Guidance for industry: pathologic complete response in neoadjuvant treatment of high-risk early-stage breast cancer: use as an endpoint to support accelerated approval. Draft guidance. 2012. Available at: http://www.fda.gov/downloads/Drugs/GuidanceComplianceRegulatoryInformation/Guidances/UCM305501.pdf. Accessed on October 26, 2017.

28. Corben AD, Abi-Raad R, Popa I, et al. Pathologic response and long-term follow-up in breast cancer patients treated with neoadjuvant chemotherapy: a comparison between classifications and their practical application. Arch Pathol Lab Med 2013; 137(8):1074–82.

29. Campbell JI, Yau C, Krass P, et al. Comparison of residual cancer burden, American Joint Committee on Cancer staging and pathologic complete response in breast cancer after neoadjuvant chemotherapy: results from the I-SPY 1 TRIAL (CALGB 150007/150012; ACRIN 6657). Breast Cancer Res Treat 2017;165(1):181–91.

30. Romero A, Garcia-Saenz JA, Fuentes-Ferrer M, et al. Correlation between response to neoadjuvant chemotherapy and survival in locally advanced breast cancer patients. Ann Oncol 2013;24(3):655–61.

31. Sheri A, Smith IE, Johnston SR, et al. Residual proliferative cancer burden to predict long-term outcome following neoadjuvant chemotherapy. Ann Oncol 2015;26(1):75–80.

32. Lee HJ, Park IA, Song IH, et al. Comparison of pathologic response evaluation systems after anthracycline with/without taxane-based neoadjuvant chemotherapy among different subtypes of breast cancers. PLoS One 2015;10(9):e0137885.

33. Liu MC, Symmans WF, Yau C, et al. Residual cancer burden (RCB) with veliparib/carboplatin in the I-SPY2 Trial. Paper presented at: San Antonio Breast Cancer Symposium. San Antonio, Texas, December 8–12, 2015.

34. Hatzis C, Gould RE, Zhang Y, et al. Predicting improvements in survival based on improvements in pathologic response rate to neoadjuvant chemotherapy in different breast cancer subtypes (abstract P6-06-37). Paper presented at: San Antonio Breast Cancer Symposium. San Antonio, Texas, Dec 10–14, 2013.

35. Peintinger F, Sinn B, Hatzis C, et al. Reproducibility of residual cancer burden for prognostic assessment of breast cancer after neoadjuvant chemotherapy. Mod Pathol 2015;28(7):913–20.

36. Naidoo K, Parham DM, Pinder SE. An audit of residual cancer burden reproducibility in a UK context. Histopathology 2017;70(2):217–22.

37. Thomas JSJ, Provenzano E, Hiller L, et al. Central pathology review with two-stage quality assurance for pathological response after neoadjuvant chemotherapy in the ARTemis trial. Mod Pathol 2017;30(8):1069–77.

38. Ellis MJ, Tao Y, Luo J, et al. Outcome prediction for estrogen receptor-positive breast cancer based on postneoadjuvant endocrine therapy tumor characteristics. J Natl Cancer Inst 2008;100(19):1380–8.

39. Penault-Llorca F, Radosevic-Robin N. Biomarkers of residual disease after neoadjuvant therapy for breast cancer. Nat Rev Clin Oncol 2016;13(8):487–503.

40. Dowsett M, Nielsen TO, A'Hern R, et al. Assessment of Ki67 in breast cancer: recommendations from the International Ki67 in Breast Cancer working group. J Natl Cancer Inst 2011;103(22):1656–64.

.

Printed and bound by CPI Group (UK) Ltd, Croydon, CR0 4YY

03/10/2024

01040384-0020